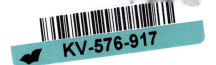

Preface

This book is principally aimed at the undergraduate dental student, although we hope it will also be of use to general dental practitioners with an interest in orthodontics and those at the start of their postgraduate training. It has been written to compliment the book *Diagnosis of the orthodontic patient*, by the same authors, and therefore assumes the reader has progressed down the path of orthodontic diagnosis and is in the process of formulating a treatment plan. Such planning requires the orthodontist to have a sound understanding of the biological principles of tooth movement, as well as an awareness of the treatment ideals and limitations. In addition, knowledge of the various types of orthodontic appliances, their design and likely mode of action is also essential. Closely linked to this, advances in materials science have led to great changes in orthodontic clinical practice in recent years. A chapter on orthodontic materials is therefore included. With increasing specialization there is a need to call upon the services of colleagues from other specialties in treating complex cases and so multidisciplinary treatments are also covered. Finally, because of the litigious environment most clinicians find themselves in, it is also essential that the potential damage that can be caused is also considered.

Bath   AJI
London   FM
March 2003

Acknowledgements

As with so many aspects of clinical work, we are indebted to many colleagues for their assistance during the preparation of this book. They include the Departments of Medical Illustration of both the Royal United Hospitals, Bath, and at the GKT Medical Institute, Kings College, London; Nabeel Abu Mezeir, Dirk Bister, David Brown, Alex Cash, Graham Cordall, Nigel Harradine, Tom Hartridge, Mary Hudd, Helen Knight, John Metcalf, Riz Parbatani, Steve Robinson, Francis Scriven, Chris Stephens, Helen Travess, Alison Williams, John Williams, and last, but not least, our respective long-suffering families.

The Orthodontic Patient:
Treatment and Biomechanics

A. J. Ireland
Consultant/S~ ·
Departme
Bristol De
and Consu
Royal Unit

and

Fraser Mc
Professor of
Honorary C(
King's Coll(
Orthodont
Orthodon

OXFORD
UNIVERSITY PRESS

OXFORD

UNIVERSITY PRESS

Great Clarendon Street, Oxford OX2 6DP

Oxford University Press is a department of the University of Oxford.
It furthers the University's objective of excellence in research, scholarship,
and education by publishing worldwide in

Oxford New York
Auckland Bangkok Buenos Aires Cape Town Chennai
Dar es Salaam Delhi Hong Kong Istanbul Karachi Kolkata
Kuala Lumpur Madrid Melbourne Mexico City Mumbai Nairobi
São Paulo Shanghai Taipei Tokyo Toronto

Oxford is a registered trade mark of Oxford University Press
in the UK and in certain other countries

Published in the United States
by Oxford University Press Inc., New York

© Oxford University Press, 2003

British Library Cataloguing in Publication Data
(Data available)

Library of Congress Cataloging in Publication Data

ISBN 0 19 851048 9

10 9 8 7 6 5 4 3 2

02

Typeset by EXPO Holdings, Malaysia
Printed in Great Britain
on acid-free paper by Biddles Ltd, King's Lynn, Norfolk

Contents

Abbreviations

APC	adhesive precoat
BMP	bone morphogenetic protein
cAMP	cyclic adenosine monophosphate
Cbfa-1	core-binding factor alpha-1
CP	cysteine proteinase
CSAG	Clinical Standards Advisory Group
CT	computed tomography
DEGDMA	diethylene glycol dimethacrylate
DPT	dental panoramic tomograph
EOA	extraoral anchorage
EOT	extraoral traction
FA	facial axis
FR	functional regulator
GMA	glycidyl methacrylate
HEMA	hydroxyethyl methacrylate
IGF	insulin-like growth factors
IL	interleukins
IMF	intermaxillary fixation
LACC	long axis of the clinical crown
LED	light-emitting diode
MBT	McLaughlin, Bennett, and Trevisi (bracket prescriptions)
MIM	metal injection moulded
MMP	matrix metalloproteinases
MRI	magnetic resonance imaging
OPG	osteoprotegerin
OPGL	osteoprotegerin ligand
PAR	Peer Assessment Rating
PDGF	platelet-derived growth factors
PI	phosphoinositide
PTH	parathyroid hormone
TEGDMA	triethylene glycol dimethacrylate
T_g	glass transition temperature
TGF	transforming growth factors
TIMP	tissue inhibitor of metalloproteinase

TMA	titanium–molybdenum alloy
TMD	temporomandibular dysfunction
TTR	temperature transition range
UDMA	urethane dimethacrylate

1 Basic biological principles

CONTENTS

There are two main biological mechanisms that need to be considered in relation to orthodontic treatment:
- growth of the craniofacial skeleton; and
- the localized tissue response in relation to tooth movement.

Growth of the craniofacial skeleton and orthodontics will be considered in Chapter 4, with particular reference to functional appliances where orthodontic loads affect structures distant to their point of action. Conversely, when a load is applied to a tooth there is an immediate and localized tissue response in and around the periodontal ligament. This chapter aims to deal with the tissue and cellular changes that occur with the application of an orthodontic load, both locally within the periodontium and more generally in the craniofacial skeleton.

1.1 CONNECTIVE TISSUE ANATOMY

There are two basic skeletal tissues involved in the overall growth and development of the craniofacial skeleton—bone and cartilage—both of which are specialized forms of connective tissue with specific roles. In general terms, bone is a supportive element, whilst cartilage is found in regions of joints allowing relatively easy movements of one bone over another.

The specific terms relating the type of tissue connecting one to another are:
- **Synchondrosis**   Bone connected to bone with a layer of cartilage
- **Syndesmosis**   Bone connected to bone with connective tissue
- **Synostosis**   Bone connected to bone by a bridge of calcified tissue

The connective tissue of the periodontal ligament is the principal site where the specialty of orthodontics has an affect. Without orthodontically induced changes in this tissue the teeth would not move during treatment. The periodontal ligament is a specialized form of joint connecting teeth to bone. Precise details of the histology and biochemistry of this tissue can be found in other specialized texts.[1]

During the skeletal development the interaction between these connective tissues is highly complex. Their precise anatomical arrangement is discussed briefly in other textbooks.[2-5] Further genetic and evolutionary details of the cells/tissues described in this chapter are to be found in ref. 6.

The specialty of orthodontics is intimately involved with the turnover of the skeleton under the influence of the loads generated by orthodontic appliances. It is by understanding the cellular biology of the craniofacial skeleton that the possibility of maximizing treatment mechanics, without producing unwanted iatrogenic problems such as root resorption, can hopefully be achieved. In particular, osteoclasts, the cells responsible for removing bone substance, cannot differentiate between alveolar bone and dentine and/or cementum. Once dental tissue is lost, there is no biological mechanism by which it can re-form. Reports of an increase in root length are a combination of measurement error and continued development of an immature root apex.[7]

For these reasons the basic cellular responses to mechanical loading will be discussed. The development of the craniofacial skeleton will be briefly described elsewhere in Chapters 7 and 9 with respect to functional appliances and patients with cleft lip and palate.

1.2 CARTILAGE

Cartilage is composed of a chondroitin-rich matrix with typical uninuclear cells called 'chondrocytes' (Fig. 1.1). There are no vascular channels within cartilage, and substances such as oxygen and glucose are transported into the matrix by diffusion. Conversely, breakdown products of glycolysis (bicarbonate and hydrogen ions) passively diffuse out of the cartilage along their own concentration gradient.

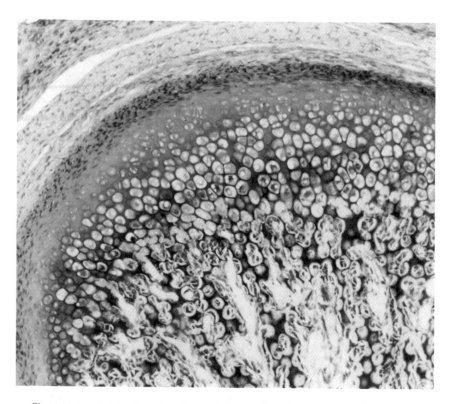

Fig. 1.1 A histological section of a condylar cartilage demonstrating the unique layers of the condylar cartilage. The area of endochondral ossification (EC) is marked by vascular invasion and chondrocytes (C) depositing extracellular matrix. In addition, the articular surface (AS) is visible. (Reproduced with kind permission of Oxford University Press (1987). The effect of articular function on the mandibular condyle of the rat. *European Journal of Orthodontics*, **9**, 87–96.)

Cartilaginous growth plates and synchondroses constitute an important part of the growth mechanism of the skeleton as a whole. Following cessation of growth, the original cartilaginous skeleton is reduced so that it ultimately only covers the articular surfaces of synovial joints. The main areas of cartilage that need to be considered during orthodontic treatment are those which have a direct influence on the facial skeleton, including:

- at the base of the skull, namely the sphenoccipital synchondrosis (see Fig. 4.4);
- the nasal septum;
- the mandibular condylar cartilage.

All other sites of cartilage in the facial skeleton have usually fused by the age of 8–9 years or have negligible effects on overall growth at the time of orthodontic treatment. Usually, treatment commences at around 12 years of age when the permanent dentition has erupted.

The cartilage-forming cells, called 'chondroblasts', have typical phenotype characteristics, and there is evidence to suggest that the bone morphogenetic proteins (BMP) induce these cells to produce characteristic types of tissue such as cartilage nodules and type II collagen.[8] It is possible that such proteins might be used as an adjunct for supporting orthodontic treatment, for ex   ample supplementing cartilaginous or endochondral bone formation. However, there is currently insufficient detailed knowledge of the true mode of action of these substances to make them realistic therapeutic adjuncts at present.

The major loading of cartilage during orthodontic treatment occurs at the condylar cartilage of the temporomandibular joint, particularly during treatment with functional appliances. Many research groups have likened the condylar cartilage to epiphyseal growth cartilages, but there are clear differences both in the histochemistry and behaviour of condylar cartilage.[9,10] The muscles of mastication influenced by these functional appliances appear to load the condylar cartilage, which then undergoes cellular changes such as an increase in cell number and increased cellular activity, followed by production of extracellular matrix and subsequent bone deposition.

1.3   BONE

Bone is composed of an organic component (collagen, non-collagenous proteins and cells) and an inorganic component (mainly hydroxyapatite). The major feature of interest in bone is the cellular component, as it is this which essentially maintains bone as a 'living' structure capable of change. Four different cell types are found in bone, namely:

- osteoblasts
- osteocytes
- osteoclasts
- bone lining cells

These will be discussed in turn.

1.3.1   Osteoblasts

These cells are defined more in terms of their function rather than their specific histological appearance, and they have many unique characteristics,[11] including:

(1) an ability to produce high levels of alkaline phosphatase;
(2) the production of type I collagen, which is necessary for calcification; and
(3) the production of osteocalcin.

Osteoblasts are also able to demonstrate an increase in the level of the intracellular messenger, cyclic adenosine monophosphate (cAMP), when stimulated with parathyroid hormone (PTH) (Fig. 1.2).

They can readily revert back to the fibroblast phenotype if the local environmental conditions are not appropriate.

Cell culture studies have also shown that BMPs stimulate the expression of phenotypic markers in osteoblasts;[12] this might be another reason why BMPs could act as therapeutic agents in orthodontic treatment, although this is still purely speculative.

Osteoblasts are derived from mesenchymal (stromal) stem cells, which are connective tissue cells found within the bone marrow cavity. They can also differentiate into other cells, including fibroblasts, adipocytes, chondroblasts, and myoblasts. Many regulators exist for the differentiation of cells, but a major factor is core-binding factor alpha-1 (Cbfa-1).[13] The osteoblasts function solely to construct the extracellular matrix of bone: type I collagen (a material which constitutes approximately 90% of the organic matrix of bone), proteoglycans, and attachment proteins. In addition to the organic matrix, bone contains many growth factors helpful in the coordination of bony activity. These factors can be produced by a number of cell types, but it is considered that they are laid down in the bony matrix by osteoblasts. These factors include insulin-like growth factors (IGFs), transforming growth factors (TGFs), platelet-derived growth factors (PDGFs), and the previously mentioned BMP molecules. The osteoblast not only promotes bone mineralization but its major function is the control of osteoclast function (see Section 1.3.3).

1.3.2   Osteocytes

Osteocytes are osteoblasts that have become surrounded by the calcified matrix of bone. Each osteocyte occupies a space or lacuna, interconnected to adjacent cells by thin cytoplasmic processes that form gap junctions. These processes, in turn, run in small canals or canaliculi in the bone and further communicate with the larger vascular channels (Volkmann and Haversian canals). It is possible that these cells act as mechanoreceptors or mechanosensors, identifying the loads placed on the individual bones and establishing the nature of such loads.[14]

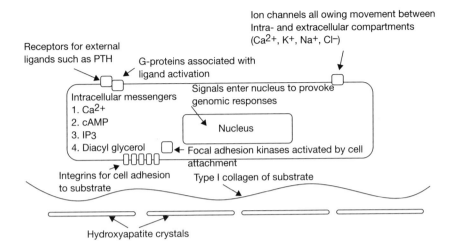

Fig. 1.2 A diagrammatic representation of an osteoblast indicating some of the signalling pathways currently recognized. PTH, parathyroid hormone; cAMP, cyclic adenosine monophosphate; IP_3, inositol triphosphate.

1.3.3 Osteoclasts

Osteoclasts are large multinucleated cells whose function is to resorb calcified cartilage and bone. They are found in well-defined pits known as 'Howship's lacunae'. The cells are derived from mononuclear-precursor stem cells in the bone marrow and travel, via the blood vessels, to the sites of activity where they can fuse with other similar cells. The cells are activated by a series of intercellular signalling molecules referred to as 'cytokines', produced by a variety of cells (including osteoblasts), and include inter-leukins (IL-1, IL-6, IL-11, IL-18), osteoprotegerin (OPG) and osteoprotegerin ligand (OPGL)[15] (Fig. 1.3).

1.3.4 Bone lining cells

Bone lining cells are flat, elongated cells covering bone surfaces. They are inactive and have a high nucleus to cytoplasmic ratio. Little is known regarding their function, but they have been considered to act as a mem-brane that controls the passage of ions into and out of the skeleton. In this way, by perhaps coordinating the remodelling of bone, these cells will have a major impact on calcium metabolism within the body.[16]

1.4   COUPLING OF BONE RESORPTION AND FORMATION

All connective tissues undergo continual breakdown and rebuilding, a process known as 'remodelling'. The skeleton is continuously remodelled

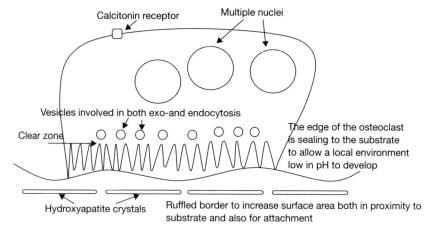

Fig. 1.3 A diagrammatic representation of an osteoclast indicating some of the functional requirements currently recognized. Receptor numbers are in the order of magnitude of 10^6.

throughout life with the resorption of old bone by osteoclasts and the subsequent formation of new bone by osteoblasts (Fig. 1.4). Internal remodelling limits the resorption and formation of bone to one location without changing its external or macroscopic form. This is in contrast to changes induced during growth involving all the bony structures. Bone remodelling is an essential part of the localized response to orthodontic forces, which permits tooth movement. Remodelling is known to occur more generally in the craniofacial skeleton during functional appliance therapy, as well as locally around the teeth.

The normal relationship between bone resorption and deposition changes throughout life; three distinct phases are known:

1.   *Phase I—The growing skeleton* (up to the age of the mid-twenties)—During this phase there is an increase in bony mass. The bodily maturation growth curves (see Scammon curves in ref. 17, Fig. 4.3) clearly show the differing rates of growth in the different tissues of the body. However, the underlying trend is always for an increase in skeletal mass. The amount of bone deposited in the skeleton at this time is far in excess of the amount lost. This can be reflected by the recommended daily amount of calcium required in constructing skeletal structures. Young children are particularly prone to poor development if the 'building blocks' of their skeleton are deficient. Tissue remodelling in these individuals, such as during orthodontic treatment, is less damaging than in other patients, and there is an overall 'intention' of the body to build skeletal form. Most tissues are well perfused and the risk of tissue damage is minimal.

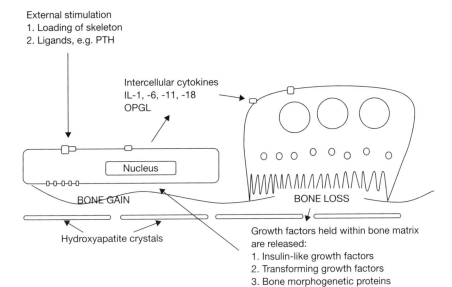

A diagrammatic representation of the interaction (coupling) of an osteoclast with an osteoblast.

Fig. 1.4 The interrelationship between osteoblasts and osteoclasts coordinating bone loss with bone gain. PTH, parathyroid hormone; IL, interleukin; OPGL, osteoprotegerin ligand.

2.   *Phase II—The adult skeleton* (the mid-twenties to late forties)—During this stage of skeletal maturation the amount of bone lost is equal to the amount of bone formed. In this way the two processes of bone loss and bone deposition are said to be 'coupled'. The skeleton appears stable provided excessive forces are not applied. There is a reduction in tissue perfusion to the skeleton in this phase and it is easy to exceed the envelope of therapeutic load to produce damage.

3.   *Phase III – The older skeleton* (beyond the late forties)—At this stage the skeleton begins to reduce in mass, there being an increase in loss of bone over bone deposition. This leads to an uncoupling of the balance between bone formation and bone resorption, and, in extreme cases, can result in the dramatic reduction of bone mass as characterized by the disease osteoporosis.

1.5   REGULATION OF BONE REMODELLING

Changes can be seen in the remodelling processes of bone with age, but what controls the whole process? Bone remodelling, which depends on a continuous supply of osteoclasts and osteoblasts, is regulated by systemic hormones (e.g. parathyroid hormone and calcitonin being the major calcium-regulating hormones) and by local factors such as the growth factors and cytokines discussed earlier.[18] Systemic hormones exert their effect by controlling the production and/or action of local mediators. In turn, these local mediators influence the cells of both the osteoclast and osteoblast lineages in a number of ways, namely:

- by stimulating the proliferation of undifferentiated precursor cells, which in turn can become osteoblasts or osteoclasts;
- by recruiting such cells to sites of remodelling activity; and
- by regulating not only their differentiation into osteoblasts or osteoclasts but also their function.

Osteoclasts have a limited life span of approximately 12.5 days, whilst that of the osteoblast is approximately 3 months. Therefore the progression of bone remodelling requires the continual addition of osteoclasts and, to a lesser extent, osteoblast precursor cells.

1.6   MECHANICALLY INDUCED STRAIN

Whenever a force is applied to bone, two prinicipal effects can be described, namely a localized cellular effect and a more generalized tissue response.

1.6.1   Cellular effects

The subject of mechanical deformation is of interest in many areas of medicine, but especially so in orthodontics. Generally, mechanical deformation leads to immediate, intermediate and long-term cellular responses.

Immediate response (within 1–2 seconds)
The first-onset change in skeletal cells includes the activation of ion channels,[19-21] leading to a change of membrane permeability and possible depolarization. This is a consequence of potassium ions leaving the cell and a much smaller number of calcium ions entering the cell. Other theories exist related to streaming potentials or piezoelectric effects; but whilst these are actual physical phenomena, the possible signals within an *in vivo* situation are questionable.[22] Potassium stretch-activated channels are a common mechanism by which most non-excitable cells respond to stretch.[23] The influx of calcium ions acts as a major second messenger, activating many pathways within the cytoplasm of the cell and subsequent nuclear pathways.

Mechanical deformation of bone cells was originally thought to be mediated via prostaglandin production and the cAMP pathway.[24,25] However, subsequent research showed that, in addition to cAMP, the phosphoinositide (PI) pathway was also activated and that the activation of adenylate cyclase was relatively small.[26] Another second messenger involved in mediating the effects of mechanical deformation is calcium (Ca^{2+}). Ca^{2+} is mobilized from intracellular stores in the endoplasmic reticulum secondary to activation of the PI pathway, leading to inositol triphosphate production and activation by such a messenger.[27] It appears likely that the Ca^{2+} changes reported by Harell et al.[25] occur as the result of a Ca^{2+} flux through stretch-activated ion channels in the cell membrane; clear evidence has linked G-proteins with this phenomena in a time scale that supports ion-channel activation.[21] Changes in cell shape, induced by changes in an individual cell skeleton (actin), can also produce a range of effects, including exposure of parts of the cell membrane (binding sites; integrins and focal adhesion kinase) to the substrate or exposure of receptor sites for specific ligands.

The actual mechanics of this response involve either physical deformation of the membrane or the activation of kinases associated with proteins attaching the cell to its substrate, especially the integrins. In addition, the activation of specific pathways may lead to caspase activation and programmed cell death (apoptosis), thus further modifying the functional response of a tissue.

Theories relating external loading of cells to bone remodelling include those of electrical effects, locally induced cellular mediators, stress and strain, and fluid flow/distribution changes; each of which is discussed further.

1. *Electrical effects*:
    (a) Piezoelectric—this is a short-lived change in potential (<3 mV over 1–2 ms) due to deformation of the inorganic components of bone (hydroxyapatite crystals).
    (b) Streaming potentials—this effect is produced by deforming a polar molecule/ion in fluid and again produces a short-lived change in potential difference.
    Both these theories are almost certainly overwhelmed by changes in the membrane potential of excitable tissues (muscles and nerves). The most overwhelming changes are produced by the muscles of mastication. The muscle is striated in form and requires an action potential change before it can contract; the normal masticatory frequency is 32–40 cycles a minute. In this way changes of 100 mV are frequently evoked, which in turn overwhelm the changes at the bone surface.[28]

2. *Locally induced cellular mediators*—The stimulation of cells to produce local messengers and/or metabolites is almost certainly an 'outcome' measure of cellular activity. However, these theories describe the consequence of mechanical loading and not the relationship.

3. *Stress and strain*[29]—This theory tries to relate the external load to the signal by considering bone in a manner similar to an engineering structure, and tries to relate the changes to either a compressive or a tensile load/strain. However (see later), the direct relationship of deformation to loading has to be questioned at a cellular level.

4. *Fluid flow/distribution changes*—As discussed later, all cells require adequate tissue perfusion, and small changes in perfusion lead to major changes in

cellular activity. The pressures within blood vessels are such that loads induced by orthodontic treatment can easily induce such changes.

However, all these theories are a 'false categorization': several theories belonging to and having an effect on another category of theory.

Intermediate response

The intermediate changes occur within 1–60 minutes of loading and involve many biochemical cytosolic messengers, including: cAMP, inositol trisphosphate, diacylglycerol, tyrosine kinase, cyclic adenosine ribose, and many more.[30] All these molecules ultimately establish a signalling mechanism, passing from the cell cytosol to within the nucleus to produce the long-term effects of mechanical loading with increased protein production and/or gene expression.

Long-term response

Changes in gene expression can occur following mechanical deformation, ranging from early-onset genes to specific protein-constructing genes such as those encoding collagen I and osteocalcin. In addition, either cell proliferation or cellular development of precursor cell populations may be activated, which in turn can increase the quantity of bone present.

1.6.2   Tissue effects

The cellular changes induced by loading (strain) are complex and not fully understood, but we are all aware of the bodily changes that occur on a more generalized scale as a result of repeated loading. Mechanically induced strain generated by physical exercise and mechanical loading is a major determinant of the structure and remodelling of the skeleton. There is a large body of evidence[31–33] to relate increases in load with an increase in the dimensions of skeletal structures. Conversely, astronauts who have limited external loading due to the diminished gravitational demands have a reduced skeletal structure and a generalized decrease in body calcium.[34,35] It can be demonstrated that a decrease in loading results in a reduction of total body calcium as the skeleton is resorbed. To overcome this loss of bone, simple mechanical stimulation is necessary. Thus astronauts undertake a period of exercise and bedridden patients have forms of physiotherapy to stimulate the skeletal structures. Basic studies on bone have clearly identified the minimum stimulation needed to maintain skeletal mass.[36] This work determined that a minimum of 30 cycles of loading during a 24-hour period is appropriate. Whilst this is sufficient to prevent loss, the experiments also established that continuous loads lead to the formation of porous bone and with a reduction in mass. This will be considered further when discussing changes induced during tooth movement.

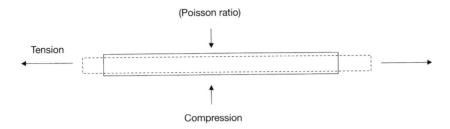

(Poisson ratio)

Tension

Compression

Fig. 1.5 The Poisson's effect of deforming a material clearly demonstrates that whilst there are distinctions between tensile and compression loads, applying one style of loading effectively loads the material with both types of load.

1.7 COMPRESSION LOADING VERSUS TENSION LOADING

There is much controversy regarding which loads activate cells most efficiently. The current level of confusion can clearly be seen in the literature by examining the reported techniques used by surgeons in assisting skeletal manipulation. The use of compression plates has been recommended for some fractures of the facial skeleton, with the consideration that this loading will enhance bone repair.[37] The latest technique, discovered serendipitously, is 'distraction osteogenesis'.[38] This stimulates bone deposition by tension, which is diametrically opposed to the concept of compression.

However, the answer to this complex problem must come from considering cells as a material, in which case it can be deduced that the cells are unable to differentiate between compression and tension. The Poisson's ratio of any material states that for the elongation of a material in one plane, there is a reduction in the dimension of the material in the plane normal to that in which the load was applied (Fig. 1.5). Therefore if cells behave in the same manner however they are deformed they will demonstrate compression in one plane and tension in another plane, and vice versa. That is, as a cell is stretched in one direction it is constricted in another.

When tooth movement occurs, there is said to be compression in the periodontal ligament in the direction of tooth movement and tension on the opposite side. Bone is said to be laid down in the areas of tension and lost in areas of compression (Fig. 1.6). This is the converse of the orthopaedic argument when misaligned fractures respond by bone addition in sites of compression and bone loss in sites of tension. However, unlike bone fractures, in orthodontics there is a specialized, soft and flexible tissue, namely the periodontal ligament. In the case of a fractured limb, soft tissues are present (e.g. the periosteum) but they surround the fracture site. Loading of either of these soft tissues will, however, modify the blood flow within them

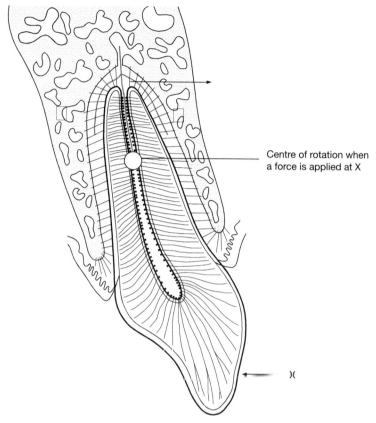

Centre of rotation when
a force is applied at X

Fig. 1.6 Diagram of the cross-section of a tooth indicating the compressive (C) and tensile (T) sites.

and in so doing, modify cellular activity. With this in mind, consider once again the periodontal ligament. In areas of compression there will be a reduced blood supply and hence minimal or no bone deposition, whilst in areas of tension there will be good perfusion, which in turn will lead to bone deposition.[39]

1.8   REGULATION OF RESORPTION

Bone resorption is a complex process involving both the removal of the mineral and the organic basis of the bone matrix. Osteoclasts are the cells responsible for this process, which occurs in the subosteoclastic resorption zone, a specialized extracellular compartment bounded by the ruffled border of the cell and the mineralized matrix (see Fig. 1.3). Osteoclasts acidify the subosteoclastic resorption zone leading to mineral dissolution, while the organic matrix is degraded by proteolytic enzymes, especially the matrix metalloproteinases (MMPs) and cysteine proteinases (CPs). It is not known how resorption sites are determined, although binding of the osteo-clast to a substrate is an essential first stage.[40] This in turn provokes an intracellular response. However, in addition to their role in directly regu-lating osteoclast formation and function, osteoblasts play an accessory role in resorption. They are first involved by retracting to expose the non-mineralized surface layer of the bone and secondly by releasing MMPs that degrade the surface layer of osteoid, thus facilitating access of osteo-clasts to the mineralized matrix. Figure 1.7 represents a hypothetical model of the cellular interactions and molecular mechanisms involved in this complex sequence of events.

Resorption is brought about by resident connective tissue cells and by infiltrating inflammatory cells. Tissue remodelling is usually tightly regu-lated by a complex interplay of cell–cell and cell–matrix interactions involv-ing the production of enzymes, activators, inhibitors, and regulatory mole-cules such as cytokines and growth factors. MMPs function at neutral pH and can digest all the structural molecules in bone matrix. Biochemical and molecular studies indicate the presence of three major groups: the specific collagenases that cleave interstitial collagens; the gelatinases which not only degrade types IV, V, VII, and XI collagens but also act synergistically with collagenases by degrading denatured collagens (gelatins); and the stromelysins, which have broader substrate specificity and can degrade naturally occurring inhibitors. TIMPs (tissue inhibitors of metalloprotein-ases) are important extracellularly in controlling the actions of MMPs.

1.9   THE PERIODONTAL LIGAMENT

This is composed of fibroblasts and fibres, collagen being the most prevalent, although elastic tissues also exist. It is the loading of the periodontal liga-ment and the induction of tissue remodelling changes that invoke the cascade of events that allow teeth to move through the alveolus. It is also an understanding of these remodelling changes and the duration of the events with respect to the patient's biological age that determine retention regimens, particularly the time taken for the tissues to adapt to the new position of the dentition (see later).

Detailed descriptions of the histology of tooth movement[41–43] have high-lighted the basic changes seen at tissue level: that is, the traditional com-pression of the ligament leading to bone loss, and tension leading to bone deposition. These previous descriptions have also identified such phenomena as 'undermining resorption' following the application of excessive loads. Another identifiable change within the periodontium associated with excess-ive loading is that of hyalinization, i.e. an amorphous ground-glass appear-ance lacking cellular or fibrous form. This area of acellular appearance is described as taking a considerable time to remodel, vascular invasion and perfusion being protracted. If this is induced it is said that 'undermining

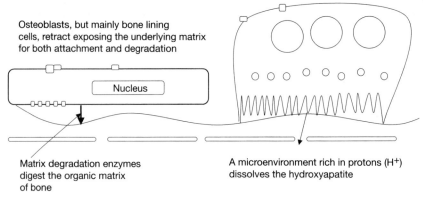

Osteoblasts, but mainly bone lining
cells, retract exposing the underlying matrix
for both attachment and degradation

Nucleus

Matrix degradation enzymes
digest the organic matrix
of bone

A microenvironment rich in protons (H$^+$)
dissolves the hydroxyapatite

A diagrammatic representation of the interaction of an osteoclast with
an osteoblast in degrading bone.

Fig. 1.7 A representation of how the osteoblast assists in the degradation of the
bone matrix.

resorption' occurs, which leads to no movement of the tooth until sudden-
ly there is resorption of the cortical plate (lamina dura of the periodontal
ligament) and the tooth can rapidly move. However, there is clear evidence
that hyalinization to varying degrees is commonplace[44] and we must aim to
minimize this rather than eliminate it completely.

Changes identified in the periodontal ligament following orthodontic loading
The following occur on the **compression side**:
- compression of blood vessels
- attraction of osteoclasts
- resorption of bone (Howship's lacunae)
- production of fibrous tissue in the Howship's lacunae;

while those on the **tension side** lead to:
- stretching of periodontal ligament fibres
- stimulation of osteoblasts on the bone surface
- deposition of bone.

The concept of an 'efficient' loading range
As a result of these considerations the concepts of an optimum tooth load
during orthodontic treatment have been developed. Forces that are too light
produce no effect; forces between a specific range of loads allow the appropriate cellular response; whilst loads above an excessive amount induce

abnormal/possible damaging tissue changes as described previously. This has been supported at the cellular level when cells were examined for the immediate consequences of ionic change; if they were excessively loaded no ionic change was observed, i.e. there appears to be an upper physiological limit beyond which the cells do not make the immediate response.[45] Clinically, this has to be considered with respect to teeth of differing root surface areas provoking differing responses:

- Very high loads lead to the induction of minimal movement of molar teeth (high loads on small, single-rooted teeth can lead to pathological change).
- Smaller loads will induce local bone remodelling allowing the teeth to move.

Tissue changes with respect to retention

Teeth that have been derotated during treatment have a high tendency to rotational relapse, either as a result of stretching of the collagen fibres within the periodontal ligament,[46,47] or as a result of stretching the gingival tissues as a whole. The correction of rotations can occur early on in treatment with fixed appliances;[48] provided the standard of oral hygiene is good, consideration should be given to carrying out pericision[49] on initially, very rotated teeth. Here, the supragingival principal fibres of the periodontium are severed to allow for the release of any tension in the soft tissues. Pericision has been shown to reduce the degree of rotational relapse many years postretention[50].

Orthodontic loads

These are often erroneously referred to as 'continuous loads'. The *in vivo* situation has to be considered at all times and loading can be either intermittent or continuous. For example, the loading characteristics of stainless-steel archwires used with fixed appliances are consistent with heavy initial loads followed by a period of load decay over 14–20 days. Conversely, with the modern flexible wires made of nickel–titanium alloys loads are more continuously applied and over a protracted period (Fig. 1.8) (see also Chapter 7). The application of forces generated by the appliances can be considered to be either inter- or intramaxillary:

- *Intermaxillary loads* (applied between the maxilla and mandible)—The major forms of either Class II or Class III interarch mechanics (intermaxillary elastics or functional appliances) typically utilize cyclic loading generated by the oral musculature. The appliances are placed in the mouth and examined, often statically, but once the patient leaves the surgery normal muscular function is reinstated and the appliances begin to interact with dynamic loads.

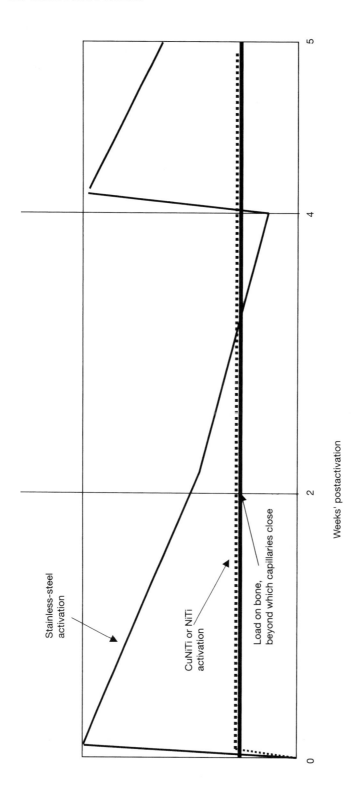

Fig. 1.8 The loads induced by stainless-steel technology and flexible nickel–titanium wire.

- *Intramaxillary loads* (loads generated within one arch; either the maxilla or mandible)—These are loads used for space closure or opening. Continuous loading will occur when nickel–titanium coil springs are used, whilst intermittent loading will be seen when space is closed using an elastic chain (see Chapter 7). Similarly, intermittent loading will occur with removable appliances used to move teeth.

It should be remembered that all these loading regimens are superimposed over the loads generated during mastication.

Blood flow

All cells require some access to a circulation, be it a micro- or macrocirculation, in order to transport the compounds necessary for aerobic respiration or to eliminate the waste products of that respiration. In the case of cartilage, nutrition is delivered via diffusion from the joint space, whilst bone cells acquire their nutrition from vascular channels within the structure. In addition, the bone lining cells previously mentioned can act as a filtering membrane controlling the exchange of ions from the inorganic part of the skeleton. The vessels from the surrounding alveolar bone generally enter the periodontal ligament space close to the apical foramen to supply the cells of the periodontal ligament. However, there are other sites all along the interface of alveolus and ligament through which blood vessels enter.

The general microcirculation of the vasculature ensures that the cells are supplied with nutrients, and that the breakdown products are removed. The continuous forming and reabsorption of tissue fluid, originally described as Starling's hypothesis,[51] has yet to be superseded by a more logical concept. For this reason a brief overview of tissue microcirculation is included here.

Arteries (arterioles) (Fig. 1.9)

The pressure is said to be 40 mmHg at the arteriolar end of the capillary. Plasma proteins (manufactured by the liver), which are too large to leave the capillary, produce an inward directed pressure of 25 mmHg. Thus at the arteriolar end of the capillary, there is an outward driving force equivalent to 15 mmHg. Cells of the blood vascular system are also too large and seldom leave the capillary, although it is now generally accepted that the diameter of capillaries is less than that of red blood cells and so there is distortion of both endothelium and erythrocytes as the cells pass along the capillaries.

Veins (venules)

At the venous end the hydrostatic pressure (that due to pressure within the fluid) is 15 mmHg, while the pressure due to the proteins remains at 25 mmHg. Therefore there is a net influx pressure of 10 mmHg, dragging the fluid back into the microcirculation together with the waste products of cellular respiration. The balance of 5 mmHg (hydrostatic minus the influx

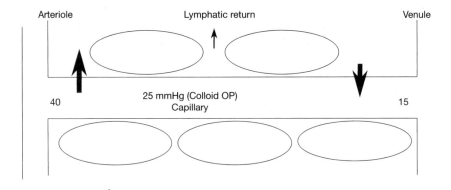

Fig. 1.9 Starlings hypothesis establishes variations in the fluid pressure throughout the vascular system but especially in the region of the capillaries. OP, outward pressure.

pressure) disappears into the lymphatic system. Whilst this is an oversimplification, it does detail the outline of what is happening around every cell supplied by a vascular supply.

Is the vascular supply important?

Studies on the rat tibia[52] have shown that by modifying the blood supply in a chronic manner, i.e. over a period of 3–6 weeks, the amount of bone present is dependent on the blood supply. A reduction in blood supply resulted in a decrease in bone mass, whilst an increase in the blood supply led to an increase in bone both in terms of quantity and density. A parallel can be seen with regard to tooth movement and age; in young patients with a highly vascularized facial skeleton there can be rapid movement, whilst in older patients there is a slower response, especially in the mandible.[53]

Anchorage

This term is used extensively in orthodontics and often in association with extraction space. Anchorage is essentially the reaction of other tissues to the forces applied by an appliance to achieve the appropriate tooth movement. It is a function of the root surface area; the larger the root surface area, the greater the load required to move the tooth. The loading has very many biological variations, and it is important to realize that what can be considered the correct level of loading on one tooth may be considered anchorage on others. For example, a heavy load applied (either with a fixed or removable appliance) to an upper central incisor may be so great that it invokes high levels of hyalinization in the periodontal ligament space, thus preventing its movement. The reaction in the remaining buccal segment teeth, with their increased root surface area, would allow them to readily move mesially (Fig. 1.10).

Conversely, a light force in the incisor will allow it to move, but its distribution over the buccal segment teeth will not allow movement. Equally the stage of development of the occlusion has major effects on the anchorage balance; younger patients with incomplete apices and a highly vascular skeleton will have differing envelopes of loading than adult patients with poor skeletal vascularity and complete apices.

It is essential for the understanding of orthodontic appliance treatment that anchorage is considered in all three spatial planes:

1. *Anteroposterior*—This is the classical consideration of anchorage and serves to illustrate the situation. Also the opposite effect (impacted mandibular premolars adjacent to mandibular second molars can be moved mesially whilst traction to the lingual arch distalises the second molar.

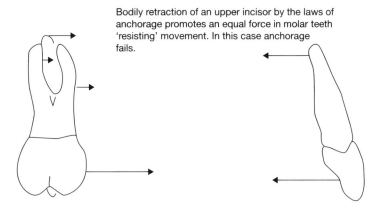

Bodily retraction of an upper incisor by the laws of anchorage promotes an equal force in molar teeth 'resisting' movement. In this case anchorage fails.

Root **surface** area is high:
Load applied per unit area is low **but at threshold**.
The tooth therefore moves mesially.

Root surface area is low:
Load applied per unit area is high **above threshold.**
The tooth therefore does not move.

Fig. 1.10 A diagrammatic representation to indicate how a heavy load applied to teeth with a small root surface area may exceed the physiological load for these teeth and prevent their movement. However, the reaction dissipated throughout the anchor teeth with a larger root surface area will approach the 'ideal' loading to induce movement.

2. *Vertical*—A lack of understanding of anchorage is often seen in this dimension when considering impacted maxillary canines. The fixed appliances, using flexible archwires, often only allow the lateral incisor and first premolar to be used as a base unit to extrude the maxillary canine. In this case the canine will remain stationary and the adjacent teeth will be intruded. Either a removable appliance or a fixed appliance with a rigid base archwire, but incorporating all the maxillary teeth, will help to redress the balance (Fig. 1.11).

3. *Transverse*—Often reciprocal; closing a median diastema, or rapid maxillary expansion.

Biology of the mechanically deformed periodontium

When a load is applied to a tooth, after deformation of the calcified structures of the tooth, the load is passed on to the vessels of the periodontal ligament and apical vessels. As described in Starling's hypothesis, there is only a small pressure within thin-walled vessels of the microcirculation, which can readily be overcome by the external forces. This initial loading provokes stasis within the periodontal ligament, reduces pulpal blood flow (intrusive forces demonstrating a mild transient reduction,[54]) and presumably must induce an environment of anaerobic respiration. Eventually a form of reactive hyperaemia develops[55] and the blood flow is restored. During this time many cells are activated to promote the production of locally active agents (interleukins, etc.—mentioned earlier), which in turn promote the activation of osteoclasts leading to bony resorption. In addition, the many degradative enzymes of the periodontal ligament (collagenase, stromelysin, etc.) begin digesting the structural proteins of the periodontal ligament.

SUMMARY

1. Tissues involved in skeleton that may be involved in growth of the face include:
   - Cartilage tissue   Sphenoccipital synchondrosis
                         Nasal septum
                         Condylar cartilage
   - Bone
2. There are four different cell types are found in bone:
   - Osteoblasts—produce high levels of alkaline phosphatase, type I collagen, osteocalcin, and respond to PTH
   - Osteocytes—mechanosensors
   - Osteoclasts—resorb bone
   - Bone lining cells—ion filters
   Osteoclasts and osteoblasts activity is coordinated—coupling.

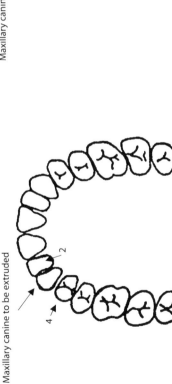

Maxillary canine to be extruded

Placement of a fixed appliance on to the whole dentition
Will put the lateral (2) and first premolar (4) at risk of intrusion.
The only root surfaces resisting intrusion are (2) and (4)

Maxillary canine to be extruded

Using a removable appliance with acrylic palate or a fixed
appliance to all teeth but with a rigid base wire will help
reduce the tendency for intrusion. Arrows indicate teeth
resisting intrusion. The palatal acrylic includes the palate
in the anchorage equation.

Fig. 1.11 The vertical consideration of anchorage to understand why it is not always possible to extrude a maxillary canine by means of a fixed appliance.

3. Three phases of skeleton
   • Phase I—The growing skeleton (up to the age of the mid-twenties)
   • Phase II—The adult skeleton (the mid twenties to late forties)
   • Phase III—The older skeleton (beyond the late forties)
   There are several theories of remodelling; electrical, local induced cellular mediators, stress and strain, and fluid flow/distribution changes.
   Compression has similar effects to tensile loading.

REFERENCES

1. Kessel, R. (1998). *Basic medical histology*. Oxford University Press.
2. Berkovitz, B. K., Moxham, B. J., and Newman, H. N. (1995). *The periodontal ligament in health and disease* (2nd edn). Mosby Wolfe, London.
3. Berkovitz, B. K. B., Holland, G. R., and Moxham, B. J. (2002). *Oral anatomy, histology and embryology* (3rd edn). Mosby, London.
4. Berkovitz, B. K. B. and Moxham B. J. (2002). *Head and neck anatomy: a clinical reference*. Martin Dunitz, London.
5. Scott, J. H. and Symons, N. B. B. (1977). *Introduction to dental anatomy*. Churchill Livingstone, London.
6. Meikle, M. C. (2002). *Craniofacial development, growth and evolution*. Bateson Publishing, Norfolk
7. Mavragani, M., Boe, O. E., Wisth, P. J., and Selvig, K. A. (2002). Changes in root length during orthodontic treatment: advantages for immature teeth. *European Journal of Orthodontics*, **24**, 91–7.
8. Asahina, I., Sampath, T. K., Nishimura, I., and Hauschka, P. V. (1993). Human osteogenic protein-1 induces both chondroblastic and osteoblastic differentiation of osteoprogenitor cells derived from newborn rat calvaria. *Journal of Cell Biology*, **123**, 921–33.
9. Copray, J. C., Jansen, H. W., and Duterloo, H. S. (1986). Growth and growth pressure of mandibular condylar and some primary cartilages of the rat *in vitro*. *American Journal of Orthodontics and Dentofacial Orthopedics*, **90**, 19–28.
10. Yamashiro, T. and Takano-Yamamoto, T. (1998). Differential responses of mandibular condyle and femur to oestrogen deficiency in young rats. *Archives of Oral Biology*, **43**, 191–5.
11. Meikle, M. C., Bord, S., Hembry, R. M., Compston, J., Croucher, P. I., and Reynolds, J. J. (1992). Human osteoblasts in culture synthesize collagenase and other matrix metalloproteinases in response to osteotropic hormones and cytokines. *Journal of Cell Science*, **103**, 1093–9.
12. Vukicevic, S., Luyten, F. P., and Reddi, A. H. (1989). Stimulation of the expression of osteogenic and chondrogenic phenotypes *in vitro* by osteogenin. *Proceedings of the National Academy of Science, USA*, **86**, 8793–7.
13. Ducy, P. (2000). Cbfa1: a molecular switch in osteoblast biology. *Developmental Dynamics*, **219**, 461–71.
14. Mullender, M. G. and Huiskes, R. (1997). Osteocytes and bone lining cells: which are the best candidates for mechano-sensors in cancellous bone? *Bone*, **20**, 527–32.
15. Kong, Y. Y., Yoshida, H., Sarosi, I., Tan, H. L., Timms, E., Capparelli, C., Morony, S., Oliveira-dos-Santos, A. J., Van, G., Itie, A., Khoo, W., Wakeham, A., Dunstan, C. R., Lacey, D. L., Mak, T. W., Boyle, W. J., and Penninger, J. M. (1999). OPGL is a key reg-

ulator of osteoclastogenesis, lymphocyte development and lymph-node organogenesis. *Nature*, **397**, 315–23.

16. McDonald, F. (2000). *Bone homeostasis: extracellular calcium levels and their control*; *MacMillan Life Science Encyclopaedia*, Article 2004. MacMillan, London.

17. Sinclair, D. and Dangerfield, P. (1998). *Human growth after birth* (6th edn). Oxford University Press.

18. Manolagas, S. C. (2000). Birth and death of bone cells: basic regulatory mechanisms and implications for the pathogenesis and treatment of osteoporosis. *Endocrine Reviews*, **21**, 115–37.

19. McDonald, F. and Houston, W. J. B. (1992). The affect of mechanical deformation on the distribution of potassium ions across the cell membrane of sutural cells. *Calcified Tissue International*, **50**, 547–52.

20. Leeves, M. A. and McDonald, F. (1995). The effect of mechanical deformation on the distribution of ions in fibroblasts. *American Journal of Orthodontics and Dento-facial Orthopaedics*, **107**, 625–32.

21. McDonald, F., Somasundaram, B., McCann, T. J., Mason, W. T., and Meikle, M. C. (1996). Calcium waves in fluid flow stimulated osteoblasts are G protein mediated. *Archives of Biochemistry and Biophysics*, **326**, 31–8.

22. McDonald, F. (1993). Electrical effects at the bone surface. *European Journal of Orthodontics*, **15**, 175–83.

23. Ypey, D. L., Weidema, A. F., Hold, K. M., Van der Laarse, A., Ravesloot, J. H., Van Der Plas, A., and Nijweide, P. J. (1992). Voltage, calcium, and stretch activated ionic channels and intracellular calcium in bone cells. *Journal of Bone and Mineral Research*, **7**(Suppl. 2), S377–S387.

24. Rodan, G. A., Bourret, L. A., Harvey, A., and Mensi, T. (1975). Cyclic AMP and cyclic GMP: mediators of the mechanical effects on bone remodeling. *Science*, **189**, 467–9.

25. Harell, A., Dekel, S., and Binderman, I. (1977). Biochemical effect of mechanical stress on cultured bone cells. *Calcified Tissue Research*, **22**, S202–S207.

26. Sandy, J. R., Meghji, S., Farndale, R. W., and Meikle, M. C. (1989). Dual elevation of cyclic AMP and inositol phosphates in response to mechanical deformation of murine osteoblasts. *Biochimica Biophysica Acta*, **1010**, 265–9.

27. McCann, T. J., Keyte, J. W., Terranova, G., Papaioannou, S., Mason, W. T., Meikle, M. C., and McDonald, F. (1998). An analysis of calcium release by DGEA: mobilisation of two functionally distinct internal stores in Saos-2 cells. *American Journal of Physiology: Cell Physiology*, **275**, C33–C41.

28. McDonald, F. and Houston, W. J. B. (1990). An *in vivo* assessment of muscular activity and the importance of electrical phenomena in bone remodelling. *Journal of Anatomy*, **172**, 165–75.

29. Epker, B. N. and Frost, H. M. (1965). Correlation of bone resorption and formation with the physical behaviour of bone. *Journal of Dental Research*, **44**, 33–41.

30. Sandy, J. R., Farndale, R. W., and Meikle, M. C. (1993). Recent advances in understanding mechanically induced bone remodeling and their relevance to orthodontic theory and practice. *American Journal of Orthodontics and Dentofacial Orthopedics*, **103**, 212–22.

31. Currey, J. D. (1979). Mechanical properties of bone tissues with greatly differing functions. *Journal of Biomechanics*, **12**, 313–19.

32. Goodship, A. E., Lanyon, L. E., and MacFie, H. (1979). Functional adaptation of bone to increased stress. *Journal of Bone and Joint Surgery*, **61A**, 539–46.

33. Rubin, C. R. (1984). Skeletal strain and the functional significance of bone architecture. *Calcified Tissue International*, **36**, S11–S18.

34. Loomer, P. M. (2001). The impact of microgravity on bone metabolism *in vitro* and *in vivo*. *Critical Reviews in Oral Biology and Medicine*, **12**, 252–61.

35. Heer, M., Kamps, N., Biener, C., Korr, C., Boerger, A., Zittermann, A., Stehle, P., and Drummer, C. (1999). Calcium metabolism in microgravity. *European Journal of Medical Research*, **4**, 357–60.

36. Lanyon, L. E. and Rubin, C. T. (1984). Static vs dynamic loads as an influence on bone remodelling. *Journal of Biomechanics*, **17**, 897–905.

37. Zachariades, N., Mezitis, M., and Rallis, G. (1996). An audit of mandibular fractures treated by intermaxillary fixation, intraosseous wiring and compression plating. *British Journal of Oral and Maxillofacial Surgery*, **34**, 293–7.

38. Ilizarov, G. A. (1989). The tension-stress effect on the genesis and growth of tissues: Part II. The influence of the rate and frequency of distraction. *Clinical Orthopedics*, **239**, 263–85. Also see: Ilizarov, G. A. (1989). The tension-stress effect on the genesis and growth of tissues. Part I. The influence of stability of fixation and soft-tissue preservation. *Clinical Orthopedics*, **238**, 249–81.

39. Wright, K. W. and Yettram, A. L. (1979). An analytical investigation into possible mechanical causes of bone remodelling. *Journal of Biomedical Engineering*, **1**, 41–9.

40. Lakkakorpi, P. T., Wesolowski, G., Zimolo, Z., Rodan, G. A., and Rodan, S. B. (1997). Phosphatidylinositol 3-kinase association with the osteoclast cytoskeleton, and its involvement in osteoclast attachment and spreading. *Experimental Cell Research*, **237**, 296–306.

41. Rygh, P. (1974). Elimination of hyalinized periodontal tissues associated with ortho-dontic tooth movement. *Scandinavian Journal of Dental Research*, **82**, 57–73.

42. Rygh, P. and Reitan, K. (1972). Ultrastructural changes in the periodontal ligament incident to orthodontic tooth movement. *Transactions of the European Orthodontic Society*, pp. 393–405.

43. Sims, M. R. (1976). Reconstitution of the human oxytalan system during ortho-dontic tooth movement. *American Journal of Orthodontics*, **70**, 38–58.

44. Brudvik, P. and Rygh, P. (1995). Transition and determinants of orthodontic root resorption–repair sequence. *European Journal of Orthodontics*, **17**, 177–88.

45. McDonald, F. and Yettram, A. L. (1995). The loading of cells and a possible upper limit of load response with respect to strain energy density. *Journal of Biomedical Materials Research*, **29**, 1577–85.

46. Reitan, K. (1958). Tissue rearrangement during retention of orthodontically rotated teeth. *Angle Orthodontist*, **29**, 105–13.

47. Edwards, J. G. (1968). A study of the periodontium during orthodontic rotation of teeth. *American Journal of Orthodontics*, **54**, 441–61.

48. Redlich, M., Rahamim, E., Gaft, A., and Shochan, S. (1996). The response of supraalveolar gingival collagen to orthodontic rotation movement in dogs. *American Journal of Orthodontics and Dentofacial Orthopedics*, **110**, 247–55.

49. Edwards, J. G. (1970). A surgical procedure to eliminate rotational relapse. *American Journal of Orthodontics*, **57**, 35–46.

50. Edwards, J. G. (1988). A long-term prospective evaluation of circumferential supracrestal fiberotomy in alleviating orthodontic relapse. *American Journal of Orthodontics and Dentofacial Orthopedics*, **93**, 380–7.

51. Ganong, W. F. (1998). *A review of medical physiology*. Lange Medical Publications, Los Altos, California.

52. Singh, M. and Brookes, M. (1971). Bone growth and blood flow after experimental venous ligation. *Journal of Anatomy*, **108**, 315–22.

53. Bradley, J. C. (1972). Age changes in the vascular supply of the mandible. *British Dental Journal*, **132**, 142–4.

54. Ikawa, M., Fujiwara, M., Horiuchi, H., and Shimauchi, H. (2001). The effect of short-term tooth intrusion on human pulpal blood flow measured by laser Doppler flowmetry. *Archives of Oral Biology*, **46**, 781–7.
55. McDonald, F. and Pitt Ford, T. R. (1994). Blood flow changes in permanent maxillary canines during retraction. *European Journal of Orthodontics*, **16**, 1–9.

2 Dentofacial classification and ideals

CONTENTS

Orthodontic treatment is performed for three main reasons, namely to improve:
- dentofacial aesthetics
- function
- health.

Function and health are controversial reasons for carrying out orthodontic treatment. These are covered extensively in other texts and in the *Index of orthodontic treatment need (dental health component)* for deciding whether a patient would benefit from orthodontic treatment (see Suggested reading). Aesthetics is certainly the main reason for orthodontic treatment, but what are the boundaries of the aesthetic ideals to which orthodontic treatment can be planned? In other words what can be considered to be normal, and when normal is not present can orthodontics bring the dentofacial complex back towards what can be considered to be an acceptable norm? In order to explore these questions it is worth considering the current description and classification of normal and abnormal occlusion or malocclusion. Similarly, the description and classification of the extraoral structures of the jaws and soft tissues will be discussed in this chapter.

2.1   OCCLUSAL IDEALS

In an **ideal** occlusion the patient will have the following features:
- 28 or 32 occluding teeth that are of normal size and shape.
- The teeth are perfectly aligned buccolingually and occlusogingivally.
- There are no rotations.
- There is no crowding or spacing.
- Each tooth is at the correct inclination (Fig. 2.1(a)) and angulation (Fig. 2.1(b)) with respect to its neighbour.
- The occlusal plane has limited Curves of Spee (anteroposterior) and Monson (transverse).
- Each upper tooth occludes with its opposing number in the lower arch and the one distal to it, with the exception of the upper third permanent molar. There is therefore a Class I buccal segment relationship (canine and molar) (see later).
- The upper teeth occlude buccal/labial to the lower arch teeth. The lower incisors therefore occlude on the palatal surfaces of the upper incisors in a Class I incisor relationship (see later). The buccal cusps of the lower molars and premolars occlude in the fossae of the upper buccal segment teeth.
- The upper and lower centrelines are coincident with each other and the facial midline. Even small deviations of the dental centreline from the facial midline can have a marked influence on the perceptions of dentofacial attractiveness.[1]
- The dental arches are symmetrical.

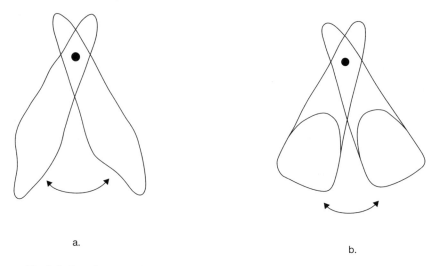

a.

b.

Fig. 2.1 Line drawings illustrating (a) inclination and (b) angulation of an upper central incisor.

A **normal** occlusion can be considered to be present when there are very minor deviations from this ideal, such as a small rotation or malalignment of a tooth. Andrews, in developing the Pre-adjusted Edgewise fixed appliance (Straight-wire® appliance), studied the occlusions of 120 so-called non orthodontic normals and came up with his six keys to normal occlusion.[2] These are listed below and discussed further in Chapter 6:

(1) correct molar relationship—the distal surface of the upper first permanent molar distobuccal cusp occludes with the mesiobuccal cusp of the lower second permanent molar;
(2) correct crown angulation (mesiodistal crown tip);
(3) correct crown inclination (labiolingual/buccolingual crown tip);
(4) no rotations;
(5) tight approximal contacts;
(6) flat occlusal plane—considered to be a desirable overcorrection as the Curve of Spee can be expected to increase with continued mandibular growth.

There is no precise definition of 'normal', and so what would be considered to be normal and acceptable to one patient may be considered abnormal and unacceptable to another. In addition, 'normal' could be considered a theoretical concept; the majority of the population do not have normal occlusions.

2.1.1 Classification of occlusion and malocclusion

The first classification of occlusion and malocclusion was developed by Angle in 1899[3] and is still widely used to describe the molar and canine relationships.

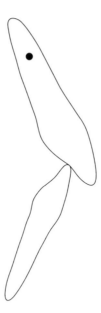

Fig. 2.2 In this Class I incisor relationship the lower incisor occludes with/lies directly below the cingulum plateau of the upper incisor.

The incisor classification is:
1. Class I—The lower incisor edges occlude with or lie directly below the cingulum plateau of the upper incisors (Fig. 2.2).
2. Class II—The lower incisor edges occlude with or lie directly palatal to the cingulum plateau of the upper incisors (Fig. 2.3). This is subdivided into:
   (a) Division 1:   the upper central incisors are of average inclination or proclined.
   (b) Division 2:   the upper central incisors are retroclined.
3. Class III—The lower incisor edges occlude with or lie directly anterior to the cingulum plateau of the upper incisors (Fig. 2.4).

In the normal occlusion the incisor relationship is Class I and the overjet measures 2–4 mm. The overbite is such that the upper incisors cover one-quarter to one-third of the lower incisors in occlusion.

The canine classification is:
1. Class I—The upper canine occludes in the buccal embrasure between the lower canine and lower first premolar (Fig. 2.5).
2. Class II—The upper canine occludes anterior to the buccal embrasure between the lower canine and lower first premolar.
3. Class III—The upper canine occludes posterior to the buccal embrasure between the lower canine and lower first premolar.

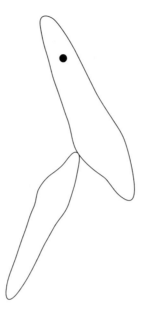

Fig. 2.3 In this Class II division 1 incisor relationship the lower incisor occludes with/lies palatal to the cingulum plateau of the upper incisor.

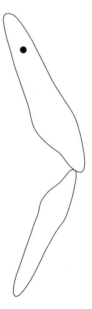

Fig. 2.4 In this Class III incisor relationship the lower incisor occludes with/lies anterior to the cingulum plateau of the upper incisor.

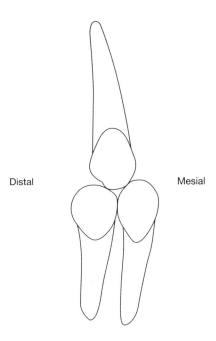

Fig. 2.5 A Class I canine relationship.

It is usual to describe how far Class II or Class III the canine relationship is from the Class I position by describing the distance in quarters of a single tooth unit (premolar width), e.g. a quarter of a unit Class II (Fig. 2.6).

The Angle's molar relationship is determined by the occlusal relationship of the mesiobuccal cusp of the upper first permanent and the anterior buccal groove of the lower first permanent molar. The molar classification is:

1. Class I—The mesiobuccal cusp of the upper first permanent molar occludes in the anterior buccal groove of the lower first permanent molar (Fig. 2.7).
2. Class II—The mesiobuccal cusp of the upper first permanent molar occludes anterior to the anterior buccal groove of the lower first permanent molar (Fig. 2.8).
3. Class III—The mesiobuccal cusp of the upper first permanent molar occludes posterior to the anterior buccal groove of the lower first permanent molar (Fig. 2.9).

As with the canine relationship, it is usual to describe how far Class II or Class III the molar relationship is from the Class I position by describing the distance in quarters of a single tooth unit (premolar width), e.g. a quarter of a unit Class II (Fig. 2.10). The Andrews' classification is more generally used today to describe molar relationships, with the important relationship being that of the distal surface of the upper first permanent molar disto-buccal cusp occluding with the mesiobuccal cusp of the lower second

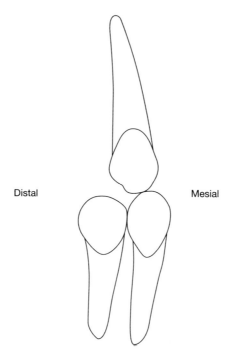

Distal   Mesial

Fig. 2.6 A ¼ unit Class II canine relationship.

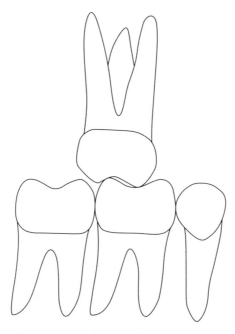

Fig. 2.7 Class I molar relationship. In this Angle's Class I molar relationship the mesiobuccal cusp of the upper first permanent molar occludes in the anterior buccal groove of the lower first permanent molar. Compare this with Andrews' Class I relationship in Fig. 2.11.

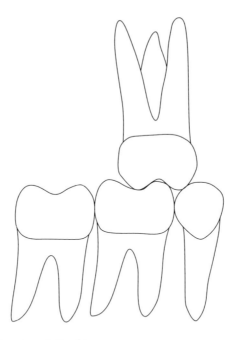

Fig. 2.8 Class II molar relationship.

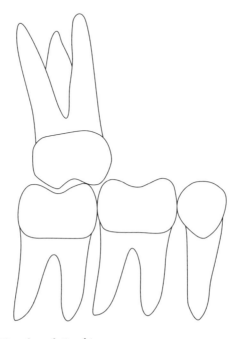

Fig. 2.9 Class III molar relationship.

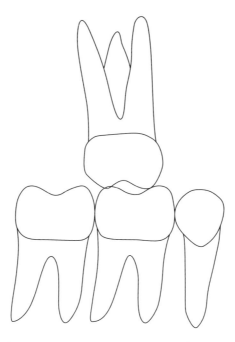

Fig. 2.10 A ¼ of a unit Class II molar relationship.

permanent molar. This is described as Class I (Fig. 2.11). Once again, in Class II the upper molar is anterior and in Class III posterior to this position, with quarter-unit descriptors added where appropriate.

When referring to a malocclusion the most important feature in the description is the incisor relationship. However, the terms 'malocclusion' and 'incisor relationship' are often used synonymously. When Angle first described the classification of malocclusion, the relationship of the first permanent molars was thought to be all important and would be reflected in the incisor relationship. It is now known that the incisor relationship, although often associated with a specific type of molar relationship, e.g. Class III incisors and Class III molars, can be totally independent of the molar relationship. The latter often being affected by the amount of crowding/spacing present.

2.2   FACIAL IDEALS

Facial ideals can be subdivided into skeletal ideals and into soft tissue ideals. These will be discussed in turn.

2.2.1   Skeletal ideals

Skeletal ideals can be further subdivided into anteroposterior, vertical, and transverse ideals.

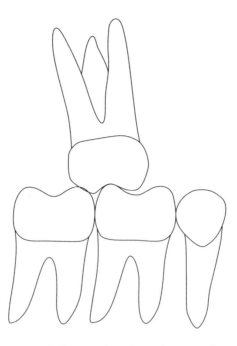

Fig. 2.11 In this Andrews' Class I molar relationship notice how the upper first permanent molar is more mesially angulated and its distobuccal cusp occludes with the mesiobuccal cusp of the lower second permanent molar.

Anteroposterior

This can be assessed both clinically and radiographically (see Suggested reading). Clinically, the maxilla will be seen to be just in advance of the mandible in a normal relationship when the teeth are in occlusion. By performing a simple cephalometric analysis and measuring the angle ANB (Fig. 2.12), the position of the maxilla can be determined numerically with respect to the mandible. An average value and a range in degrees for the angle ANB for this normal or Class I skeletal relationship is 3° ± 1°. A malrelationship, outside the range of normal, can be classified as Class II or Class III and is seen when the angle ANB is greater than 4° degrees or less than 2°, respectively (Figs 2.13(a) and (b)). Deciding whether an anteroposterior skeletal relationship is abnormal and therefore understanding the impact this will have on any proposed treatment is relatively straightforward when it is at one extreme or another, i.e. Class II or Class III. The difficulty comes when the anteroposterior skeletal pattern is only slightly outside the range of normal. For example, the angle ANB might measure 5° and so the case can definitely be classified as a Class II skeletal pattern. However, clinically it may be difficult to decide whether it is Class I or mild Class II; similarly, for Class III skeletal patterns.

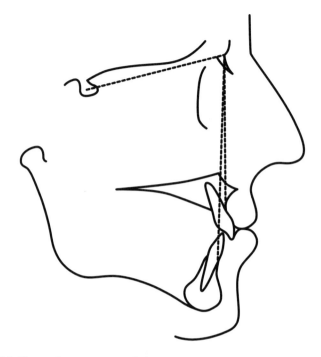

Fig. 2.12 The angle ANB on a cephalometric analysis. This is a Class I skeletal relationship.

A normal occlusion can be seen with a Class I normal anteroposterior skeletal relationship, but can also be seen in cases where the skeletal pattern differs from Class I tending towards Class II and Class III. By the same token, malocclusion can be seen in Class I cases. This is fortunate for the orthodontist, since a malocclusion can be treated to produce an ideal or normal occlusion not only in cases with a Class I skeletal pattern, but also in many Class II and Class III cases. However, as a general rule, unless there is already dentoalveolar compensation present (Fig. 2.14), the further away from normal the skeletal pattern, the more the orthodontist has to work to overcome the skeletal malrelationship in order to produce a normal occlusion.

Whether such dentoalveolar compensation is present or not, there are limiting factors which will determine how much further the orthodontist can adapt the position of the teeth to produce a normal occlusion. These include:

- *The alveolar bone and its ability to further remodel during tooth movement*— Generally bone is more able to remodel in the younger, growing patient (see Chapter 1).
- *Related to the alveolar bone will be the gingival attachment, particularly labial to the lower incisors*—When the attachment is thin, there is a risk that proclining the lower incisors may lead to gingival recession. The likelihood of

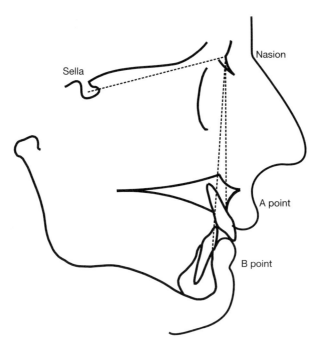

Fig. 2.13(a) In this cephalometric analysis the angle ANB exceeds 4° and so is a Class II skeletal pattern.

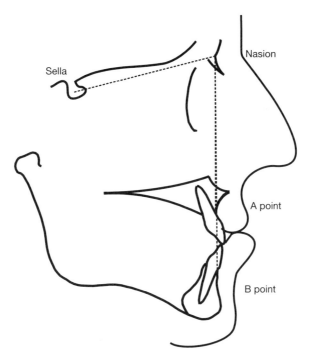

Fig. 2.13(b) In this cephalometric analysis the angle ANB is less than 2° and so is a Class III skeletal pattern.

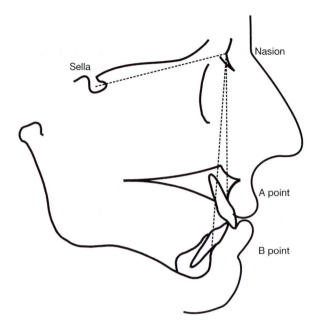

Fig. 2.14 In this cephalometric analysis the angle ANB is greater than 4° and so there is a Class II skeletal pattern, but the incisor relationship is Class I due to dentoalveolar compensation in the form of proclination of the lower incisors.

this happening is probably age-related, being more likely in adult patients. Research suggests it does not occur in children or adolescents, since the alveolus and attached gingivae can more effectively remodel during tooth movement in these patients.[4] However, this does not mean the lower incisors can be proclined with impunity, and a limit of 2–3 mm proclination is probably the maximum that is acceptable.[5]

- *The position of soft tissue balance*[6]—For example, proclining the lower incisors into the lower lip and out of soft tissue balance is likely to be unstable and lead to relapse.
- *Aesthetics*—Although it may be possible to move the teeth to produce an occlusion, at what might be considered to be one end of the range of normal, both intraoral and/or extraoral aesthetics might be compromised (Figs 2.15(a) and (b)).

Although normal anteroposterior skeletal relationships have been described there are many variations on the theme of normal, which are dependent on sex, age, and race. For example, the male anteroposterior relationship tends more towards Class III than the female, and the Afro-Caribbean face usually demonstrates a greater mean value for the angle ANB with both the upper and lower jaws being more prognathic than in the Caucasian face.[7] These variations are important considerations when treating to the so-called normal face.

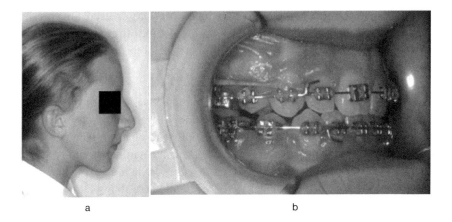

a   b

Fig. 2.15 (a) The lower part of the face of this patient demonstrates a retrusive mandible and yet the intraoral view (b) of the fixed appliance prior to debond shows there is a Class I incisor relationship.

Vertical

Vertical facial dimensions can be described angularly in degrees, as a linear measurement, or perhaps most simply in proportions (Fig. 2.16). The patient may therefore be described as having a normal, long or short face, but there is a continuous range from one extreme to the other. Although a

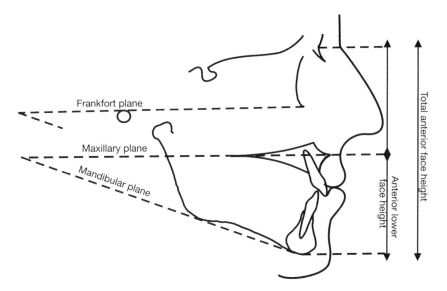

Fig. 2.16 Vertical facial dimensions can be measured as angles between two planes (e.g. between the maxillary and mandibular planes), as linear measurements (e.g. anterior lower face height), or as a ratio or percentage of one measurement to another (e.g. anterior lower face height to total face height).

long face may be associated with a reduced overbite or even an anterior open bite, and a short face with a deep and sometimes traumatic overbite, a normal occlusion can also be seen in all these facial forms.[8]

Transverse

Transverse skeletal relationships are really only assessed clinically. This is because radiographic landmark determination, and therefore any measurements made from a posteroanterior radiograph of the face and jaws, is unreliable. Almost everyone has some degree of facial asymmetry and so it can be considered to be normal. In extreme cases, which can obviously be described as being outside the range of normal, there may be an effect on the occlusion in the form of a crossbite (Fig. 2.17). Fortunately this is unusual. In most patients the transverse discrepancies are small and a normal occlusion is often seen or is readily attained with orthodontic treatment. If there is any doubt that the asymmetry may get worse with continued facial growth then serial records, photographs, and study models can be obtained in the first instance. If it is found to be progressive then a referral for further investigations, such a radioisotope scan for active growth sites, may be appropriate.

It is important to realize that the range of what can be perceived to be normal can be large, and within a population will blend seamlessly away from the normal towards either extreme. Normal may also be different between different racial groups, between the sexes, and between patients of differing ages.

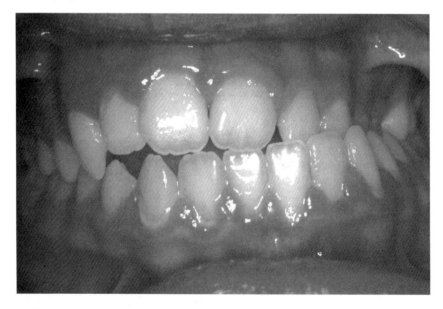

Fig. 2.17 The skeletal asymmetry of this patient is evident as a crossbite intraorally.

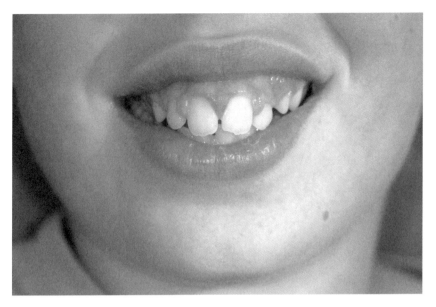

Fig. 2.18 Patients with a gummy smile showing excessive tooth and gingivae on smiling.

2.2.2   Soft tissue ideals

It is usual during the examination of a patient to assess the soft tissue form and function, particularly of the lips. Clinically this includes:
- lip competence
- lip length
- degree of protrusion or retrusion.

All three are closely related. Competent lips can be considered to be normal and are desirable for three reasons:
- *Aesthetics*—Incompetent lips, particularly if there is a short upper lip, can lead to the appearance of the patient showing too much upper incisor tooth and gingival tissue, particularly on smiling; the so-called gummy smile (Fig. 2.18).
- *Function*—It provides the patient with a lip-to-lip anterior oral seal during swallowing.
- *Health*—Competent lips will help to prevent gingival drying, which can be associated with gingival hyperplasia and gingivitis.[9] During normal development it is not unusual for a child to have incompetent lips, which become competent during adolescence. This is either due to soft tissue growth or because it is socially more acceptable to have competent lips, or at least incompetent lips that are habitually held together. Lip length changes dramatically during normal facial growth and affects both the lower and the upper lip.[10]

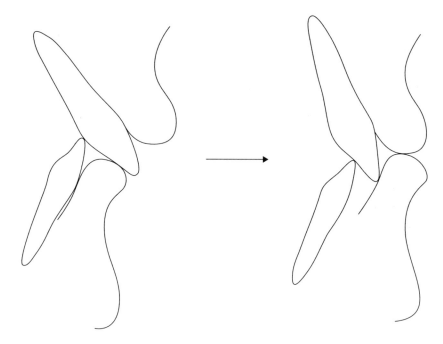

Fig. 2.19(a) Following treatment the upper incisors should be within lower lip control.

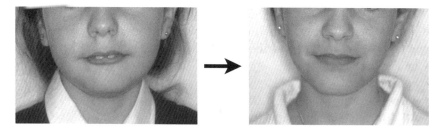

Fig. 2.19(b) In this patient the upper incisors have been retracted within lower lip control.

Placing the upper incisors within the control of the lower lip is well recognized as an important aid to long-term stability, particularly following orthodontic treatment of a Class II division 1 incisor relationship (Figs 2.19(a) and (b)). It is desirable that the lower lip covers the incisal third of the upper incisors at rest. The upper lip should meet the lower lip and therefore cover the gingival two-thirds of the crown of the upper incisors.

In the absence of orthodontic treatment the soft tissues are thought to play an important part in establishing a normal occlusion via dentoalveolar compensation in cases where there is a skeletal discrepancy, as described in Section 2.2.1 (Skeletal ideals). Only when this skeletal discrepancy becomes more marked might dentoalveolar compensation be unable to establish a normal occlusion. In such cases, if the lips are incompetent and the lower

lip does not cover the upper incisors at rest, the upper incisors become proclined, leading to the development of a Class II division 1 incisor relationship. Conversely, if the lower lip is high relative to the crowns of the upper
incisors it can lead to retroclination of these teeth and the development of
a Class II division 2 incisor relationship.

So far the vertical position of the lips has been discussed. What about
their anteroposterior position? There have been many attempts to quantify
the degree of soft tissue protrusion or retrusion in the ideal face.
Cephalometric radiographs can be used to measure various soft tissue
profiles in an attempt to describe this feature, and also as an aid to treat-
ment planning (Fig. 2.20). Such measurements include the:
- E or [a]esthetic line[11]
- H or harmony line[12,13]
- S or Steiner S line[14]
- NLA or nasolabial angle.

There are numerous limitations of such measurements, e.g. racial variations, changes with growth, and what is actually considered to be normal.
For example, what may be considered to be a normal anteroposterior position of the lips in an Afro-Caribbean patient may be considered to be protrusive in a Caucasian patient and *vice versa*. The measurements will vary

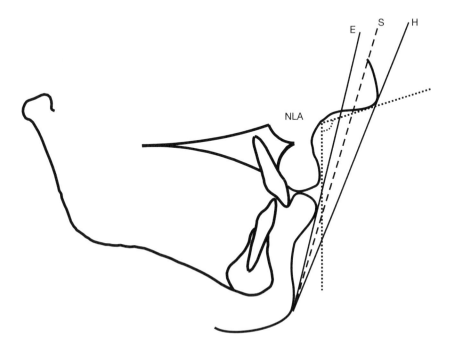

Fig. 2.20 Some soft tissue measurements used in orthodontic treatment
planning. H, harmony line; S, Steiner S line; E, esthetic line; NLA, nasolabial
angle.

with age, particularly in male patients where soft tissue and nose growth may continue beyond 18 years of age.[10]

If soft tissues are so important, why is there no accurate and commonly used method of soft tissue assessment for orthodontic diagnosis and treatment planning, as is the case with dental and skeletal relationships? There are a number of reasons why. To begin with, unlike teeth and bone, soft tissue position and form is constantly changing and so any radiographic, photographic, or laser scanning record is merely a snapshot in time and will be subject to obvious limitations.[15] In addition, the physiological measurement of facial muscle activity shows poor reproducibility, since the recruitment of motor units varies with the tone of the muscles throughout any 24-hour period. The position, and hence activity, of the facial soft tissues is highly dependent on the emotional state of the patient. Angle, nearly 100 years ago,[16] proposed that if the teeth were placed in the optimal occlusion then good facial harmony would result. It is certainly known that orthodontic treatment can affect the degree of protrusion or retrusion of the lips, as well as the nasolabial angle.[17] The difficulty is that the effect of planned tooth movements on soft tissue position is often very variable and cannot be reliably predicted. For instance, it has been proposed that in order to achieve the ideal profile of the lips, the lower incisors should be moved to lie 0–2 mm anterior to a line drawn on a lateral cephalometric radiograph between the A point and the pogonion[18] (Fig. 2.21). However, far from producing a reproducible lip position it has been shown to produce a variation in lip protrusion of up to 10 mm.[19] It has also been shown that positioning the lower incisors in relation to this A–pogonion line is not related to the long-term anteroposterior stability of these teeth. In view of the 10 mm variation in soft tissue protrusion perhaps this is not so surprising.[20]

It would seem that we all have our own opinions as to what constitutes a normal or soft tissue ideal in terms of dentofacial aesthetics. However, recording what constitutes normal or abnormal and how it is affected by orthodontic treatment is far from simple, particularly on such an animated object as the face. This has more been more succinctly put by Peck and Peck[21] who stated, 'Obviously, there is no such thing as an equation for facial beauty. No numbers or devices can totally express the complexity of facial aesthetics.'

2.3   THE ASSESSMENT OF ORTHODONTIC TREATMENT RESULTS

So far, dental, skeletal, and soft tissue ideals have been discussed and it can be seen that a normal or ideal occlusion can be readily described and classified as such, whereas a normal or ideal soft tissue pattern cannot. Skeletal

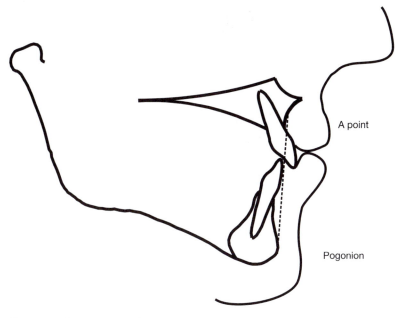

A point

Pogonion

Fig. 2.21 The A–pogonion line.

and soft patterns might vary slightly from their ideals even though the occlusion is normal. In judging the success of orthodontic treatment it is important the teeth are placed in a stable position, which is functional and not detrimental to their long-term health. The patient should be happy with the overall dentofacial aesthetic result. However, such an assessment is somewhat subjective and in a modern healthcare setting a more measurable quality of outcome is becoming important. Although it is not possible to objectively assess soft tissue outcome with any degree of accuracy, it is possible to assess skeletal outcome in the anteroposterior and vertical planes using a before- and after-treatment cephalometric analysis (Figs 2.22(a) and (b)). This might be appropriate where functional appliances or orthognathic surgery had been used. For the vast majority of orthodontic treatments such an approach would be of limited value, in that only the inclinations of the incisor teeth, the overjet, and overbite could be assessed. In any case, these last two features could be more easily assessed using study models without the risks associated with additional radiographs. A system that adds to our perceptions of ideal is to score before- and after-treatment study models using an index known as the 'Peer Assessment Rating' or 'PAR[22] index'. However, this must be seen as an adjunct and not a replacement for other methods of assessment.

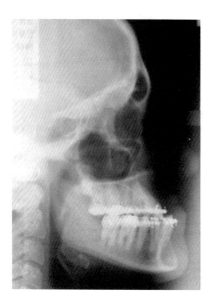 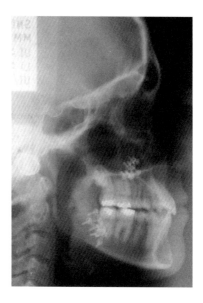

Fig. 2.22(a) Before and after treatment lateral cephalograms of an osteotomy patient.

2.4   THE PEER ASSESSMENT RATING (PAR) INDEX

The occlusal features of the study models that are assessed in order to come up with pre- and post-treatment PAR scores are:
- upper and lower anterior segments
- left and right buccal occlusion
- overjet
- overbite
- centreline.

Each of these is scored as follows:
- **Upper and lower anterior segments**—Crowding, spacing, and tooth impactions are assessed from the mesial of the canine to canine in the upper and lower labial segments. This is undertaken by measuring the contact point displacements. The scoring system is:

Contact point displacement	PAR score
0.0–1 mm	0
1.1–2 mm	1
2.1–4 mm	2
4.1–8 mm	3
> 8 mm	4
Impacted teeth	5

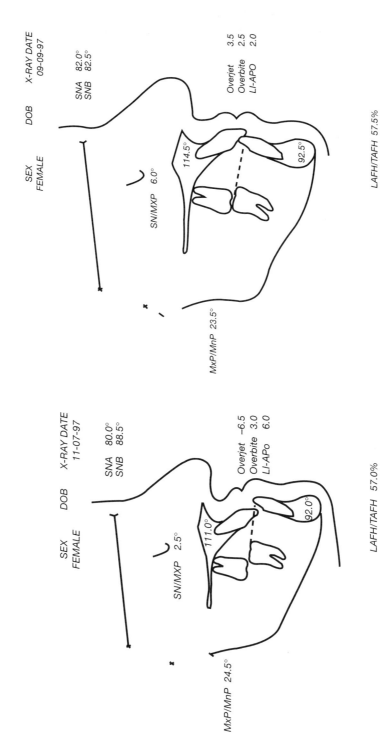

Fig. 2.22(b) Before and after treatment tracings of the lateral cephalograms of an osteotomy patient.

- **Left and right buccal occlusion**—This is assessed in all three planes of space, anteroposteriorly, vertically and transversely as follows:

Anteroposterior	PAR score
Full unit interdigitation I, II, or III	0
Less than ½ unit discrepancy	1
½ unit discrepancy	2

Vertical	
No open bite	0
Open bite of >2 mm on 2 or more teeth	1

Transverse	
No crossbite	0
Crossbite tendency	1
Single tooth crossbite	2
>1 tooth in crossbite	3
>1 tooth in scissors bite	4

- **Overjet**—The overjet measurement and any anterior crossbites are recorded as follows:

Overjet	PAR score
0–3 mm	0
3.1–5 mm	1
5.1–7 mm	2
7.1–9 mm	3
> 9 mm	4

Anterior crossbites	
No crossbite	0
1 or more teeth edge to edge	1
1 tooth in crossbite	2
2 teeth in crossbite	3
>2 teeth in crossbite	4

The total score for overjet and anterior crossbites is then multiplied by a weighting factor of 6.

- **Overbite**—Aims to measure the worst vertical overlap or open bite of the incisor teeth and the scoring is:

Overbite	PAR score
≤ one-third coverage of the lower incisor	0
>one-third but <two-thirds coverage of the lower incisor	1
>two-thirds coverage of the lower incisor	2
≥ a full lower incisor tooth coverage	3

Open bite	
No open bite	0
Open bite Ė 1 mm	1
1.1–2 mm open bite	2
2.1–3 mm open bite	3
≥ 4 mm open bite	4

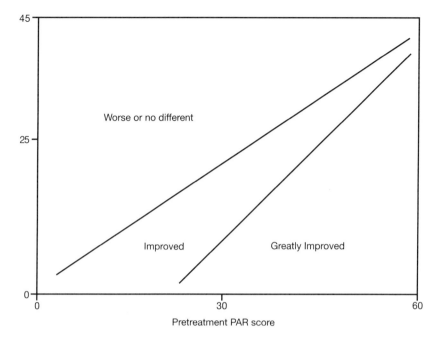

Fig. 2.23 The PAR nomogram. Reproduced with kind permission from Shaw *et al.* (1991). *British Dental Journal,* **170**, 107–12.

The total score here is multiplied by a weighting factor of 4.

- **Centrelines**—The discrepancy between the upper and lower dental mid-lines is noted in quarters of a lower incisor width and scored as follows:

Centreline	PAR score
0–¼ lower incisor width discrepancy	0
¼–½ lower incisor width discrepancy	1
>½ lower incisor width discrepancy	2

The total score here is also multiplied by a weighting factor of 4.

Once all the scores and their weightings have been determined the start PAR score can be calculated as their sum. The whole procedure is repeated for the post-treatment study models in order to arrive at an end-of-treatment PAR score. By knowing the pre- and post-treatment PAR scores the change due to treatment can be presented in one of two ways:

1. The percentage reduction in PAR score can be used in combination with the actual reduction in PAR score.
2. A nomogram can be used, in which the pretreatment PAR score is plotted on the x-axis and post-treatment is plotted on the y-axis. The case is then assigned one of three outcomes: worse—no different, improved, or greatly improved (Fig. 2.23).

The PAR index therefore provides numerical data on treatment outcome and how close the final occlusal result is to the occlusal ideal. However, it is worth remembering that the index as currently designed does have some obvious shortcomings. For example, the exclusive use of study models takes no account of axial inclinations of the teeth, of torque in the labial segments, or of possible iatrogenic damage. Also the weightings used mainly favour alignment in the labial segments, with less emphasis on buccal segment relationships.

2.5   SUMMARY OF DENTOFACIAL CLASSIFICATION AND IDEALS

1. The main reasons for performing orthodontic treatment are:
   - dentofacial aesthetics
   - function
   - health.
2. The dentofacial ideals are:
   - occlusal ideals
   - skeletal ideals
   - soft tissue ideals—this is the most difficult to describe.
3. The assessment of orthodontic treatment results is most easily made using the Peer Assessment Rating (PAR) index in conjunction with radiographic assessment and clinical observation. The PAR index gives a weighted score for the pre- and post-treatment occlusion.

2.6   OBJECTIVES

1. List the occlusal ideals.
2. Describe the skeletal ideals in all three dimensions.
3. Describe the problems with determining soft tissue ideals.
4. List the five main categories comprising the PAR index and their relative weightings.

FURTHER READING

McDonald, F. and Ireland, A. J. (1998). *Diagnosis of the orthodontic patient*, Chapter 7: *Health considerations*, pp. 130–48. Oxford University Press, Oxford.

REFERENCES

1. Johnston, C. D., Burden, D. J., and Stevenson, M. R. (1999). The influence of dental to facial midline discrepancies on dental attractiveness ratings. *European Journal of Orthodontics*, **21**, 517–22.
2. Andrews, L. F. (1972). The six keys to normal occlusion. *American Journal of Orthodontics*, **62**, 296–309.
3. Angle, E. H. (1899). Classification of malocclusion. *Dental Cosmos*, **41**, 248–264; 350–7.
4. Ruf, S., Hansen, K., and Pancherz, H. (1998). Does orthodontic proclination of lower incisors in children and adolescents cause gingival recession? *American Journal of Orthodontics and Dentofacial Orthopedics*, **114**, 100–6.

5. Ackerman, J. L. and Proffit, W. R. (1997). Soft tissue limitations in orthodontics: treatment planning guidelines. *Angle Orthodontist*, **67**, 327–36.
6. Proffit, W. R. (1978). Equilibrium theory revisited. *Angle Orthodontist*, **48**, 175–86.
7. Connor, A. M. and Moshiri, F. (1985). Orthognathic surgery norms for American black patients. *American Journal of Orthodontics and Dentofacial Orthopedics*, **87**, 119–34.
8. Bishara S. E. and Jakobsen J. R. (1985). Longitudinal changes in three normal facial types. *American Journal of Orthodontics and Dentofacial Orthopedics*, **88**, 466–502.
9. Wagaiyu, E. G. and Ashley, F. P. (1991). Mouthbreathing, lip seal and upper lip coverage and their relationship with gingival inflammation in 11–14 year-old schoolchildren. *Journal of Clinical Periodontology*, **18**, 698–702.
10. Blanchette, M. E., Nanda, R. S., Currier, G. F., Ghosh, J., and Nanda, S. K. (1996). A longitudinal cephalometric study of the soft tissue profile of short- and long-face syndromes from 7 to 17 years. *American Journal of Orthodontics and Dentofacial Orthopedics*, **109**, 116–31.
11. Ricketts, R. M. (1960). A foundation for cephalometric communication. *American Journal of Orthodontics*, **46**, 330–57.
12. Holdaway, R. A. (1983). A soft tissue cephalometric analysis and its application in orthodontic treatment planning. Part 1. *American Journal of Orthodontics and Dentofacial Orthopedics*, **84**, 1–28.
13. Holdaway, R. A. (1984). A soft tissue cephalometric analysis and its application in orthodontic treatment planning. Part 2. *American Journal of Orthodontics and Dentofacial Orthopedics*, **85**, 279–93.
14. Steiner, C. C. (1953). Cephalometrics for you and me. *American Journal of Orthodontics*, **39**, 729–55.
15. Bishara, S. E, Cummins, D. M, Jorgensen, G. J., and Jakobsen, J. R. (1995). A computer assisted photogrammetric analysis of soft tissue changes after orthodontic treatment. Part I: Methodology and reliability. *American Journal of Orthodontics and Dentofacial Orthopedics*, **107**, 633–9.
16. Angle, E. H. (1906). *Malocclusion of the teeth*. S. S. White, Philadelphia.
17. Cummins, D. M., Bishara, S. E., and Jakobsen, J. R. (1995). A computer assisted photogrammetric analysis of soft tissue changes after orthodontic treatment. Part II: Results. *American Journal of Orthodontics and Dentofacial Orthopedics*, **108**, 38–47.
18. Williams, R. (1969). The diagnostic line. *American Journal of Orthodontics*, **55**, 458–76.
19. Park, Y. C, Burstone, C. J. (1998). Soft-tissue profile—fallacies of hard-tissue standards in treatment planning. *American Journal of Orthodontics and Dentofacial Orthopedics*, **90**, 52–62.
20. Houston, W. J. B. and Edler, R. (1990). Stability and relapse of dental arch alignment. *British Journal of Orthodontics*, **17**, 235–41.
21. Peck, H. and Peck, S. (1970). A concept of facial esthetics. *Angle Orthodontist*, **40**, 284–317.
22. Richmond, S. (1990). A critical evaluation of orthodontic treatment in the general dental services of England and Wales. Unpublished PhD Thesis, University of Manchester, UK.

3 Removable appliances

CONTENTS

Removable appliances have been used extensively in orthodontics for many years. However, their use is often brought into disrepute due to a lack of understanding of their mode of action and the limitations this imposes. Fixed appliances are capable of three-dimensional tooth movements, whilst removable appliances are largely limited to straightforward tipping.

3.1 GENERAL PRINCIPLES OF REMOVABLE APPLIANCES

3.1.1 Tooth movements

A removable appliance induces tipping of a tooth around a point known as the 'centroid', 'centre of resistance', or 'centre of rotation', which is said to be located between 30 and 40% from the root apex when considering the whole length of the tooth (Fig. 3.1).[1-3]

Typically, the force application necessary to tip a single-rooted tooth has been quoted as being around 30 g. However, this might be a somewhat simplistic outlook; the true loads can be as high as 3 kg[4] in the case of some

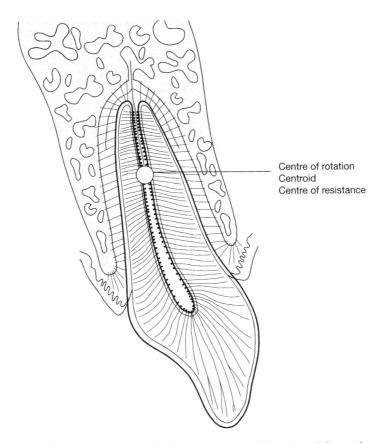

Centre of rotation
Centroid
Centre of resistance

Fig. 3.1 The centroid, centre of resistance or centre of rotation of the tooth, about which the incisor will rotate when a force is applied to the crown.

fixed appliances, such as the quadhelix, used for palatal expansion. Teeth are in fact designed to withstand much heavier loads, with the loads applied during mastication easily exceeding this figure.[5] Therefore the traditional 30 g figure is almost certainly not a wholly realistic, nor clinically expedient figure, but more a figure that has been adopted into orthodontics by convention. A number of factors will determine the optimum force for tooth movement, including the root surface area of the tooth and the type of movement (tipping versus bodily movement, intrusion versus extrusion). There will also be variation between individuals. Certainly excessive force application is one possible cause of iatrogenic damage (see Chapter 9).

3.1.2 Appliance wear

Removable appliances are generally worn for 23 hours and 50 minutes of every 24-hour period. In other words, they are worn full time and only removed for cleaning. This time is reduced, as directed by the clinician, when the patient begins the phase of retention whilst waiting for the soft tissues to remodel (see Chapter 1). Studies on functional appliances and compliance show that most patients wear appliances half as much as they admit to.[6,7] Therefore, in order for treatment to be successful and efficient it is essential that the importance of correct wear is stressed to the patient at the commencement of treatment. There is clear evidence that patients retain only a limited amount of the verbal information provided to them at the chairside. Simple reinforcement in the form of a printed information leaflet and calendar should therefore also be given when the appliance is fitted and has certainly been shown to be effective in this respect.[8]

Once treatment is proceeding it is essential to ensure that the overall duration is kept as short as possible for two main reasons:

1. If the removable appliance is used as a precursor to fixed appliance treatment, prolonging the removable phase may use up a large proportion of the patient's finite level of compliance. The treatment may therefore never reach completion.

2. The longer the treatment, the greater the risk of iatrogenic damage, in particular root resorption.[9,10]

3.1.3 Appliance hygiene and care

The simplest and easiest way to maintain an appliance in a 'clean' state is to gently clean it with a toothbrush and toothpaste, with particular attention being paid to the fitting surface of the appliance. However, excessive brushing should be avoided as the abrasive present within the toothpaste may easily damage the soft acrylic in the longer term. Specialized cleaning agents and solutions are not required. If the clinician instructs the patient to wear the appliance part time, then instructions must also include the necessity for keeping the appliance moist. Being partly manufactured from acrylic and in close association with wet plaster or stone, the dimensional stability of the appliance depends on a degree of moisture.[11] If this moisture is lost, stresses are released and the appliance distorts.

3.2   REMOVABLE APPLIANCE DESIGN

The three basic elements of a removable appliance are:
• force
• fixation
• framework.
Each of these will be dealt with in turn.

3.2.1   Force

Components of removable appliances

Those used to apply force to the teeth are:
• Springs   usually made from 0.5, 0.6, or 0.7 mm-diameter stainless steel wire
• Bows   usually made from 0.5 or 0.7 mm-diameter stainless steel wire
• Screws   opening 0.2 mm per ¼ turn
• Elastics

Springs

Typical springs used on removable appliances include:
• Z-spring—typically made from 0.5-mm stainless-steel wire on a single tooth and 0.6 mm on two adjacent teeth (Fig. 3.2(a));
• T-spring—typically made from 0.5-mm stainless-steel wire (Fig. 3.2(b));
• palatal canine retraction spring—made from 0.5-mm stainless-steel wire (Fig. 3.2(c));
• buccal canine retraction spring—made either from supported 0.5-mm or 0.7-mm unsupported stainless-steel wire (Fig. 3.2(d)).
These springs, by definition, have to be flexible with the appropriate wire characteristics for tooth movement. If too flexible, the wires are easily distorted by the patient (activated beyond their elastic limit, leading to permanent deformation). To protect these delicate springs a guide wire may be provided and the acrylic formed into a 'box' overlying the spring, i.e. boxed and guarded (Fig. 3.3), or supported by additional sleeving.

Great emphasis is sometimes placed on the manner in which coils are bent up in some of these springs. Namely, should the wire be bent in such a way that the coil tightens up when the appliance is fitted and uncoils as the tooth moves, or vice versa (Fig. 3.4)? Although theoretically it may be important, in clinical practice it makes little, if any, difference.

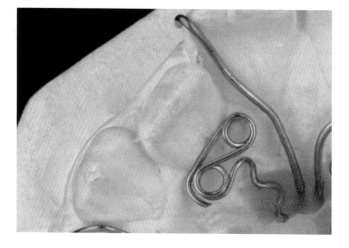

a

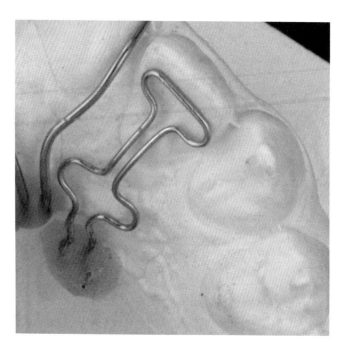

b

Fig. 3.2 Photographs of commonly seen springs. (a) Z-spring used to procline teeth; (b) T-spring to move molars buccally.

Bows

These types of components are used for both overjet reduction and for providing anterior fixation. An example of a bow used for overjet reduction is the Roberts Retractor made from 0.5-mm stainless steel with supporting

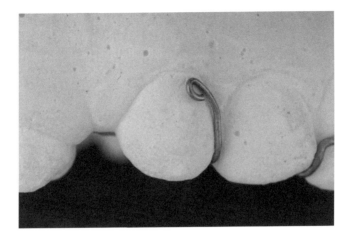

c

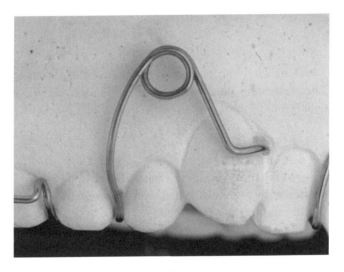

d

Fig. 3.2 (*continued*) (c) palatal canine retraction spring to move canines distally; (d) buccal canine retraction spring to move a canine palatal and distally.

buccal sleeving. Anterior fixation can also be provided by bows such as the Hawley bow (made from 0.7-mm wire), but this function will depend on the proclination of the upper incisors and therefore the degree of undercut present that will resist displacement of the appliance (see Southend clasp, below).

Elastics

These have been used in conjunction with removable appliances in order to retract the upper labial segment. However, their action is poorly controlled,

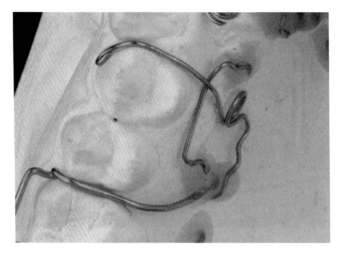

Fig. 3.3 A boxed and guarded spring assisting in the control of wire flexibility.

which can lead to flattening of the arches and possible stripping of the gingivae. The main advantage is, however, aesthetics, elastics being less obtrusive (Fig. 3.5).

Screws

These can be used to move teeth:
(1) transversely—for the correction of posterior crossbites;
(2) anteroposteriorly—for moving teeth over the bite, especially if more than one incisor needs to be moved (Fig. 3.6).

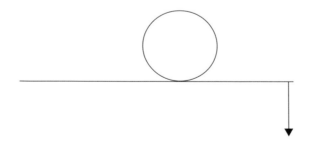

a

Fig. 3.4 The incorrect design of springs will lead to poor activation of the appliance and a reduction in the apparent effectiveness of orthodontic therapy. If the coil is placed so the spring is activated by opening of the coil it is mechanically more efficient (a and b).

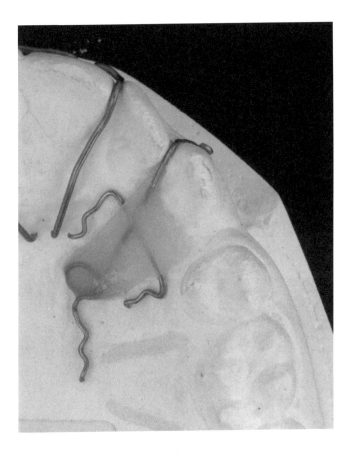

b

Fig. 3.4(b)

Ideal tooth movement is achieved by turning the screw a quarter of a turn every 3–7 days (0.2 mm). Rapid maxillary expansion is a variation on this type of expansion and normally relates to fixed appliances. However, it is possible to use a removable appliance to deliver this type of force if the appliance is well constructed and the patient is very cooperative, and in these circumstances the midline screw is turned twice a day.

Force and tooth movement

Anteroposterior tooth movement

Moving teeth anteriorly

This is typically undertaken in Class III cases to eliminate an anterior mandibular displacement. It is necessary to ensure there is a positive overbite to retain the tooth movements after treatment. However, it is easy to inadvertently reduce the overbite during treatment due to:

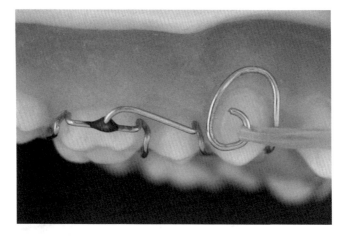

a

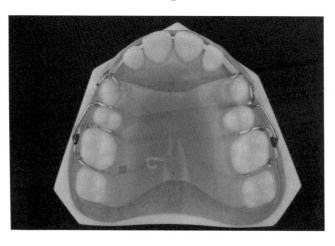

b

Fig. 3.5 Elastics attached by the means of hooks (a) can be used to retract the labial segment but can be difficult to manage (b).

(1) rotation of the upper incisor(s) about its fulcrum, leading to a relative intrusion of the incisal edge (Fig. 3.7(a));

(2) the application of a spring on a sloping surface, leading not only to the wanted anteroposterior force vector but also an unwanted intrusive force vector (Fig. 3.7(b));

(3) elimination of an anterior displacement, leading to a backward rotation of the mandible and so reducing the overbite (Chapter 4).

Single tooth movements can be undertaken with either a T-spring or a Z-spring made from 0.5-mm stainless-steel wire. Two teeth can be moved using a double Z-spring made from 0.6-mm wire. All four upper incisors can be moved using a 0.9-mm recurved spring (Chapter 4, Fig. 4.15).

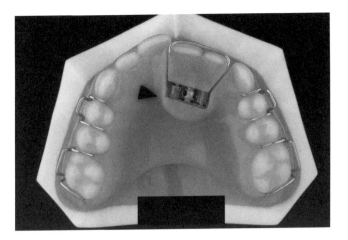

Fig. 3.6 The use of a screw to move two incisors labially.

Moving teeth posteriorly

Canine retractors, whether approaching from the buccal or the palatal, have been classically described to retract maxillary canine teeth. In order for their use to be successful it is important the canine is mesially angulated prior to treatment. This is because the removable appliance will only tip the tooth about its centroid. Use of a removable appliance, where the canine is of normal angulation or is already distally angulated prior to treatment, will lead to an unsightly distally angulated tooth at completion of treatment. It

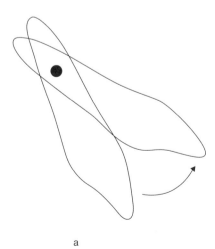

a

Fig. 3.7(a) The intrusion of a tooth due to rotation about its axis leading to an apparent movement of the incisal edge superiorly.

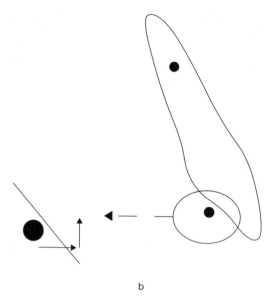

b

Fig. 3.7(b) The placement of a spring on the palatal surface of the tooth will not only result in a vector of movement labially but also one in an intrusive direction.

is because of this and the greater control afforded by fixed appliances, that the use of removable appliances for canine retraction is declining. If a canine is inadvertently made distally angulated with a removable appliance, correction with a subsequent fixed appliance is certainly more complicated than if all the treatment had been performed with a fixed appliance. This is because of the extrusive effect of the archwire in combination with the distoangular tooth and the slot in the canine Straight-wire® bracket (Fig. 3.8) (see section 6.2.4 overbite reduction).

Distal movement of molars
An appliance that has become popular for moving the maxillary first molars distally in conjunction with headgear, prior to the use of a fixed appliance, is variously known as the Tucker, nudger, or Ten Hoeve[12] appliance. Whilst the headgear is worn for 14–16 hours a day, the appliance is worn 23 hours and 50 minutes of every day, helping to maintain the distalized molar in its corrected position when the headgear is not being worn. However, a disadvantage of this appliance is that if headgear wear is poor, then the spring acting against the mesial surface of the first molar will ultimately end up proclining the upper labial segment and increasing the overjet. This is an unwanted reciprocal force effect. Also, if the headgear is improperly adjusted then the molar merely tips about its centroid; which may give the clinical appearance of an improved molar relationship. However, when fixed

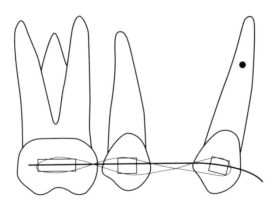

Fig. 3.8 The distal angulation of the canine forces the archwire in an occlusal direction anteriorly, thereby extruding the labial segments and worsening the overbite.

appliances are then fitted at a later stage in treatment, the early aligning archwires will rapidly upright the molar causing the crown to tip mesially.

Vertical tooth movement

Intrusive vertical tooth movements are very difficult to achieve in a controlled manner. Intrusion of an individual tooth is very precise and demands a high degree of technical ability to ensure the correct vector of movement. It is important the tooth is intruded within the confines of the labial and lingual cortical plates of alveolar bone, which can be difficult to achieve with a removable appliance.

On the other hand, removable appliances are very good for tooth extrusion, both individually (as in the case of an unerupted solitary tooth) or as a group (usually by relative inhibition of the normal overeruption of other teeth). The classic example of the latter is the flat anterior biteplane, which prevents the labial segment from overerupting but allows overeruption of the posterior buccal segments (Fig. 3.9). In allowing this, one of the treatment goals of Andrews' six keys is achieved, producing a flat Curve of Spee.[13] The posterior buccal segment overeruption can result in a transient change in the anterior lower face height measurement (see Fig. 4.8, Chapter 4). Although this may permit occlusal correction, such an increase in anterior lower face height, especially in a growing child, will be unstable and inevitably revert back to type with time. The exception to this is where the anterior lower facial height is already increased and the patient demonstrates a posterior growth rotation of the mandible. Here the anterior lower facial height may continue to increase.

Although true intrusion with an anterior biteplane can be difficult, it appears to be more effective with posterior biteplanes. By discluding the posterior teeth and effectively stretching the pterygomasseteric sling with its

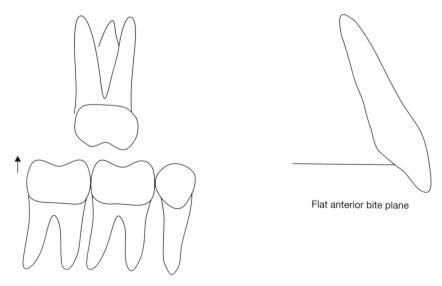

Flat anterior bite plane

Fig. 3.9 A diagrammatic representation of how the overeruption of the posterior buccal segments occurs following the placement of a removable appliance with a flat anterior bite plane. In so doing the curve of Spee if flattened.

striated masticatory muscles, the posterior teeth appear to intrude. This effect is commonly seen with some functional appliances (see Chapter 4).

Extrusion of an individual tooth

The acrylic baseplate of an upper removable appliance, in contact with the palate, provides a great deal of vertical anchorage against which to extrude either a maxillary incisor (Fig. 3.10) or a maxillary canine tooth. Thus because the surface area of bone, resisting the forces of anchorage generated by the tooth to be extruded (i.e. the tooth socket), is substantially smaller than that of the palate against which the appliance is pushing, there will be extrusion of the correct teeth and limited intrusion of anchorage teeth. In the case of both an erupted or unerupted tooth, traction can be applied from the removable appliance via a wire ligature or gold chain affixed to a bracket on the tooth.

Transverse tooth movement

Transverse movement is commonly used to correct a unilateral crossbite with an associated displacement. This feature of a malocclusion is commonly seen where there has been a digit sucking habit. When a number of teeth are to be moved as in this case, then a screw type of appliance should be used. The pitch of screws used in removable appliances is usually 0.2 mm and patients are asked to turn the key a quarter of a turn once or twice a

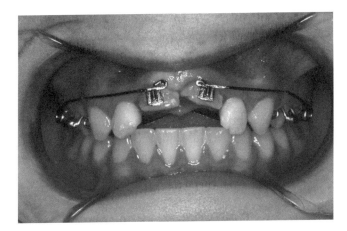

Fig. 3.10 An appliance to extrude two maxillary central incisors.

week until the crossbite is corrected. It is important that patients are instructed to turn the screw with the supplied key when the appliance is out of the mouth in order to prevent the key from being inhaled or ingested. Following activation, the patient should put the appliance back in the mouth and push it firmly into place. If they don't, the teeth will not move. Instead, the appliance will fit less and less well as the screw is opened more and more. Eventually the appliance will no longer fit at all clinically. This not only wastes time but also valuable patient cooperation. It is also worth remembering that as the teeth will be moving transversely the addition of a posterior bite platform may not always be required; the teeth spend the majority of their time out of occlusion and the molar teeth in particular may have a crown morphology with very 'flat' cusps.

Teeth can be selectively moved or not moved by ensuring the acrylic of the baseplate is only in contact with the teeth that need to be moved. This is particularly important if potential scissors-bite relationships of buccal teeth are to be avoided. Individual teeth can be moved with the use of a single T-spring rather than a screw.

3.2.2   Fixation

A number fixation mechanisms are used to retain removable appliances in the mouth. These include:

- Adams' cribs   0.7 mm-diameter stainless steel
- C-clasps   0.7 mm-diameter stainless steel
- Southend clasp   0.7 mm-diameter stainless steel
- Fitted labial bows   0.7 mm-diameter stainless steel

- Reverse U-loop labial bow   0.7 mm-diameter stainless steel
- Hawley bow   0.7 mm- or 0.8 mm-diameter stainless steel

Active forces from the springs, bows, screws, and elastics may well displace the removable appliance from the mouth, rendering their action less efficient and effective. A loose-fitting appliance will also be uncomfortable for the patient, and if it is continually moving in the mouth will lead to fatigue failure of one or more of the metal components. This will mean the patient will either not wear the appliance, or it may be out of the mouth on a number of occasions in order to be repaired, during which time the teeth will not be moving; in clinical circumstances with very unstable tooth movements the teeth will actually relapse to the position at the beginning of treatment. Good fixation is required to prevent, or at least minimize, such problems. The two commonest fixation devices used on removable appliances will now be discussed (others are discussed later in this chapter).

1.   *Adams' cribs*—Described by Adams,[14] these are prepared to fit into undercuts on the mesial and distal embrasures of first permanent molars and made from 0.7 mm-diameter stainless-steel wire (Fig. 3.11). They are also commonly used to gain retention from both premolar teeth and primary molars. In the case of the first deciduous molars they are commonly made from 0.6 mm wire.

2.   *Southend clasps*—This is a variation of a crib for anterior teeth and has been extensively described.[15] The clasp is constructed around the gingival

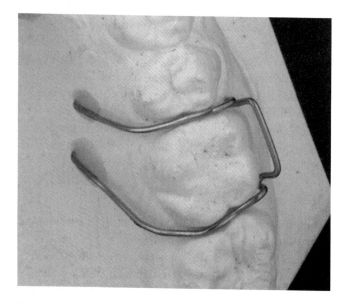

Fig. 3.11 An Adams' universal crib for retaining an appliance.

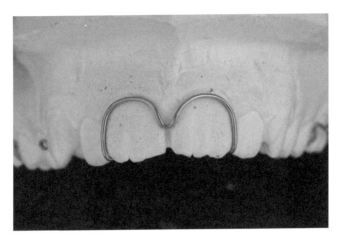

Fig. 3.12 A southend clasp used for anterior retention. The commonest site of fatigue failure is at the incisal edge.

margin of the maxillary central incisors; it is only necessary to use this when there is a limited undercut, that is when the upper incisors are not proclined. If this is not observed then the clasp is flexed unnecessarily during placement and removal of the appliance and will frequently fracture. If the clasp fails it is usually at the region of reflection of the clasp (Fig. 3.12) where the wire has been work-hardened to the greatest amount.

Anchorage

Anchorage comes from considering the number of teeth included in the appliance to resist the active/force components of the appliance. This concept should be considered in the anterior/posterior direction and the vertical and the transverse planes.

Anteroposterior anchorage is the type of anchorage often described in standard teaching. However, it must also be considered as not only acting in all three planes of space but also in all directions in each dimension, i.e. for example, when moving incisors either labially or palatally.

Simply considered in the case of a Hawley appliance (Fig. 6.46) with an activated labial bow, the force is induced by the retraction of the upper labial segment. This provokes a reciprocal response in the posterior teeth (the first molars) to move these teeth mesially, enhancing the tendency for the teeth to move mesially with physiological mesial drift.

The converse is seen in the appliance proclining a maxillary incisor over the occlusion. The forces generated by the active component (Z-spring, T-spring, or screw) anteriorly produces a reciprocal force on the posterior teeth leading to their distal movement (Fig. 3.13).

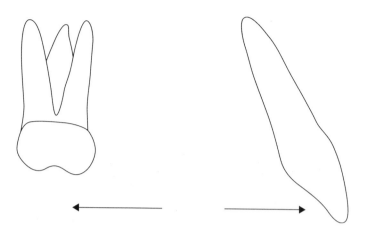

Fig. 3.13 Reciprocal forces to procline an upper maxillary incisor will effectively distalize the buccal segments.

Aspects of the appliance that resist unwanted tooth movements include wire work and acrylic, especially where the latter contacts the vault of the palate.

3.2.3 Framework

The material most often used is cold-cure acrylic (see Materials, Chapter 7), and this connects all aspects of the appliance. Care must be exercised with cold-cure acrylic, to ensure laboratory processing has eliminated as much residual monomer as possible. Failure to do this can lead to mucosal irritation from monomer leaching out of the appliance.[16] This typically appears like denture stomatitis and is limited to the mucosa in contact with the baseplate.

There is no justification, mechanically, for including strengtheners in acrylic. All that these wires achieve is a reduction in the effective cross-sectional area of the acrylic and they act as a means of stress concentration; this weakens the acrylic.

It is possible to modify these appliances to include bite platforms; these may be posterior or anterior. Anterior bite platforms are required for overbite reduction and are usually constructed behind the upper incisors and canines sufficient to prop the occlusion approximately 4–5 mm in the premolar regions. As the overbite reduces and the separation of the premolars reduces, additional acrylic can be added to continue overbite reduction as necessary. When fitting an appliance with an anterior biteplane it is essential that at least two lower incisors are in contact with the acrylic when in occlusion, otherwise if only one tooth is in contact this can lead to a high loading on the tooth making it very painful and thus possibly limiting the patient's compliance. However, if all the incisal edges of the four lower incisors are not level at the commencement of treatment and an aim is to rectify this, then it is important that they are allowed to differentially erupt in order to achieve level incisal edges. If all four incisors contact the biteplane and are of irregular heights at the beginning of treatment, they will also be like this at the end of treatment.

Posterior biteplanes are usually used when teeth are being pushed over the bite. For the patient's comfort in this case, it is important that the occlusion of the lower posterior teeth is even on the biteplane. Here, the height of the biteplane needs only to be sufficient for the teeth being moved to be free from occlusal interference with the opposing teeth. Whilst children are generally adaptable, it is better to adjust the posterior biteplanes to obliterate the Freeway space to aid compliance. If there is still some vertical overlap of the incisal edges after the first increase in face height, then time should be allowed for neurophysiological adaptation (about 3–4 weeks) and the thickness of the posterior bite platforms increased again. In this way patient compliance will be supported.

3.3   STANDARD DESIGNS OF CONTEMPORARY REMOVABLE APPLIANCES

3.3.1   Removable retainer (Hawley)

Indications

Used for retention of corrected tooth position following orthodontic treatment. Protocols vary, but a minimum is usually 3 months' full-time wear, i.e. 23 hours and 50 minutes in every 24 hours.

Design

- Cribs positioned on the upper first molars (may be on the second molars if appropriate) (0.7-mm wire).
- Labial bow from upper left canine to upper right canine attached (0.7-mm wire).
- Acrylic baseplate saddled posterior to the first molars.

3.3.2   Posterior expansion appliance

Indications

Used for correction of a unilateral crossbite in the mixed dentition/permanent dentition associated with a mandibular displacement.[17,18]

Design

- Cribs positioned on both the first maxillary molars (0.7-mm wire) and either the first primary/deciduous molars (0.6-mm wire) or first premolars (0.7-mm wire).
- Midline expansion screw to be turned either once every 3 days (0.2 mm per turn; retention/fixation of the appliance has to be good and the acti-

vation of the screw should not displace the appliance), or once every 7 days depending on the degree of expansion required.
- Posterior biteplanes designed to eliminate any interfering contacts with the lower arch. If this capping is not present then it essential that the intermolar distance of the **lower** dentition is measured during the follow-up visits; it is not sufficient to merely examine the teeth in occlusion. (see section 3.5.3)

3.3.3   Anterior crossbite

Indications

For use with an anterior crossbite in the mixed dentition/permanent dentition associated with a mandibular displacement.

Design

- Cribs placed on both the first maxillary molars (0.7-mm wire) and either the first primary/deciduous molars (0.6-mm wire) or first premolars (0.7-mm wire).
- Either a T- or Z-spring (0.5-mm wire) used to procline the required anterior teeth.
- Posterior capping is used to eliminate any interfering contacts with the lower arch (Fig. 3.14). If the thickness of acrylic within the posterior biteplanes is greater than the patient's Freeway space to clear the anterior teeth, then the patient must be allowed to adapt to this new position. At a subsequent visit acrylic is added to the bite platforms to increase their height.

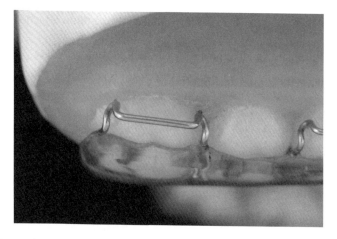

Fig. 3.14 The association of posterior capping over the occlusal surfaces of the buccal teeth to assist in the correction of a crossbite.

- An alternative design is to have cribs on the upper first molars (0.7-mm wire), a Southend clasp (0.7-mm wire) on the two adjacent upper incisors, usually the upper central incisors, and an anterior screw which provides the force to move the upper incisors over the bite. Posterior biteplanes will still be required.

3.3.4　Space maintainer

Indications

Indications for this appliance are limited because of the types of occlusions that require space maintainers. Particular cases with a high caries rate do not benefit from an appliance used long term in the oral cavity; this in turn can provoke more disease.

Table 3.1 Suggested treatment visits for patients with a Hawley retainer

Visit		Clinical procedures
1.		Examine, diagnose, and radiographically assess the dentition if the patient is aged 8 years or above. Upper and lower alginate impressions and an occlusal record should also be taken. A removable appliance should be constructed.
2.	1–2 weeks later	Fit the appliance, instruct the patient in the care of the appliance, the number of hours of wear anticipated, the amount and duration of discomfort, the duration of salivary excess and speech disturbances. Instruct the patient that if there is any loss or breakage of the appliance they should contact the practitioner as soon as convenient to determine if any repairs are necessary. Loss of the appliance requires attention on the next available working day.
3.	4–6 months later	Review the patient's speech with the appliance in place, and observe the patient removing the appliance. Examine the general condition of the appliance. Consider moving to a part-time regimen.
4.	6–12 months later	Consider the occlusion and determine if further treatment is necessary. Final impressions can be taken as a record of the final occlusion.

Table 3.2 Suggested treatment visits for correction of a unilateral crossbite with a displacement

Visit		Clinical procedures
1.		Examine, diagnose, and radiographically assess the dentition if the patient is aged 8 years or above. Upper and lower alginate impressions and an occlusal record should also be taken. A removable appliance should be constructed.
2.	1–2 weeks later	Fit the appliance, instruct the patient in the care of the appliance, the number of hours of wear anticipated, the amount and duration of discomfort, the duration of salivary excess and speech disturbances, and demonstrate the activation of the appliance. Adjust the posterior bite platform so that even occlusal contact is made.
3.	4–5 weeks later	Review the patient's speech with the appliance in place, examine the wear facets of the posterior bite platforms and observe the patient removing the appliance. Measure the space in the midline of the appliance; if necessary, turn the screw in the opposite direction to determine how many turns of the screw have occurred. Examine the dentition for any signs of pathology (hard or soft) and, with the mandible in the retruded contact position, examine the posterior segment. If the crossbite has been corrected remove the posterior bite platforms, ensuring the edges are left smooth and do not irritate the lingual mucosa. If not, instruct the patient to continue turning the screw for a further 4 weeks.
4.	4–5 weeks later	As in visit 3. Crossbite should normally be corrected by this stage. If it has been fully corrected, remove the biteplanes and stop turning the screw. If the intercuspation is satisfactory then a night-time regimen of wear can be instigated. Ensure the patient is aware of the need to keep the appliance in clean water when not in place intraorally.

Table 3.2 Suggested treatment visits for correction of a unilateral crossbite with a displacement (*continued*)

Visit		Clinical procedures
5.	4–5 weeks later or 3 months later	If crossbite is not correcting consider stopping treatment; there is a risk of reducing compliance at a later stage if 'interceptive' appliance therapy is protracted. If this visit has been preceded by 3 months of night-time wear then the appliance can be discarded and the development of the occlusion can be monitored in a continual fashion at the appropriate time interval. Final impressions can be taken as a record of the final occlusion.

Design

- Cribs positioned on both the first maxillary molars (0.7-mm wire).
- A labial bow or southend clasp is used, but care should be taken not to let the bow or clasp interfere with any desired spontaneous tooth movement or eruption of teeth.

3.4   SUGGESTED TREATMENT VISITS FOR PATIENTS WITH VARIOUS ORTHODONTIC APPLIANCES

See Tables 3.1–3.4.

3.5   COMMONEST FAILURES FOR NO TOOTH MOVEMENT

3.5.1   Anteroposterior

Reduction in overjet

The cases that progress most readily are those with already proclined incisors. Excessive retroclination of these teeth could lead to a Class II division 2 incisor relationship being created.

The overbite may be such that there is no space to retract the upper incisors; often the acrylic can reduce/prevent tooth movement. In particular, the incorrect trimming of biteplanes (in both simple removable appliance cases and fixed appliance cases) can cause delays in treatment.

Table 3.3 Suggested treatment visits for correction of an anterior crossbite with a displacement

Visit		Clinical procedures
1.		Examine, diagnose, and radiographically assess the dentition if the patient is aged 8 years or above. Upper and lower alginate impressions and an occlusal record should also be taken. In particular, the eruption of the maxillary incisors needs to be clearly assessed. There is no benefit to the patient in having an appliance to procline one incisor then another incisor once erupted leading to protracted treatment. A removable appliance should be constructed.
2.	1–2 weeks later	Fit the appliance, instruct the patient in the care of the appliance, the number of hours of wear anticipated, the amount and duration of discomfort, the duration of salivary excess and speech disturbances, and demonstrate the activation of the appliance. Adjust the posterior bite platform so that even occlusal contact is made. If there is insufficient clearance of the incisal edge(s) in occlusion, it may be appropriate to allow the patient to adapt to the appliance, the neurophysiological pathways including extra- and intrafusal fibres being capable of rapid adaptation in children, and reviewing in 2 weeks with a view to adding cold-cure acrylic to further increase the height of the bite platforms. Adjust the Z-spring by pulling forwards.
3.	4–5 weeks later	Review the patient's speech with the appliance in place, examine the wear facets of the posterior bite platforms, and observe the patient removing the appliance. Examine the acrylic on the palatal aspect to the incisor(s) being proclined. A space should be visible between the tooth and acrylic of the baseplate. Examine the dentition for any signs of pathology (hard or soft) and, with the mandible in the retruded contact position, examine the maxillary labial segment. If the anterior crossbite has been corrected remove the posterior bite platforms, ensuring the edges are left smooth and do not irritate the lingual mucosa. If not, readjust the Z-spring and review the patient in another 4–5 weeks.

Table 3.3 Suggested treatment visits for correction of an anterior crossbite with a displacement (*continued*)

Visit		Clinical procedures
4.	4–5 weeks later	As in visit 3. The crossbite should normally be corrected by this stage. If it has been fully corrected, remove the biteplanes and make the spring passive. If the incisal overbite is satisfactory then a night-time regimen of wear can be instigated. Ensure the patient is aware of the need to keep the appliance in clean water when not in place intraorally.
5.	4–5 weeks later or 3 months later	If crossbite has not corrected consider stopping treatment; there is a risk of reducing compliance at a later stage if 'interceptive' appliance therapy is protracted. If this visit has been preceded by 3 months of night-time wear then the appliance can be discarded and the development of the occlusion can be monitored in a continual fashion at the appropriate time interval. Final impressions can be taken as a record of the completed orthodontic occlusion prior to further occlusal development.

Proclining teeth over the bite

Inadequate clearance of the occlusion that enables the teeth to move anteriorly.

3.5.2 Vertical

Most often posterior or anterior bite platforms; ideally they should be of such a size to obliterate the 'Freeway space'. Once neurophysiological adaptation has taken place, then acrylic is added to increase the thickness of the biteplane as appropriate. If the biteplane is initially too thick it will be very uncomfortable for the patient and will not be worn. Insufficient height to a biteplane will mean either an overbite will not reduce or, in the case of posterior biteplanes, occlusal interferences will not be removed.

3.5.3 Transverse

Failure to activate the screw is the major problem; patients have to be instructed in the surgery and allowed to demonstrate to you that they are able to activate the appliance. Occasionally the screw itself is faulty and the appliance will not therefore work. In some circumstances, well-intercuspated

Table 3.4 Suggested treatment visits for a space maintainer

Visit		Clinical procedures
1.		Examine, diagnose, and radiographically assess the dentition if the patient is aged 8 years or above. Upper and lower alginate impressions and an occlusal record should also be taken. A removable appliance should be constructed.
2.	1–2 weeks later	Fit the appliance, instruct the patient in the care of the appliance, the number of hours of wear anticipated, the amount and duration of discomfort, the duration of salivary excess and speech disturbances, and demonstrate the activation of the appliance. Ensure the appliance is able to maintain the space for the eruption of permanent successors.
3.	4–5 weeks later	Review the patient's speech with the appliance in place, examine the acrylic of the appliance; it should appear matt if it has been cleaned correctly. Observe the patient removing the appliance. Examine the dentition for any signs of pathology (hard or soft) and especially monitor the level of oral hygiene. These appliances may well have to be worn for several years awaiting the eruption of the permanent dentition and it is imperative that levels of oral hygiene are such that caries is not enhanced. This is essential in patients who may well have lost buccal teeth due to carious attack.
4.	3 months later	As in visit 3. If the intercuspation is satisfactory then a night-time regimen of wear can be instigated. Ensure the patient is aware of the need to keep the appliance in clean water when not in place intraorally.
5.	6 months later	Continue monitoring the development of the occlusion and, in particular, ensure the space maintainer is not compromising eruption of teeth. If this visit has been preceded by 3 months of night-time wear then the appliance wear can be reduced even further, such as to alternate nights. Final records, including impressions, can be taken as a record of the final occlusion and to assess the need for further treatment.

lower molars will expand at the same rate as the upper molars; clinically there will appear to be no change in crossbite. Measurement of the lower intermolar distance will help to identify this at the chairside.

3.5.4 Patient compliance

As previously stated, this has a major impact on the success of the appliance. Patient compliance is improved by providing a well-designed, well-fitting, and retentive appliance, and by unambiguously explaining to the patient in simple straightforward terms how to care for and wear the appliance.

3.6   SUMMARY

1. General principles of removable appliances:
   - tooth movements
   - appliance wear
   - appliance hygiene and care.
2. Removable appliance design:
   - **force**: springs, bows, screws, elastics
     (a) *anterior posterior tooth movement*:
       (i)   moving teeth anteriorly
       (ii) moving teeth posteriorly
       (iii) distal movement of molars
     (b) *vertical tooth movement:*
       (i)   extrusion of an individual tooth
     (c) *transverse tooth movement*
   - **fixation**: Adam's cribs, C-clasps, Southend clasp, fitted labial bows, reverse U-loop labial bow, Hawley bow
   - **anchorage**
   - **framework**.
3. Standard designs of contemporary removable appliances:
   - removable retainer (Hawley)
   - posterior expansion appliance
   - anterior crossbite
   - space maintainer.
4. Commonest failures for no tooth movement:
   - anteroposterior
   - vertical
   - transverse
   - patient compliance.

3.7 OBJECTIVES

1. Appreciate that removable appliances are complex and potentially damaging to the dentition.
2. Identify the types of tooth movements the appliances are capable of achieving.
3. Be able to design simple removable appliances for specific clinical goals.

REFERENCES

1. Yettram, A. L., Wright, K. W., and Houston, W. J. (1977). Centre of rotation of a maxillary central incisor under orthodontic loading. *British Journal of Orthodontics*, **4**, 23–7.
2. Stephens, C. D. (1979). The orthodontic center of rotation of the maxillary central incisor. *American Journal of Orthodontics*, **76**, 209–17.
3. Williams, K. R. and Edmundson, J. T. (1984). Orthodontic tooth movement analysed by the Finite Element Method. *Biomaterials*, **5**, 347–51.
4. Jones, S. P. and Waters, N. E. (1989). The quadhelix maxillary expansion appliance. Part I: Mechanics. *European Journal of Orthodontics*, **11**, 169–78.
5. Waltimo, A. and Kononen, M. (1993). A novel bite force recorder and maximal isometric bite force values for healthy young adults. *Scandinavian Journal of Dental Research*, **101**, 171–5.
6. Bartsch, A., Witt, E., Sahm, G., and Schneider, S. (1993). Correlates of objective patient compliance with removable appliance wear. *American Journal of Orthodontics and Dentofacial Orthopedics*, **104**, 378–86.
7. Sergl, H. G. and Zentner, A. (1998). A comparative assessment of acceptance of different types of functional appliances. *European Journal of Orthodontics*, **20**, 517–24.
8. Cureton, S. L., Regennitter, F. J., and Yancey, J. M. (1993). The role of the headgear calendar in headgear compliance. *American Journal of Orthodontics and Dentofacial Orthopedics*, **104**, 387–94.
9. Sameshima, G. T. and Sinclair, P. M. (2001). Predicting and preventing root resorption. Part II: Treatment factors. *American Journal Orthodontics and Dentofacial Orthopedics*, **119**, 511–15.
10. Sameshima, G. T. and Sinclair, P. M. (2001). Predicting and preventing root resorption. Part I: Diagnostic factors. *American Journal Orthodontics and Dentofacial Orthopedics*, **119**, 505–10.
11. Murphy, K. M., Carter, J. M., Johnson, R. R., and Sorensen, S. E. (1985). Determination of residual stresses in denture base polymers using the layer removal technique. *Journal of Biomedical Materials Research*, **19**, 971–80.
12. Cetlin, N. M. and Ten Hoeve, A. (1983). Nonextraction treatment. *Journal of Clinical Orthodontics*, **17**, 396–413.
13. Andrews, L. F. (1972). The six keys to normal occlusion. *American Journal of Orthodontics*, **62**, 296–309.
14. Adams, K. F. (date). *A manual of removable appliances*. Oxford University Press, Oxford.
15. Stephens, C. D. (1979). The Southend clasp. *British Journal of Orthodontics*, **6**, 183–5.
16. Fernstrom, A. I. and Oquist, G. (1980). Location of the allergenic monomer in warm-polymerized acrylic dentures. Part I: Causes of denture sore mouth, incidence of allergy, different allergens and test methods on suspicion of allergy to denture material—a survey of the literature. Case report, allergenic analysis of denture and test casting. *Swedish Dental Journal*, **4**, 241–52.

17. Sonnesen, L., Bakke, M., and Solow, B. (1998). Malocclusion traits and symptoms and signs of temporomandibular disorders in children with severe malocclusion. *European Journal of Orthodontics*, **20**, 543–59.

18. Nilner, M. and Petersson, A. (1995). Clinical and radiological findings related to treatment outcome in patients with temporomandibular disorders. *Dentomaxillofacial Radiology*, **24**, 128–31.

4 Functional appliances

CONTENTS

Functional, or myofunctional appliances as they are also known, are appliances that utilize forces generated by the orofacial soft tissues in order to move the teeth. They are constructed in such a way as to posture the mandible away from the rest position, with the forces being generated by the resultant soft tissue stretch (Fig. 4.1). In addition to moving the teeth, functional appliances have also been used with a view to modifying facial growth. This is particularly so in the case of Class II skeletal relationships and, to a lesser extent, Class III skeletal relationships. Before describing how functional appliances work it is worth briefly reconsidering the mechanisms involved in normal facial growth.

4.1 GROWTH OF THE FACE

It is known that the human facial skeleton constitutes approximately one-ninth of the size of the head at birth, with the rest being composed of the neural skeleton. By the time of adulthood and skeletal maturity, this proportion has increased, so that the face represents approximately one-quarter of the size of the head (Fig. 4.2).[1] What happens in the intervening years will be of great interest to the orthodontist. For if functional appliances are to be used to modify facial growth, it would follow that they should be used during periods of active growth. The pace of growth from birth to adulthood is not constant but occurs more rapidly at certain times

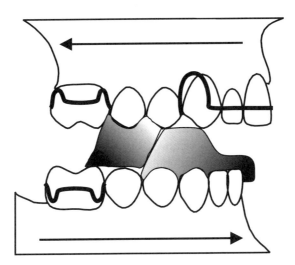

Fig. 4.1 This diagram illustrates a functional appliance in place used to treat a Class II division 1 incisor relationship. The arrows indicate the direction of the forces applied to the teeth in each arch as a result of the intermaxillary traction effect exerted by the appliance.

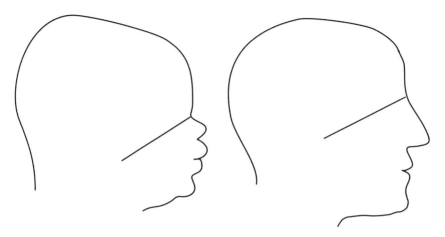

Fig. 4.2 Diagram of an infant and adult head in profile. Although they have been drawn the same size, notice the differences in facial proportions as a percentage of overall head size.

and within certain tissues. This is illustrated well by the Scammon curves,[2] which map the rate of growth against age for somatic (including the facial skeleton), neural, and lymphoid tissues (Fig. 4.3).

The controlling mechanisms in facial growth are thought to be primarily genetic, but it has been known for centuries that skeletal growth can be altered by environmental factors. Examples of such environmental alteration include foot binding and head binding. The Chinese practised foot binding in women for over 1000 years to produce what was considered to be the attractive, small 'lotus' foot. Head binding, performed in order to produce an elongated head, which was thought to be associated with great intelligence, has been practised in many parts of the World including Africa, the South Pacific Islands, and Normandy in France. Whereas such practises are performed over many years, functional appliances are worn for perhaps 15–18 months and not usually full time. An exception to this more usual part-time wear is seen with the Herbst appliance, which is bonded to the teeth and so cannot be removed by the patient (see Section 4.5.6). Certainly full-time wear of functional appliances has been demonstrated to lead to condylar growth in animals,[3,4] affecting both condylar size and shape[5] as well as stimulating adaptive remodelling of the glenoid fossa.[6]

In orthodontics, functional appliances are traditionally used at the beginning of the pubertal growth spurt when the facial skeleton is growing rapidly, which in girls is 10–12 years of age and in boys approximately 2 years later, at 12–14 years.[7] More recently there has been a move towards treatment at an earlier age, in the hope of attaining a lasting orthopaedic rather than just an orthodontic effect. For the orthodontist there are basic questions to be answered:

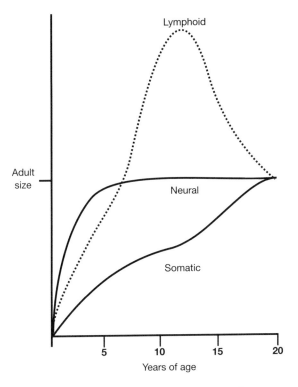

Fig. 4.3 Scammon growth curves for lymphoid, neural, and somatic tissues.

1. Do we have the mechanics capable of modifying craniofacial growth?
2. Is the change we produce a 'clinically' significant change beyond normal growth and biological variation?
3. Is the change stable after cessation of treatment and growth?
4. Do we produce any 'harm' to the patient?

Growth affects the relationship between the mandible and maxilla in all three spatial planes: anteroposteriorly, vertically, and transversely. This three-dimensional jaw relationship is normally affected by growth at a number of sites:

• *Base of the skull*—The cartilaginous synchondroses between the bones of the skull base act as primary growth centres. These include the frontoethmoidal, sphenoethmoidal, spheno-occipital, and the basioccipital synchondroses. Of these the sphenoethmoidal (fused by 6 years of age) and the spheno-occipital synchondroses (fused by 14 years of age)[8] (Fig. 4.4) are of importance to the orthodontist. As a result of growth at these sites, the glenoid fossa, and hence the mandible, will move backwards with respect to the maxilla. This will affect both the anteroposterior and vertical relationships of the jaws.

• *Mandibular condyles*—The condylar growth cartilages may lead to the backwards, upwards, and outwards growth of each condyle (Fig. 4.5). They

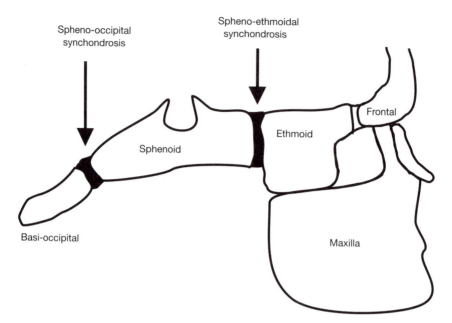

Fig. 4.4 Cross-section of the anterior part of the skull base illustrating the two major synchondroses.

are important in both increasing mandibular length, from the condylar head to the bony chin, and also increasing the intercondylar width. The anteroposterior relationship of the mandible to the maxilla is therefore maintained at a time when backward movement of the two glenoid fossae is occurring as a result of growth at the synchondroses. Condylar growth also maintains the transverse relationship of the articulation between the mandible and the maxilla, at a time when the distance between the glenoid fossae is also increasing. Growth at the condyle is not always in the general direction of the ramus, but can be upwards and backwards, or upwards and forwards, with a variation of up to 45 degrees[9] (Fig. 4.6).

• *Maxillary sutures*—Growth occurs at both the circumaxillary suture system and the mid-palatal suture up until the early to mid-teens.[10] Sutures are no longer regarded as primary growth centres, unlike the synchondroses at the base of the skull, but are thought to deposit bone in response to the bone displacement created as a result of growth in other tissues. For example, it has been postulated that normal downwards and forwards growth of the maxilla is due to growth of the orbital contents, the nasal septum, and, possibly, soft tissue stretch associated with growth in the vertebral column. In the case of the latter, vertebral growth results in the head being moved away from the shoulders, which in turn is thought to lead to tension in the suprahyoid tissues. It is this soft tissue stretch which then exerts the downward displacing force on the maxilla. Whatever the mechanism, as the

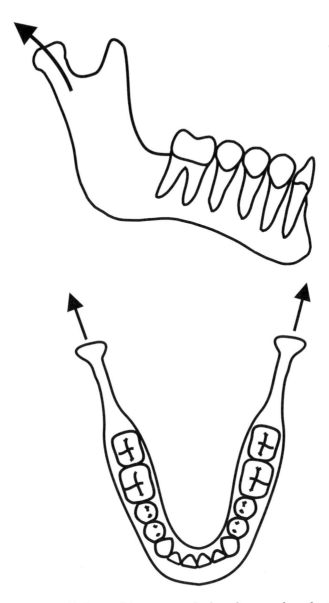

Fig. 4.5 The mandibular condyles can grow backwards, upwards, and outwards in order to maintain the relationship between the mandible and maxilla.

maxilla moves downwards, sutural growth takes place to keep the bones closely approximated.

• *Surface deposition and resorption*—In addition to growth at the synchondroses, sutures, and condyles, both the maxilla and mandible undergo surface remodelling. Bone deposition occurs on some surfaces and resorption takes place on others. This not only leads to changes in size but also in the

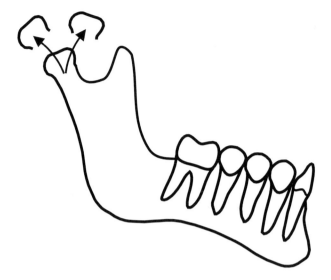

Fig. 4.6 The condyle can grow posteriorly or anteriorly.

form of both jaws, and can therefore modify the effects of growth elsewhere (see Growth rotations, below).

4.1.1 Growth rotations

Although growth of the mandible and maxilla is generally considered to be in a downwards and forwards direction, in reality it is much more complex than this. Not only do both jaws show rotational growth, but this is further modified by surface remodelling. Deposition and resorption of bone occurs at the surface of both the mandible and maxilla and may lessen or increase the overall effect of growth. In the late 1950s and early 1960s, implant studies were performed by Björk.[11,12] Either three or four subperiosteal metallic implants were placed in the mandible and the maxilla of children, and the growth changes from 4 to 24 years of age were monitored with the aid of lateral skull radiographs. Using these markers, which were placed in such a way that they remained in a stable position within the bone and their position could be verified, it was subsequently noted that both the mandible and maxilla could show rotational growth with respect to the cranial base, rather than just downward and forwards. This is known as a '**true rotation**'[13] (Fig. 4.7), the centre of which can vary from individual to individual. However, there is also an '**apparent rotation**', which is the angular change between the lower border of the mandible and the cranial base (Fig. 4.8). This is what is normally measured on a lateral skull radiograph. When the values for the true rotation and the apparent rotation are compared they are often very different. The true rotation might perhaps

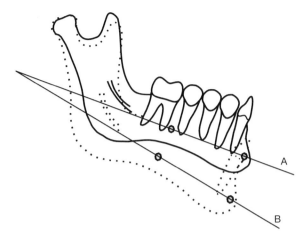

Fig. 4.7 A true rotation of the mandible. Note the subperiosteal implants (circles) and the inferior dental canal used as stable markers. As the mandible grows downwards and forwards (from the solid to the dotted line) there is a true clockwise rotation relative to the anterior cranial base from line A to line B.

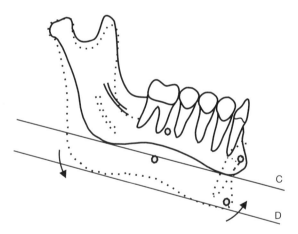

Fig. 4.8 An apparent rotation of the mandible. This diagram is a copy of Fig. 4.7, except that the lower border of the mandible has remodelled. The angle of the mandible has remodelled downwards and the lower border of the chin has remodelled upwards (look at the arrows). The mandibular plane has therefore apparently remained unchanged with respect to the anterior cranial base (lines C to D) even though the angle between the implants (true rotation) has changed greatly.

measure 10° and yet the apparent rotation might be minus 5°. The apparent rotation can therefore negate 50% of the true rotation. This difference is due to '**angular remodelling**' at the lower border of the mandible. The same true and apparent rotations, with angular remodelling, can occur at

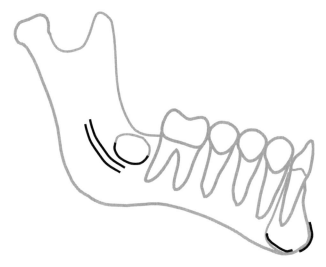

Fig. 4.9 Mandibular reference points.

the posterior border of the ramus of the mandible and also within the max-illa. In the latter case, the angular remodelling occurs at the hard palate and floor of the nose[14] and the true rotation, which in the maxilla is less than that seen in the mandible, can be anterior or posterior. By the use of posteroanterior radiographs and subperiosteal implants, the maxilla has also been shown to undergo transverse rotations, often widening posteriorly and narrowing anteriorly.

Although the rotations mentioned above were only realized with the use of subperiosteal markers, it was also demonstrated that the following refer-ence points could act as stable reference markers, substituting to some extent for the implants. These reference points are:[15]

- *Mandible* (Fig. 4.9):
  - anterior surface of the symphysis
  - the inner surface the symphysis at its lower border
  - any distinct trabeculae in the symphysis
  - inferior dental canal
  - the lowest outline of unerupted molar tooth germs prior to root formation;
- *Maxilla*:
  - the anterior surface of the zygomatic process.[14]

By convention, with a lateral skull radiograph facing to the right, a posterior growth rotation of the mandible occurs in a clockwise direction and an anterior rotation occurs in an anticlockwise direction. The opposite is true for maxillary growth rotations (Fig. 4.10).

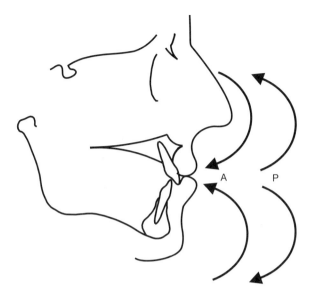

Fig. 4.10 Anterior (A) and posterior (P) growth rotations in the mandible and maxilla.

What is the relevance of these growth rotations to the orthodontist?

These rotations are of most significance where the extremes of growth are seen. Examples of these extremes are shown in Figs 4.11 and 4.12.

The extraoral and intraoral clinical signs and orthodontic consequences of anterior and posterior growth rotations are:

- *Anterior growth rotation of the mandible*:
  - a reduced anterior lower face height
  - an increased posterior lower face height
  - a convex lower border of the mandible
  - a deep overbite
  - an overbite that is difficult to reduce
  - lower incisor crowding as the mandible carries the teeth upward and forward towards the lips
  - space closure during treatment can prove difficult;
- *Posterior growth rotation of the mandible*:
  - an increased anterior lower face height
  - a reduced lower posterior face height
  - a concave lower border of the mandible
  - a reduced overbite or anterior open bite
  - lower incisor crowding as the mandible carries the teeth downward and forward towards the lips
  - rapid space loss following extractions for the relief of crowding.

It is also important to identify the trend of growth and to plan mechanics to minimize any deterioration of this growth form. For example, in a

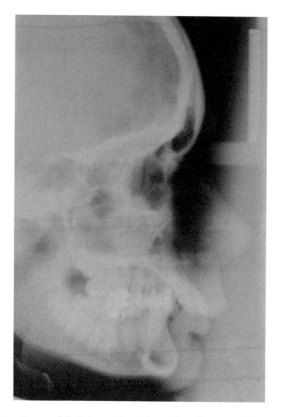

Fig. 4.11 An extreme of facial growth with a reduced anterior lower facial height and an anterior growth rotation.

high-angle case (one with an increased anterior lower face height, an increased maxillary–mandibular planes' angle, and a posterior growth rotation) treatment mechanics should be designed to prevent tooth extrusion, especially in the buccal segments. Thus functional appliances that prevent further eruption of the labial segments but allow overeruption of the buccal segments are not appropriate.

4.2 MODE OF ACTION OF FUNCTIONAL APPLIANCES

Although functional appliances are undoubtedly used with success in orthodontic treatment, in particular with Class II division 1 incisor relationships, the biggest controversy associated with their use is their mode of action. Three such mechanisms have been postulated and are best understood with reference to the treatment of a Class II division 1 incisor relationship. These are:
• skeletal changes
• dentoalveolar changes
• soft tissue changes.

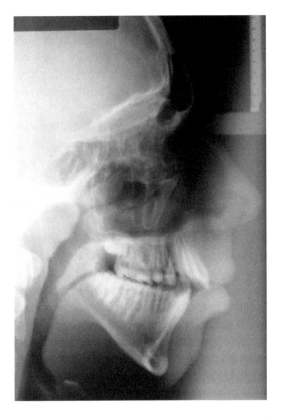

Fig. 4.12 An extreme of facial growth with an increased anterior lower facial height and a posterior growth rotation.

4.2.1   Skeletal changes

The theoretical skeletal changes that may occur as a result of wearing functional appliances can be considered in two dimensions (transverse changes are not considered due to the overall poor results from functional appliances), namely anteroposterior and vertical, and are:

(1) additional overall growth of the mandible;

(2) accelerated growth of the mandible, but not necessarily additional growth;

(3) a change in the direction of growth of the mandible;

(4) a change in the position of the mandibular condyle and glenoid fossa; and

(5) restricted growth of the maxilla.

   However, does the clinical use of a functional appliance actually result in skeletal change in orthodontic patients? The published evidence would suggest the following:

1. *Additional overall growth of the mandible*—Certainly increased growth can be demonstrated in animal studies, where the appliances are cemented

in place for a number of years.[16] Many reports have been published in which functional appliances have been found to lead to increased mandibular growth in humans, even though the appliances are not worn for such a long time.[17] However, care must be taken when interpreting the results of such studies, since they are often retrospective and the control subjects are not always well matched for factors such as age, sex, and skeletal pattern. More recently there have been a number of prospective, clinical, randomized controlled trials into the effects of functional appliances, where many of these shortcomings have been overcome.[18–20] Although some have demonstrated increased mandibular growth of around 0.5 mm/year, during the period of study lasting 12–15 months, it is questionable whether such changes are of clinical significance, even though they may be statistically significant.[19]

2.   *Accelerated growth of the mandible, but not necessarily additional growth*— Once again, controversy exists as to whether any additional growth achieved during functional appliance therapy is maintained once the functional appliance is no longer worn. This controversy exists not only between different studies, but also occasionally between reports from the same author at different times. Some studies have found that the additional growth, seen during the period of functional appliance therapy for a Class II skeletal pattern, is gradually lost at a diminished rate during the 3–4 years following treatment as the patients continue to grow,[21–23] If this is the case, mandibular size and position will be no different between individuals, whether or not they were treated with a functional appliance. Other studies have suggested that increased mandibular growth, observed during functional appliance therapy for Class II skeletal relationships is maintained in the longer term, with no reduction in subsequent growth.[24,25] It would seem that this controversy, like many others surrounding functional appliances, will persist until the longer term results of randomized control trials are published.

3.   *A change in the direction of growth of the mandible*—Those that might occur with functional appliances can be:
• a change in the overall direction from downwards and forwards to a more horizontal direction, thereby helping to correct a Class II skeletal relationship;[26–31]
• a change in direction of growth of the mandibular condyle from upward and anterior to a more posterior direction, which would once again help in the correction of a Class II skeletal relationship[32–34] (see Fig. 4.6).

4.   *A change in the position of the mandibular condyle and glenoid fossa*— Studies on primates, in which a functional appliance is cemented into position for up to 14 months (e.g. the Herbst appliance, see Section 4.5.6), have shown forward movement of the glenoid fossa through bony remodelling.[35] Such anterior repositioning will contribute a great deal to a Class II skeletal

correction. In human studies, no such extensive changes have been found using the same appliance but over a shorter 7-month period.[36] Indeed, with the more commonly used removable functional appliances and using magnetic resonance imaging (MRI) techniques, there is no such evidence of any forward remodelling of the fossa that might contribute to any correction of a Class II skeletal relationship.[37,38]

5.   *Restricted growth of the maxilla*—It has been postulated that anterior maxillary growth can be inhibited by the use of a functional appliance in the treatment of a Class II skeletal pattern.[39,40] However, a number of studies have either not demonstrated any such maxillary restraint, or the changes observed are small; it is unknown whether such small changes are then maintained in the longer term once functional appliance treatment has ceased.[41-43]

4.2.2 Dentoalveolar change

In most of the studies into the mode of action of functional appliances, the largest dimensional effect occurs as a result of induced dentoalveolar change.[44] For a Class II division 1 incisor relationship these changes include (Fig. 4.13):
(1) retraction of the upper incisors (palatal tipping);
(2) proclination of the lower incisors;
(3) overbite reduction, by reducing lower incisor eruption while permitting buccal segment tooth eruption;
(4) mesial movement of the lower buccal segment teeth, occurs because they move mesially as they continue to erupt;
(5) distal movement of the upper buccal segment teeth—in combination with mesial movement of the lower buccal segment teeth, the molar relationship can be altered, hopefully to a Class I relationship;
(6) expansion of the upper arch.
These will be dealt with in turn.

1.   *Retraction of the upper incisors (palatal tipping)*—This is usually a wanted effect of functional appliances. Many functional appliances have some form of labial bow that makes a point of contact on the labial surface of the upper incisor teeth. As a result of the distalizing force exerted by the mandible, it is easy to understand how the upper incisors undergo palatal tipping thereby reducing the overjet (Fig. 4.13). Sometimes palatal spurs are added to the appliance instead of a labial bow (Fig. 4.14). This has been shown to be effective in reduce palatal tipping of the upper incisors possibly encouraging more mandibular growth.[45]

2.   *Proclination of the lower incisors*—While retroclination of the upper incisors is a wanted effect, proclination of the lower incisors is frequently an unwanted effect except in specific malocclusions. In an attempt to minimize

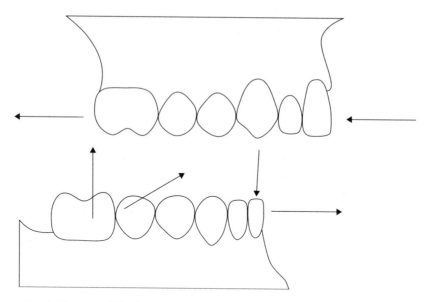

Fig. 4.13 Some of the dentoalveolar effects of a functional appliance used to treat a Class II division 1 incisor relationship (excluding possible arch expansion).

this proclination, functional appliances often have acrylic capping on the lower incisors, which is extended labially to come close to the labial gingival margins of the teeth (Fig. 4.14). However, even within this extensive capping, the lower incisors will still procline to some extent. There are two specific instances when lower incisor proclination within the appliance might be desirable, namely:

- if the patient previously had a thumb-sucking habit, which had the effect of retroclining the incisors; and
- where the overbite is deep and the lower incisors appear trapped in the palate; here the incisors may have retroclined as forward mandibular growth continues.

In both instances the lower incisors may have been unable to achieve a more labial yet stable position because of the habit or trapping. In such cases the acrylic on the lower incisors may only cover the incisal edges and not extend labially.

3. *Overbite reduction*—Overbite reduction can occur within a functional appliance by reducing lower incisor eruption while permitting buccal segment tooth eruption (see Fig. 4.13).

4. *Mesial movement of the lower buccal segment teeth*—As the lower buccal segment teeth erupt, not only do they move occlusally but they also erupt mesially. This will have the effect of changing the molar relationship. If it started as a Class II relationship, then mesial movement of the lower molars

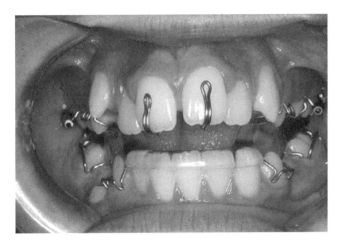

Fig. 4.14 Palatal spurs on a functional appliance can be used to minimize palatal tipping. Labial acrylic on the lower incisors is used to help reduce labial tipping.

will mean the molar relationship will progress towards Class I (see Fig. 4.13).

5.   *Distal movement of the upper buccal segment teeth*—In the case of a Class II division 1 incisor relationship, the forward posturing of the mandible by the appliance will have a distalizing effect on the upper buccal segment teeth. In combination with mesial movement of the lower buccal segment teeth, the molar relationship will hopefully progress towards a Class I relationship.

6.   *Expansion of the upper arch*—It may be necessary to expand the upper arch so that as the mandibular teeth are moved anteriorly, the upper buccal segment teeth do not go into crossbite. This can be achieved in a number of ways. With a two-part functional appliance such as the Clark twin block,[46] where one appliance fits the lower arch and one fits the upper arch, it is possible to expand the upper by incorporating a midline screw into this part of the appliance. Other functional appliances are made as a single unit and so a midline screw cannot be used, since it would have to expand both the upper and lower arches simultaneously or lead to fracture of the lower part of the appliance. Instead, it may be possible to trim the acrylic around the upper buccal segment teeth in order to encourage the teeth to erupt buccally (see Section 4.5.2). Alternatively, in the case of the Fränkel appliance there are buccal acrylic shields that hold the cheeks away from the teeth, so that the upper arch will expand under the influence of the tongue (see Section 4.5, Examples of commonly used functional appliances). If a single-part functional appliance is to be used and significant upper arch expansion is required to achieve arch coordination, then a short course of

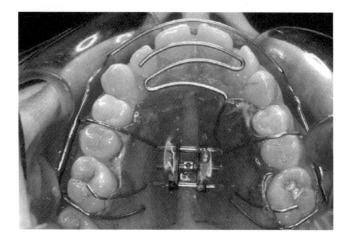

Fig. 4.15 An initial upper removable appliance can be used to expand the upper arch prior to the use of a functional appliance.

upper removable appliance therapy to expand the upper arch may be required prior to fitting the functional appliance (Fig. 4.15).

4.2.3 Soft tissue changes

The final possible mode of action of functional appliances is the long-term effect they might have on the soft tissues. For example, the functional regulator appliances devised by Fränkel (see Section 4.5.4), in combination with lip exercises, are said to alter the position of the lips and cheeks. If these soft tissues are then encouraged to be in the correct positions and function normally, it would follow that the teeth will then move to their correct positions under the influence of these soft tissues. The theory behind this mode of action of the functional regulator is therefore based on the functional matrix theory of Moss.[47-49] The reality is that, like most functional appliances, the most significant effect is achieved through dentoalveolar change.[50]

4.3   TIMING OF TREATMENT USING FUNCTIONAL APPLIANCES

As with many aspects of functional appliance therapy, the timing of treatment is the subject of some controversy. Consider the following questions:
• If functional appliances are to be used with the express aim of altering skeletal pattern, isn't it best to fit the appliance during the period of active facial growth?

- If growth can be altered, then is it perhaps the case that the earlier the functional appliance is fitted the greater will be the overall effect on the facial skeleton?
- If, however, the effects are mainly dentoalveolar, surely functional appliances can be used at any age, including adulthood?

Traditionally, functional appliances have been fitted just prior to the pubertal growth spurt as was discussed in Section 4.1 (Growth of the face). This will usually be somewhere between 10 and 12 years of age in girls and 12–14 years of age in boys. Once fitted, the overall treatment time is usually in the region of 9–12 months, depending on the size of the initial overjet. The average rate of overjet reduction is approximately 1 mm per month, but this value can vary, with overjet reduction sometimes occurring quickly at the beginning and slowing down towards the end of treatment.

In recent years the possibility of treatment starting at 8–9 years of age has been considered, and certainly there has been a shift towards two-stage treatments. These begin with an initial phase of functional appliance therapy, followed by a second fixed-appliance phase. The evidence from prospective clinical trials would seem to suggest that starting treatment with an initial functional appliance phase, followed by the second fixed-appliance phase, does not lead to clinically significant changes in the observed skeletal pattern at the end of the combined treatment, when compared to individuals who were only treated later with fixed appliances and without the initial functional phase of treatment.[51,52] Instead, the overall treatment time of the two-phased approach tends to be longer than in cases where treatment is carried out at a later stage with only fixed appliances.[53]

What about the use of functional appliances after the majority of facial growth has taken place? The little work undertaken on the effect of functional appliances in adults would seem to suggest that almost no skeletal changes occur, and that only a small degree of dentoalveolar change might be observed.[54] Functional appliances would therefore seem to be of little value in the treatment of adult patients.

4.4 CLASSIFICATION OF FUNCTIONAL APPLIANCES

There is no universally accepted classification of functional appliances. They can be classified according to:
- their component parts;[55]
- whether they are primarily tooth-borne or tissue-borne;
- the malocclusion in which they are being used, i.e. a Class II or Class III incisor relationship;
- the degree of soft tissue stretch they induce when in place.

A classification based on the latter point is one of the simplest, certainly for Class II functional appliances. Using this classification there are thought to be two basic types of functional appliance:[56]

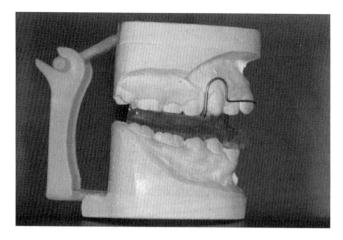

Fig. 4.16 A Harvold functional appliance. Notice how far open the bite has been taken. Acrylic has been trimmed away from the lower buccal segment teeth to permit eruption.

1. *Myotonic*—Here it is thought that the elastic recoil within the stretched soft tissues generates the forces that move the teeth. An example of such an appliance is the Harvold appliance (Fig. 4.16).
2. *Myodynamic*—In this case, it is thought the forces that move the teeth are generated by stimulation of the masticatory muscles as a result of wearing the functional appliance. Any striated muscle when stretched, via muscle spindle and Golgi tendon organ detection, will undergo a reflex contraction (e.g. the knee jerk reflex). In the jaws this may induce the force responsible for tooth movement. However, if the patient habitually postures the mandible forwards (mandibular deviation) the muscle will already be preadapted and so the forces will not be as efficiently produced and functional treatment will not be as effective. Examples of this type of appliance are the Clark twin block, Bionator, and Medium opening activator.

4.5   EXAMPLES OF COMMONLY USED FUNCTIONAL APPLIANCES

Very many types of functional appliance are available to the orthodontist. Currently the most commonly used include those discussed below.

4.5.1   Clark twin block

This can be classified as:
• tooth-borne
• myodynamic
• Class II or Class III.

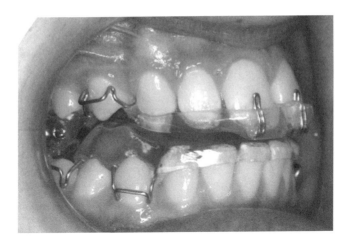

Fig. 4.17 A Clark twin-block type of functional appliance.

The twin block was devised by Clark,[57] and, as the name suggests, it has two opposing acrylic blocks on either side of the arch (Fig. 4.17). These prevent the patient closing into centric occlusion and instead force the mandible into a postured position. This will be anteriorly in Class II cases and posteriorly in Class III cases. A unique feature of the twin block is that it is composed of two separate appliances, an upper and a lower. This gives it a number of advantages over one-piece appliances, including:

- increased patient comfort;
- the ability to expand the upper arch using a midline screw;
- easy reactivation of the appliance to a more postured position by adding to the acrylic on the blocks.

There are very many designs of the twin block, but the principle of the two opposing blocks is always the same. Some are complex in order that specific tooth movements can be achieved during the functional phase of treatment. For example, proclination of the upper labial segment, converting a Class II division 2 incisor relationship into a Class II division 1 (see Section 4.6.2.). Other designs are much simpler, consisting of separate upper and lower vacuum-formed retainers in which acrylic blocks are simply embedded (Fig. 4.18). The initial design incorporated 'flying EOT' tubes in the upper appliance, into which high-pull headgear was fitted in an attempt induce maxillary intrusion. At the same time, an anterior elastic from the lower appliance, lingual to the lower anterior teeth, passing to the headgear facebow was used to promote an anterior growth rotation of the mandible in order to overcome the typical growth pattern seen in high-angle Class II skeletal cases.

At the end of a course of treatment with the twin-block appliance, whatever the precise design, it is common to see lateral open bites (Fig. 4.19) as

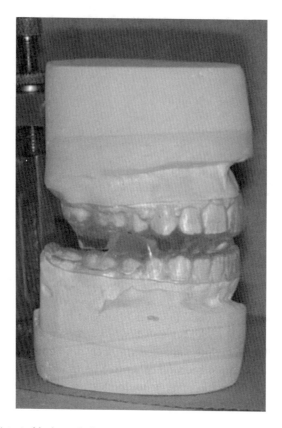

Fig. 4.18 A twin block made from vacuum-formed material and acrylic blocks.

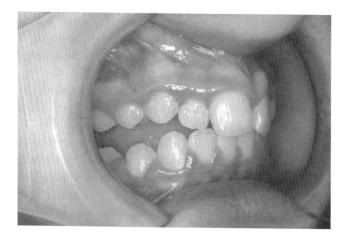

Fig. 4.19 Lateral open bites are commonly seen at the end of active treatment with a twin block.

the buccal segment teeth are prevented from erupting. The twin block has therefore been suggested for use in cases requiring functional appliance therapy, but in which there is an increased anterior lower face height. The open bites can be encouraged to close at the end of active treatment, either by reducing the height of the blocks, or by asking the patient to go on to part-time wear of the appliances.

4.5.2   Bionator

This can be classified as:
- tooth-borne
- myodynamic
- Class II.

The bionator (Fig. 4.20) is a one-piece functional appliance with limited tongue space, and as such is not as well tolerated by the patient as the twin block. It is also not as easily reactivated: it either requires a remake, or the appliance must be sectioned, advanced, and then put together again in the laboratory. Generally the bionator has no retentive components, although an Adams' crib can be added to the upper first molars, and so can be quite a loose fit for the patient. This can be useful if deciduous molars are likely to be lost in the near future. It is also meant to encourage the patient to bite into the appliance in the desired postured position, thereby helping to keep it in place and making it more comfortable to wear. The acrylic over both the lower and upper buccal segment teeth can be trimmed to allow these teeth to erupt and help reduce the overbite. It can also encourage further alteration of the molar relationship. Simply reducing the acrylic over the lower buccal segment teeth will enable them to erupt, and as they do so, they will erupt mesially. In the upper arch, the acrylic around the upper buccal segment teeth can be removed, except where it is in contact with the mesiopalatal aspect of the teeth. By leaving this area of acrylic and angling the way in which the remainder of the acrylic is trimmed, it is possible to encourage the upper buccal segment teeth to erupt both distally and buccally. Therefore, not only is the molar relationship altered, but it is also possible to get a small degree of expansion of the upper arch (see Section 4.2.2).

The bionator contains a limited amount of wirework. There is a labial bow that is extended into the form of buccal wire loops. The labial bow portion lies passively against the upper incisors, whilst the extended buccal loops are there to hold the cheeks away from the teeth. Supposedly, this is to allow expansion of the buccal segment teeth, although it is doubtful if this is ever likely to occur. This is because the wire probably does not hold the cheeks away from the teeth very effectively and the teeth cannot move buccally unless the acrylic of the appliance is trimmed, as described earlier. The second piece of wirework is the coffin spring (Fig. 4.21). In the

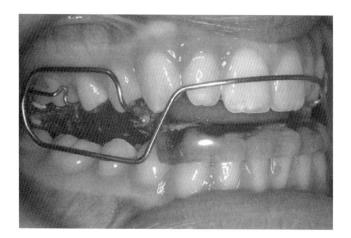

Fig. 4.20 A bionator.

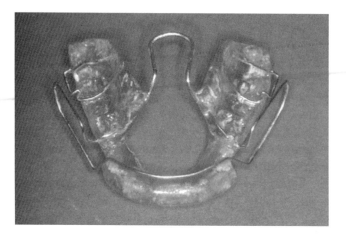

Fig. 4.21 The coffin spring in a bionator. This spring sits close to the palate.

bionator this spring cannot be used to expand the upper arch, as in the case of a simple upper removable appliance, since it would fracture the acrylic in contact with the lower arch at the midline. Its purpose is to encourage the patient to position their tongue more anteriorly within their mouth and thereby maintain a more anterior position of the mandible during treatment. Whether the coffin spring makes any difference is open to debate. Certainly a bionator without the inclusion of the coffin spring is likely to work equally well.

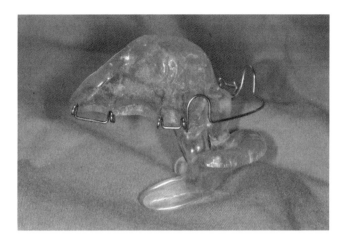

Fig. 4.22 A medium opening activator.

4.5.3 Medium opening activator

This can be classified as:
- tooth-borne
- myodynamic
- Class II.

An example of this appliance is shown in Fig. 4.22. It can be seen that it is much more skeletal in design than the bionator, although, like the bionator, it is a one-piece design. The reduced amount of acrylic, particularly in the lower arch, means it has found favour as a functional appliance that can be used simultaneously with fixed appliances and is relatively easily tolerated. It has the same limitations as a bionator, but unlike a bionator it has Adams' cribs and so is more retentive, supposedly preventing the mandible from dropping back during sleep. It is not possible to trim the upper acrylic as described with the bionator.

4.5.4 Fränkel FR-II

This can be classified as:
- tissue-borne
- myodynamic
- Class II.

The Fränkel FR-II appliance[58] (Fig. 4.23) is one of four functional appliances originally described by Fränkel. Both the FR-I and FR-II are used to treat Class II incisor relationships, the FR-III is for Class III incisor relationships, and the FR-IV is used to treat anterior open bites. FR stands for 'functional regulator' and, in addition to posturing the mandible anteriorly, the FR-II has labial acrylic pads and acrylic buccal shields. The labial pads are present

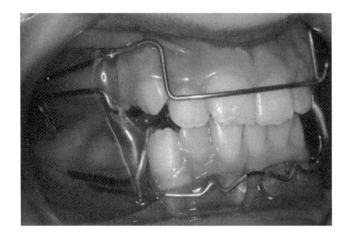

Fig. 4.23 A Fränkel FR-II appliance.

to encourage the lips to take up a more normal posture, and it is recommended that the patient performs lip exercises to maintain a competent lip posture with the appliance in place. The buccal shields are also thought to modify the behaviour of the soft tissues of the cheeks. Not only do the buccal shields permit expansion of the arches under the influence of the tongue by keeping the cheeks away from the teeth, but they are also thought to stretch the soft tissues at the base of the labial sulcus. This stretching, in turn, is thought to pull on the periosteum overlying the alveolus and promote bone deposition, thereby widening the apical basal bone into which the teeth can then move. This soft tissue mode of action (see Section 4.2.3) is theoretical and is yet to be proven in humans. Indeed, in animal studies no such bone deposition on the buccal aspect of the alveolus has been observed.[59] Moreover, the labial acrylic pads act as a lip bumper in the lower labial sulcus. These, in common with lip bumpers,[60] induce lower incisor proclination.

4.5.5 Harvold

This can be classified as:
• tooth-borne
• myotonic
• Class II.

Unlike the other functional appliances so far discussed, the Harvold appliance is myotonic. As can be seen in Fig. 4.16, not only does the Harvold appliance posture the mandible anteriorly, but the patient's mouth is also propped open by 5–6 mm beyond the freeway space.[61] The appliance is trimmed to permit eruption of the lower buccal segment teeth, whilst the upper buccal segment teeth are prevented from erupting. As well as affecting the usual dentoalveolar changes seen with functional appliances, with the design of this appliance it was hoped that maxillary growth might be restricted.[62] However, the evidence for any such clinically significant long-term skeletal effects on the maxilla is not available.

4.5.6   Herbst

This can be classified as:

- tooth-borne
- Class II or Class III
- fixed.

Unlike the functional appliances so far discussed, the Herbst appliance, which was first introduced in 1905 by Emil Herbst, (see ref. 63) cannot be removed and instead is fixed to the teeth. After the 1930s very little was published on the appliance, until it was repopularized by Pancherz in the late 1970s and early 1980s.[64,65] Essentially, a steel rod or plunger is screwed to the lower appliance in the premolar region, and fits into a steel tube screwed to the upper appliance in the upper first molar region (Fig. 4.24). As the patient closes their mouth, this plunger, in its tube, forces the mandible anteriorly in Class II cases. The method by which the plunger and tube are attached to the teeth can vary. It can either be to bands on the lower premolars and upper molars (these bands are sometimes constructed from a thicker metal than standard fixed appliance bands), which are part of an upper and a lower fixed appliance, or acrylic splints can be bonded to the teeth into which the plunger and tube are screwed. The reported advantages of the Herbst appliance include:[66]

- full-time wear;
- improved compliance compared with other functional appliances because it cannot be removed by the patient; and

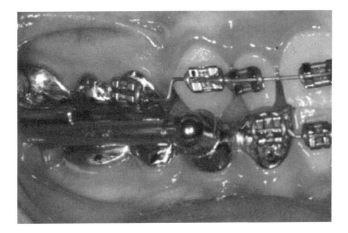

Fig. 4.24 A Herbst appliance.

- shorter treatment time.
  However, the disadvantages include:
- fracture of the premolar and molar bands;
- loosening of the premolar and molar bands;
- difficulty in ensuring there are no voids beneath the acrylic splint in the bonded version, which could lead to caries;
- removal of the adhesive at the end of treatment using the bonded version can be difficult; and
- potential long-term damage to the temporomandibular joint.

Since its reintroduction many variations of the Herbst appliance have been described in the orthodontic literature, including: a removable Herbst,[67-69] a maxillary banded or bonded appliance with a removable mandibular appliance,[70,71] or with the active part of the Herbst, namely the piston and tube, attached directly to upper and lower fixed appliances.[72] Whatever the final design, like all functional appliances the majority of the occlusal changes seen with the Herbst appliance are dentoalveolar and any skeletal changes that may be affected by the use of the appliance are usually lost in the post-treatment period.[73] The major determinant of post-treatment stability is thought to be occlusal interdigitation, and so the use of the Herbst has not been recommended for use in the mixed dentition.

4.6   FUNCTIONAL APPLIANCE CORRECTION OF CLASS II INCISOR RELATIONSHIPS

Functional appliances are most commonly used in the treatment of Class II division 1 incisor relationships on moderate to severe Class II skeletal bases. Cases on Class I or mild skeletal II bases are often more appropriately treated with removable or fixed appliances. Class II division 2 cases are also sometimes treated using functional appliances.

4.6.1   Class II division 1 incisor relationships

The classic Class II division 1 case that used to be treated with a functional appliance had the following features:
- well-aligned arches;
- spaced arches, particularly in the lower labial segment;
- upper molars that were not distally angulated;
- a molar relationship of half a unit Class II or less;
- a Class I or only mild Class II skeletal relationship.

Following functional appliance treatment such cases would not require fixed appliances to improve tooth position due to the initially well-aligned arches. The arch spacing would facilitate overjet reduction and at the same time permit the lower buccal segment teeth to erupt mesially within the functional appliance. In this way the molar relationship could be corrected and the lower incisors would not become crowded. At the same time, the fact that the upper molars were not distally angulated meant that the distalizing effect of the functional appliance on the upper buccal segment teeth would not lead to excessively tipped molars. A Class I or mild Class II skeletal pattern was considered acceptable because the functional appliance was only thought to have dentoalveolar effects. Indeed, the case scenario described above could probably just as easily be treated with an upper removable appliance to reduce the overbite and eventually reduce the overjet.

Today, functional appliances are also used in the treatment of Class II division 1 incisor relationships with crowded arches and where the skeletal pattern is a moderate to severe Class II. In the case of crowded arches the crowding is often initially ignored and the aims of the treatment are to reduce the overjet and overbite, thereby creating a Class I incisor relationship. At the same time, the molar relationship is hopefully corrected to Class I. At the end of this initial phase of treatment the case can then be treated as a Class I incisor relationship with crowding. A second phase of treatment can then be carried out using fixed appliances. When planning this second fixed appliance phase, one of the following options may also need to be considered:

• *Anchorage reinforcement*—If no additional space is required to treat the case, it is common to reinforce the anchorage in the upper arch during the fixed appliance phase. This can be in the form of a transpalatal arch or headgear to the first molar bands.

• *Distal movement of the upper buccal segment teeth*—If no space is required in the lower arch and the upper arch is only mildly crowded (i.e. less than half a tooth unit of space is required in each upper quadrant), then headgear will be required to distalize the upper buccal segment teeth (extraoral traction). Once this space has been created, it will be necessary to continue the headgear wear, with reduced hours and force levels in order to reinforce the anchorage (extraoral anchorage).

• *Extractions*—If space is required in both arches, then upper and lower arch extractions are often required. If the crowding is confined to the upper arch and is greater than half a unit in each upper arch quadrant, only upper arch extractions may be performed.

• *Extractions and anchorage reinforcement*—Anchorage reinforcement plus extractions will be required where the removal of upper first premolars will only just provide sufficient space to treat the case in this second fixed appliance phase.

• *Distal movement of the upper buccal segments and extractions*—If more than a unit of space is required in the upper arch it may be necessary to distalize the upper buccal segments in addition to upper first premolar extractions.

Management of the transition from the initial functional appliance phase to the second fixed appliance can be particularly difficult. A lateral cephalogram should be taken prior to commencing functional appliance therapy and also at the end of the functional phase. This will help in the assessment of the results of the treatment so far and the tooth movements required during the fixed appliance phase. It is for this reason that functional appliance therapy, particularly when followed by fixed appliance treatment, is best performed by a specialist in orthodontics.

4.6.2   Class II division 2 incisor relationships

Just as a Class II division 1 incisor relationship on a Class I or mild Class II skeletal base is more appropriately treated with removable or fixed appliances, rather than functional appliances, so too is a Class II division 2 incisor relationship on the same skeletal bases. However, functional appliances are also used to treat the latter on moderate to severe Class II skeletal bases. In this case the Class II division 2 incisor relationship must first be converted to a Class II division I. This can be done using an upper removable appliance, an upper fixed appliance, or a combination of the two (Fig. 4.25). Once converted to a Class II division 1 incisor relationship, the functional appliance treatment can begin, followed as necessary by a second fixed appliance phase. With a functional appliance such as the Clark twin block it is possible to perform the conversion of a Class II division 2 to a Class II division 1 incisor relationship at the same time as the functional appliance treatment is carried out (Fig. 4.26). As with Class II division 1 cases, the crowding can be dealt with following the functional appliance phase, and during the second fixed appliance phase.

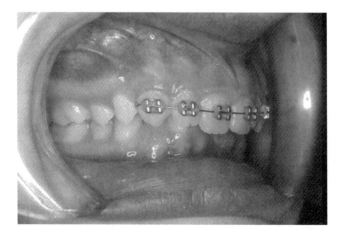

Fig. 4.25 A Class II division 2 incisor relationship converted to a Class II division 1 using a sectional fixed appliance prior to the use of a functional appliance.

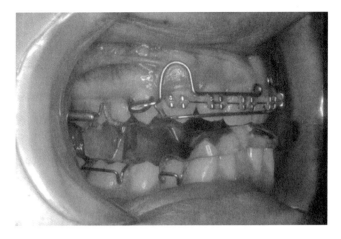

Fig. 4.26 A sectional fixed appliance and twin-block functional appliance being used simultaneously.

4.7 FUNCTIONAL APPLIANCE CORRECTION OF CLASS III INCISOR RELATIONSHIPS

Functional appliances have been used for the treatment of Class III incisor relationships with varying degrees of success. Examples of the appliances used are the Fränkel FR-III (Fig. 4.27) and the Class III twin block. The changes they affect are once again largely dentoalveolar, causing mainly retroclination of the lower incisors and somewhat less proclination of the upper incisors.[74] A concurrent downward and backward rotation of the mandible can also help to produce a positive overjet (Fig. 4.28), although an unwanted effect of this is the associated overbite reduction.[75] A positive

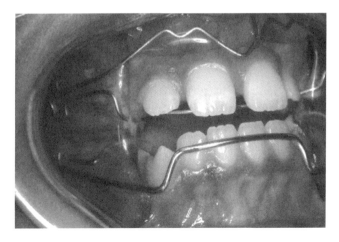

Fig. 4.27 A Fränkel FR-III appliance.

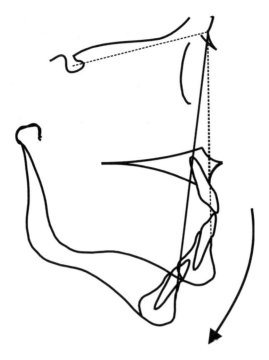

Fig. 4.28 The downwards and backwards rotation of the mandible as a result of the functional appliance in a Class III incisor relationship can result in an increased overjet, but often at the detriment of a reduced overbite.

overbite is required to maintain the acquired positive overjet at the end of treatment.

Just as dentoalveolar changes are the most significant effect seen with functional appliances in the anteroposterior direction, they are also the most significant in the transverse direction. Crossbite correction in Class III cases treated with functional appliances occurs principally as a result of tipping of the buccal segment teeth, rather than by any additional growth of the maxilla.[76]

In recent years there has been renewed interest in the treatment of Class III incisor relationships on Class III skeletal bases by orthodontic means, but not with functional appliances. Instead, the interest has been in the use of reverse pull (protraction) headgear in combination with upper arch expansion appliances. This will be discussed further in Chapter 5.

4.8   MANAGEMENT OF FUNCTIONAL APPLIANCES

The management of the stages in functional appliance therapy will now be dealt with.

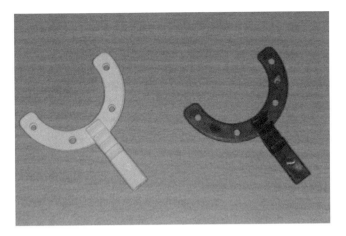

Fig. 4.29 Plastic bite-registration forks.

4.8.1   Records and bite registration

At the start of functional appliance therapy it is important to have initial records of the patient, namely details from the clinical examination, study models, and radiographs, including a lateral cephalogram with the teeth in centric occlusion. In order to construct the appliance it is necessary to take impressions for working models and a bite registration. For Class II functional appliances the bite is taken with the patient's mandible postured anteriorly. There are no hard and fast rules as to the degree of posture, but generally if the overjet is 7–8 mm it may be possible to take the bite registration with the patient postured in an edge-to-edge incisor relationship. When the overjet is greater than this, the patient can be asked to posture anteriorly as far as is comfortably possible. In addition to posturing anteriorly, the bite is usually taken with the patient's mouth open by approximately 4–5 mm in the first premolar region. The exact degree of opening may vary according to the type of functional appliance being made. The construction bite is usually made of wax, and taking it can be aided by the use of a plastic bite-registration fork (Fig. 4.29). Once the bite registration has been taken, the working models can be mounted on a planeline articulator and the appliance constructed (Fig. 4.30). For Class III functional appliances it is very difficult to get the patient to posture the mandible backwards, but the bite registration needs to be taken in centric relation and once again with the bite open.

4.8.2   Fitting the appliance

Functional appliances are quite bulky and it is best to ask the patient to get used to wearing them over a period, rather than expecting perhaps full-time wear from the beginning. A common regimen is to wear the appliance in

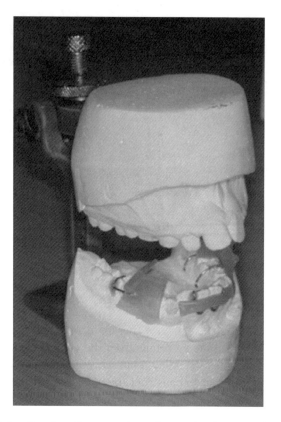

Fig. 4.30 A functional appliance constructed on a planeline articulator.

the evening and at night to begin with, before finally moving on to full-time wear, perhaps 1–2 weeks later. Patients should also be told:

- exactly how many hours per day they are eventually expected to wear the appliance. With some appliances this may only be evenings and nights, e.g. the Andresen, whilst with others it will be full time, e.g. the Clark twin block.

- how their speech will be different to begin with. They should be told to concentrate on speaking with their teeth biting into the appliance and that their speech will return to normal within a few days.

- that they may experience some degree of toothache to begin with, but that it will pass in 3–5 days.

- that if they play contact sports they should remove the appliance and wear a mouthguard. When not in the patient's mouth, the functional appliance should be placed in a tough plastic box for safekeeping.

- similarly, that if they take the appliance out for eating it should be placed in the plastic box.

- they should remove the appliance when they brush their teeth. The appliance should be cleaned with a toothbrush and toothpaste.

Obviously in the case of fixed functional appliances such as the Herbst appliance, the instructions and advice to the patient will vary from the above.

4.8.3   Monitoring treatment progress

After fitting the appliance, it is common to review progress in a couple of weeks to check that it is being worn and is comfortable. Sometimes the acrylic, particularly on the lingual of the lower appliance, causes soreness or ulceration and needs to be adjusted. After this check appointment the patient is then reviewed every 6–8 weeks. At each review appointment:

- Check that the appliance is in the mouth.
- Listen to the patient's speech. Is it normal? If it isn't, then they are unlikely to be wearing the appliance very much.
- Look at the appliance out of the mouth. Is it looking a little grubby? Intraorally is there a little gingival inflammation where the appliance is in contact with the tissues? If the answer to these questions is 'Yes', then the patient is wearing the appliance.
- Finally, with the appliance out of the mouth, ask the patient to relax so that you can gently guide the mandible back into centric relation. Now measure the overjet with the mandible in this position, with the teeth in occlusion. This overjet measurement is the definitive answer as to whether the treatment is working, and should be recorded in the patient's notes at each visit. It is usual for the overjet to reduce by approximately 1 mm/month, although it is not uncommon to see a reduction of 2 mm/month; the maxillary and mandibular dentition are being moved simultaneously. Sometimes the reduction is greater than this in the early stages of treatment. If it is less than this it is possible the patient is not wearing the appliance as instructed. If the patient has been wearing the appliance for a few months and overjet reduction has been satisfactory and then appears to slow down, either the patient is no longer wearing the appliance as instructed, or the appliance needs reactivating.
- In addition to the overjet measurement, the maximum forward postured position or maximum reverse overjet that the patient can achieve can also be measured. It has been found that the difference between the overjet in centric relation and maximum protrusion will often remain the same throughout treatment, even though the overjet is reducing. If it is found that the overjet is reducing rapidly, but maximum protrusion is not increasing as rapidly, then the patient is probably posturing when the initial overjet, in what is thought to be centric relation, is being measured. In which case a further attempt should be made to get the patient to relax, so that the mandible can be gently guided back into centric relation and the overjet correctly recorded.[77]

Monitoring treatment progress is not always easy to do, and failure to notice that the appliance is not being worn can lead to protracted and slow

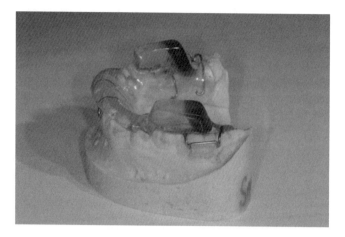

Fig. 4.31 A twin block can easily be advanced by the addition of cold-cure acrylic to the lower or upper blocks.

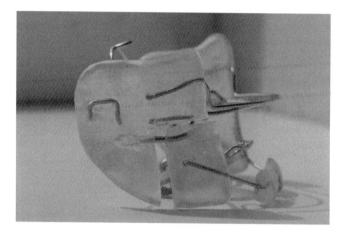

Fig. 4.32 A Fränkel FR-II appliance is advanced by moving the lower wirework mesially within the labial acrylic shields.

treatment progress. Indeed, a failure to progress at all can be as high as 34% of cases.[78]

4.8.4 Functional appliance reactivation

In the case of Class II functional appliances that need reactivation, the aim is to have the appliance make the patient posture the mandible further anteriorly. Some functional appliances lend themselves to a relatively straightforward reactivation or advancement, whilst with others the only real method of reactivation is to remake the appliance. In the case of the Clark twin block, reactivation is easily achieved by the addition of cold-cure acrylic to the distal of the lower block (Fig. 4.31). If a 3-mm further advancement of the mandible is required then 3 mm is added to each lower block. With the Fränkel FR-II, reactivation is accomplished by removing the acrylic around the lower wirework where it enters the buccal shields. This wirework is then advanced by the desired amount, before cold-cure acrylic is used to reaffix it into place. Once again the degree of activation is easily visualized (Fig. 4.32). The Herbst appliance is also easily advanced by unscrewing the piston, sliding an additional piece of steel tubing on to it and then screwing it back into position once more. Appliances such as the bionator and Harvold are not so easily advanced and usually have to be remade in the more anterior position.

Generally advancement should be considered every 2–3 months. It is better for patient compliance to underactivate the appliance when it is initially fitted, allow them to adapt, and then to reactivate the appliance a few months later.

4.8.5   Management following active functional appliance treatment

Once the overjet has been corrected, usually down to 0–2 mm in Class II cases and to a positive overjet in Class III cases, further records should be taken, namely study models and a new lateral cephalogram. The latter will help determine the treatment changes that have taken place and aid subsequent treatment planning. There are two possible treatment options from this point onwards:

1. If the arches are well aligned and the patient is satisfied with their occlusion, the functional appliance can be worn as a retainer and the patient may go on to nights'-only wear. In the case of the Clark twin block it is usual to see lateral open bites at the completion of the active phase of treatment (see Fig. 4.19). Part-time wear of the appliance will allow these open bites to close, usually over a period of 3–6 months. Subsequent to this in the growing patient, the amount of wear can be reduced further, perhaps over a period of 1–2 years. There is, as yet, no real evidence as to the best retention regimen.

2. If the overjet has been corrected but the teeth are still malaligned, then further treatment may involve the use of fixed appliances, sometimes supplemented by the use of headgear and/or extractions. The need for headgear and or extractions will depend not only the degree of crowding, but also the tooth movements that have taken place during the first, functional appliance, phase of treatment. As discussed earlier, a common and often unwanted side-effect of treatment in Class II cases is lower incisor proclination. This may be evident clinically as well as on the lateral cephalogram. If pronounced, it may be necessary to perform lower arch extractions in order to retrocline the lower incisors towards their pretreatment position. This will obviously lead to an increase in the overjet and therefore necessitate upper arch extractions, possibly with

headgear being required to reinforce the anchorage. It can be seen that the transition from functional appliances to fixed appliances can be difficult to manage and is therefore more appropriately treated by a specialist in orthodontics.

4.9   SUMMARY

1. Growth of the face
2. Growth rotations—mandible, maxilla, and relevance of these growth rotations to the orthodontist
3. Mode of action of functional appliances:
   - *skeletal effects*:
     (a) additional overall growth of the mandible;
     (b) accelerated growth of the mandible, but not necessarily addition-al growth;
     (c) a change in the direction of growth of the mandible;
     (d) a change in the position of the mandibular condyle and glenoid fossa;
     (e) restricted growth of the maxilla.
   - *dentoalveolar change*:
     (a) retraction of the upper incisors (palatal tipping);
     (b) proclination of the lower incisors;
     (c) overbite reduction;
     (d) mesial movement of the lower buccal segment teeth;
     (e) distal movement of the upper buccal segment teeth;
     (f) expansion of the upper arch.
   - *soft tissue change*
4. Timing of treatment using functional appliances
5. Classification of functional appliances:
   - component parts
   - tooth-borne or tissue-borne
   - malocclusion (Class II or Class III)
   - soft tissue stretch (myotonic or myodynamic)
6. Examples of functional appliances:
   - Clark twin block
   - bionator
   - medium opening activator
   - Fränkel regulator FR-II
   - Harvold
   - Herbst
7. Functional appliance correction of Class II incisor relationships
8. Functional appliance correction of Class III incisor relationships
9. Management of functional appliances:
   - records and bite registration

- fitting the appliance
- monitoring treatment progress
- functional appliance reactivation
- management following active functional appliance treatment

4.10 OBJECTIVES

1. Describe the sites of importance in facial growth.
2. What is meant by a 'growth rotation' and what is their relevance to the orthodontist?
3. What are the modes of action of functional appliances?
4. What malocclusions can functional appliances be used to treat and what is the best timing of this treatment?
5. How can functional appliances be classified?
6. List some functional appliances. How can each be classified?
7. Describe the management of functional appliance treatment.

REFERENCES

1. Scott, J. H. and Symons, N. B. B. (1977). *Introduction to dental anatomy.* Churchill Livingstone. London.
2. Scammon, R. E. (1930). The measurement of the body in childhood. In *The measurement of man* (ed. J. A. Harris, C. M. Jackson, D. G. Paterson, and R. E. Scammon). University of Minnesota Press.
3. Charlier, J. P., Petrovic, A., and Herrmann-Stutzmann, J. (1969). Effects of mandibular hyperpropulsion on the prechondroblastic zone of young rat condyle. *American Journal of Orthodontics,* **55**, 71–4.
4. McNamara, J. A. Jr and Carlson, D. (1979). Quantitative analysis of temporomandibular joint adaptations to protrusive function. *American Journal of Orthodontics,* **76**, 593–611.
5. Stockli, P. W. and Willert, H. G. (1971). Tissue reactions in the temporomandibular joint resulting from anterior displacement of the mandible in the monkey. *American Journal of Orthodontics,* **60**, 142–55.
6. Hinton, R. J. and McNamara, J. A. Jr. (1984). Temporal bone adaptations in response to protrusive function in juvenile and young adult rhesus monkeys (*Macaca mulatta*). *European Journal of Orthodontics,* **6**, 155–74.
7. Tanner, J. M., Whitehouse, R. H., Marubini, E., and Resele, L. F. (1976). The adolescent growth spurt of boys and girls of the Harpenden growth study. *Annals of Human Biology,* **3**, 109–26.
8. Melsen, B. (1972). Time and mode of closure of the spheno-occipital synchrondrosis determined on human autopsy material. *Acta Anatomica (Basel),* **83**, 112–18.
9. Björk, A. (1969). Prediction of mandibular growth rotation. *American Journal of Orthodontics,* **55**, 585–99.
10. Melsen, B. (1972). A histological study of the influence of sutural morphology and skeletal maturation on rapid palatal expansion in children. *Transactions of the European Orthodontic Society,* **??**, 499–507.
11. Björk, A. (1955). Facial growth in man studied with the aid of metallic implants. *Acta Odontologica Scandinavica,* **13**, 9–34.

12. Björk, A. (1963). Variations in the growth pattern of the human mandible: longitudinal radiographic study by the implant method. *Journal of Dental Research*, **42**, 400–11.

13. Solow, B. and Houston, W. J. B. (1988). Mandibular rotations: concepts and terminology. *European Journal of Orthodontics*, **10**, 177–9.

14. Björk, A. and Skieller, V. (1977). Growth of the maxilla in three dimensions as revealed radiographically by the implant method. *British Journal of Orthodontics*, **4**, 53–64.

15. Björk, A. and Skieller, V. (1983). Normal and abnormal growth of the mandible. A synthesis of longitudinal cephalometric implant studies over a period of 25 years. *European Journal of Orthodontics*, **5**, 1–46.

16. McNamara, J. A. Jr and Bryan, F. A. (1987). Long-term mandibular adaptations to protrusive function: an experimental study in *Macaca mulatta*. *American Journal of Orthodontics and Dentofacial Orthopedics*, **92**, 98–108.

17. Luder, H. U. (1981). Effects of activator treatment—evidence for the occurrence of two different types of reaction. *European Journal of Orthodontics*, **3**, 205–22.

18. Tulloch, J. F, Phillips, C., Koch, G., and Proffit, W. R. (1997). The effect of early intervention on skeletal pattern in Class II malocclusion: a randomized clinical trial. *American Journal of Orthodontics and Dentofacial Orthopedics*, **111**, 391–400.

19. Keeling, S. D., Wheeler, T. T., King, G. J., Garvan, C. W., Cohen, D. A., Cabassa, S., McGorray, S. P., and Taylor, M. G. (1998). Anteroposterior skeletal and dental changes after early Class II treatment with bionators and headgear. *American Journal of Orthodontics and Dentofacial Orthopedics*, **113**, 40–50.

20. Illing, H. M., Morris, D. O., and Lee, R. T. (1998). A prospective evaluation of Bass, Bionator and Twin Block appliances. Part I—The hard tissues. *European Journal of Orthodontics*, **20**, 501–16.

21. DeVincenzo, J. P. (1991). Changes in mandibular length before, during, and after successful orthopedic correction of Class II malocclusions, using a functional appliance. *American Journal of Orthodontics and Dentofacial Orthopedics*, **99**, 241–57.

22. Pancherz, H. and Fackel, U. (1990). The skeletofacial growth pattern pre- and post-dentofacial orthopaedics. A long-term study of Class II malocclusions treated with the Herbst appliance. *European Journal of Orthodontics*, **12**, 209–18.

23. Johnston, L. E. Jr. (1996). Functional appliances: a mortgage on mandibular position. *Australian Orthodontic Journal*, **14**, 154–7.

24. Perillo, L., Johnston, L. E. Jr., and Ferro, A. (1996). Permanence of skeletal changes after function regulator (FR-2) treatment of patients with retrusive Class II malocclusions. *American Journal of Orthodontics and Dentofacial Orthopedics*, **109**, 132–9.

25. Mills, C. M. and McCulloch, K. J. (2000). Posttreatment changes after successful correction of Class II malocclusions with the Twin Block appliance. *American Journal of Orthodontics and Dentofacial Orthopedics*, **118**, 24–33.

26. Woodside, D. G. and Linder-Aronson, S. (1979). The channelization of upper and lower anterior face heights compared to population standard in males between ages 6 and 20 years. *European Journal of Orthodontics*, **1**, 25–40.

27. Woodside, D. G. and Linder-Aronson, S. (1986). Progressive increase in lower anterior face height and the use of posterior occlusal bite block in its management. In *Orthodontics: state of the art, essence of the science* (ed. L. W. Graber), pp. 200–21. CV Mosby, St Louis.

28. Linder-Aronson, S., Woodside, D. G., and Lundstrom, A. (1986). Mandibular growth direction following adenoidectomy. *American Journal of Orthodontics*, **89**, 273–84.

29. Pearson, L. E. (1973). Vertical control through use of mandibular posterior intrusive forces. *Angle Orthodontist*, **43**, 194–200.

30. Pearson, L. E. (1978). Vertical control in treatment of patients having backward rational growth tendencies. *Angle Orthodontist*, **48**, 132–40.
31. Fränkel, R. and Fränkel, C. (1983). A functional approach to treatment of skeletal open bite. *American Journal of Orthodontics*, **84**, 54–68.
32. Williams, S. and Melson, B. (1982). Condylar development and mandibular rotation and displacement during activator treatment: an implant study. *American Journal of Orthodontics*, **81**, 322–6.
33. Birkebaek, L., Melsen, B. and Terp, S. (1984). A laminagraphic study of the alterations in the temporomandibular joint following activator treatment. *European Journal of Orthodontics*, **6**, 267–76.
34. Petrovic, A. (1974). Control of postnatal growth of secondary cartilages of the mandible by mechanisms regulating occlusion: cybernetic model. *Transactions of the European Orthodontic Society*, **50**, 69–75.
35. Woodside, D. G., Metaxas, A., and Altuna, G. (1987). The influence of functional appliance therapy on glenoid fossa remodeling. *American Journal of Orthodontics and Dentofacial Orthopedics*, **92**, 181–98.
36. Ruf, S. and Pancherz, H. (1998). Temporomandibular joint growth adaptation in Herbst treatment: a prospective magnetic resonance imaging and cephalometric roentgenographic study. *European Journal of Orthodontics*, **20**, 375–88.
37. Chintakanon, K., Sampson, W., Wilkinson, T., and Townsend, G. (2000). A prospective study of Twin-block appliance therapy assessed by magnetic resonance imaging. *American Journal of Orthodontics and Dentofacial Orthopedics*, **118**, 494–504.
38. Croft, R. S., Buschang, P. H., English, J. D., and Meyer, R. (1999). A cephalometric and tomographic evaluation of Herbst treatment in the mixed dentition. *American Journal of Orthodontics and Dentofacial Orthopedics*, **116**, 435–43.
39. Jakobsson, S. O. (1967). Cephalometric evaluation of treatment effect on Class 11, Division 1 malocclusions. *American Journal of Orthodontics*, **53**, 446–57.
40. Harvold, E. P. and Vargervik, K. (1970). Morphogenic response to activator treatment. *American Journal of Orthodontics*, **60**, 478–90.
41. DeVincenzo, J. P., Huffer, R. A., and Winn, M. W. (1987). A study in human subjects using a new device designed to mimic the protrusive functional appliances used previously in monkeys. *American Journal of Orthodontics*, **91**, 213–24.
42. Lund, D. I. (1998). The effects of twin blocks: a prospective controlled study. *American Journal of Orthodontics and Dentofacial Orthopedics*, **113**, 104–10.
43. Mills, C. M. and McCulloch, K. J. (1998). Treatment effects of the twin block appliance: a cephalometric study. *American Journal of Orthodontics and Dentofacial Orthopedics*, **114**, 15–24.
44. Pancherz, H. (1984). A cephalometric analysis of skeletal and dental changes contributing to Class II correction in activator treatment. *American Journal of Orthodontics*, **85**, 125–34.
45. Harradine, N. W. T. and Gale, D. (2000). The effects of torque control spurs in twin-block appliances. *Clinical Orthodontics and Research*, **3**, 202–9.
46. Clark, W. J. (1988). The twin block technique: a functional orthopedic appliance system. *American Journal of Orthodontics and Dentofacial Orthopedics*, **93**, 1–18.
47. Fränkel, R. (1969). The treatment of Class II, division 1 malocclusion with functional correctors. *American Journal of Orthodontics*, **55**, 265–75.
48. Fränkel, R. (1980). A functional approach to orofacial orthopaedics. *British Journal of Orthodontics*, **7**, 41–51.
49. Moss, M. L. and Salentijn, L. (1969). The primary role of the functional matrices in facial growth. *American Journal of Orthodontics*, **55**, 566–77.

50. Chadwick, S. M., Aird, J. C., Taylor, P. J. S., and Bearn, D. R. (2001). Functional regulator treatment of Class II division 1 malocclusions. *European Journal of Orthodontics*, **23**, 495–505.

51. Tulloch, J. F. C., Phillips, C., and Proffit, W. R. (1998). Benefit of early Class II treatment: progress report of a two-phase randomized clinical trial. *American Journal of Orthodontics and Dentofacial Orthopedics*, **113**, 62–72.

52. Ghafari, J. G., Shofer, F. S., Laster, L. L., Markowitz, D. L., Silverton, S., and Katz, S. H. (1995). Monitoring growth during orthodontic treatment. *Seminars in Orthodontics*, **1**, 165–75.

53. Livieratos, F. A. and Johnston, L. E. (1995). A comparison of one-stage and two-stage non-extraction alternatives in matched Class II samples. *American Journal of Orthodontics and Dentofacial Orthopedics*, **108**, 118–31.

54. McNamara, J. A. (1984). Dentofacial adaptations in adult patients following functional regulator therapy. *American Journal of Orthodontics*, **85**, 57–71.

55. Vig, P. S. and Vig, K. W. L. (1986). Hybrid appliances: a component approach to dentofacial orthopedics. *American Journal of Orthodontics and Dentofacial Orthopedics*, **90**, 273–85.

56. Graber, T. M. and Neumann, B. (1984). *Removable orthodontic appliances* (2nd edn). W. B. Saunders, Philadelphia.

57. Clark, W. J. (1982). The twin block traction technique. *European Journal of Orthodontics*, **4**, 129–38.

58. McNamara, J. A. Jr and Huge, S. A. (1981). The Fränkel appliance (FR-2): model preparation and appliance construction. *American Journal of Orthodontics*, **80**, 478–95.

59. Kalogirou, K., Ahlgren, J., and Klinge, B. (1996). Effects of buccal shields on the maxillary dentoalveolar structures and the midpalatal suture—histologic and biometric studies in rabbits. *American Journal of Orthodontics and Dentofacial Orthopedics*, **109**, 521–30.

60. O'Donnell, S., Nanda, R. S., and Ghosh, J. (1998). Perioral forces and dental changes resulting from mandibular lip bumper treatment. *American Journal of Orthodontics and Dentofacial Orthopedics*, **113**, 247–55.

61. Harvold, E. P. and Vargervik, K. (1971). Morphogenetic response to activator treatment. *American Journal of Orthodontics*, **63**, 478–90.

62. Harvold, E. P. and Vargervik, K. (1985). Response to activator treatment in Class II malocclusions. *American Journal of Orthodontics and Dentofacial Orthopedics*, **88**, 242–51.

63. Herbst, E. (1934). Dreissigjährige Erfahrungen mit dem Retentions—Scharnier. *Zahnärztliche Rundschau*, **43**, 1515–24, 1563–8, 1611–16.

64. Pancherz, H. (1979). Treatment of Class II malocclusions by jumping the bite with the Herbst appliance: a cephalometric investigation. *American Journal of Orthodontics*, **76**, 423–41.

65. Pancherz, H. (1981). The effect of continuous bite jumping on the dentofacial complex: a follow-up study after Herbst appliance treatment of Class II malocclusions. *European Journal of Orthodontics*, **3**, 49–60.

66. Pancherz, H. (1985). The Herbst appliance. *American Journal of Orthodontics*, **87**, 1–20.

67. McNamara, J. A. (1988). Fabrication of the acrylic-splint Herbst appliance. *American Journal of Orthodontics and Dentofacial Orthopedics*, **94**, 10–18.

68. McNamara, J. A. and Howe, R. P. (1988). Clinical management of the acrylic-splint Herbst appliance. *American Journal of Orthodontics and Dentofacial Orthopedics*, **94**, 142–9.

69. Howe, R. P. (1984). The acrylic-splint Herbst, problem solving. *Journal of Clinical Orthodontics*, **18**, 497–501.

70. Howe, R. P. (1982). The bonded Herbst appliance. *Journal of Clinical Orthodontics*, **16**, 663–7.

71. Valant, J. R. and Sinclair, P. M. (1989). Treatment effects of the Herbst appliance. *American Journal of Orthodontics and Dentofacial Orthopedics*, **95**, 138–47.

72. Clements, R. M. and Jacobson, A. (1982). The MARS appliance. *American Journal of Orthodontics*, **82**, 445–55.

73. Pancherz, H. (1997). The effects, limitations, and long-term dentofacial adaptations to treatment with the Herbst appliance. *Seminars in Orthodontics*, **3**, 232–43.

74. Kerr, W. J. S., Ten Have, T. R., and McNamara, J. A. Jr. (1989). A comparison of skeletal and dental changes produced by function regulators (FR-2 and FR-3). *European Journal of Orthodontics*, **11**, 235–42.

75. Ülgen, M. and Firatli, S. (1994). The effects of the Fränkel's function regulator on the Class III malocclusion. *American Journal of Orthodontics and Dentofacial Orthopedics*, **105**, 561–7.

76. Ülgen, M. and Firatli, S. (1996). The effects of the FR-3 appliance on the transversal dimension. *American Journal of Orthodontics and Dentofacial Orthopedics*, **110**, 55–60.

77. Petit, H. H. and Chate, M. (1984). The K test and the Condylar test. *Journal of Clinical Orthodontics*, **21**, 384–94.

78. Cohen, A. (1981). A study of class II division 1 malocclusions treated by the Andresen appliance. *British Journal of Orthodontics*, **8**, 159–63.

5   Headgear

CONTENTS

Headgear is a mechanism whereby structures outside the oral cavity are used to apply forces to the teeth. These forces can be classified as:
- extraoral anchorage (EOA)
- extraoral traction (EOT).

With extraoral anchorage, headgear is used to prevent untoward mesial movement of the anchor teeth. Extraoral traction is used to move the teeth. The difference between EOA and EOT is in the number of hours of wear and the force applied (duration and loading).

5.1 COMPONENTS OF HEADGEAR

Headgear consists of four major components:
1. *A head cap, of which there are a number of designs*—They are almost always made of fabric or plastic tape that passes coronally, around the occiput, and sometimes around the nape of the neck. Examples are shown in Figs 5.1, 5.2, and 5.3.
2. *A facebow or whisker that fits into the fixed or removable appliance*—This is made from stainless steel and there is usually an inner whisker that fits into the appliance and an outer whisker that passes outside the mouth (Fig. 5.4).

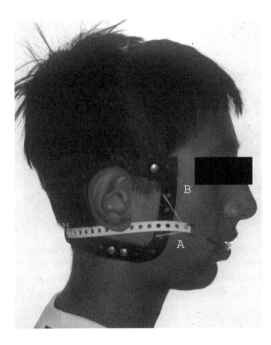

Fig. 5.1 An example of a standard form of headgear; the 'Interlandi' headgear in this case. The headgear can be attached to the straps at various positions to provide either a form of cervical or low pull (A) or a higher occipital pull (B).

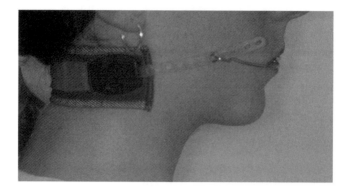

Fig. 5.2 A cervical neck strap used essentially for cases with a low maxillary/ mandibular planes' angle to achieve extrusion and thus help with a deep overbite.

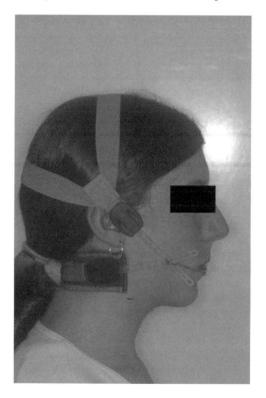

Fig. 5.3 A combination headgear using an occipital cap together with a cervical neck strap. Removing the cervical neck strap can modify the pull, so that an intrusive force is applied to molars as is required in a high maxillary/mandibular planes' angle case where there is a problem achieving any vertical overlap of the incisor teeth.

3. *A means of applying a force between the head cap and facebow*—This can be an elastic or a spring, or indeed part of the head cap may itself be elasticized (Fig. 5.5).

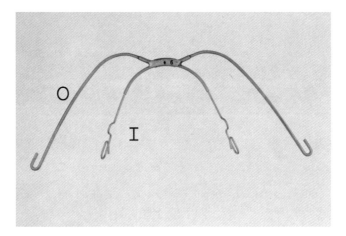

Fig. 5.4 The standard form of a facebow. This can be modified for safety. There is a rigid outer bow (O) usually made of 1.2 mm-diameter stainless steel and a more flexible inner bow (I) of 0.9 mm-diameter stainless steel.

4. *Safety mechanisms*—In recent years concerns have been raised about the use of headgear in orthodontics (see Chapter 9), particularly the risk of traumatic injury to the eyes.[1-3] As a result of which it is recommended that headgear and its facebow comprises at least two safety features.[4] The various safety components available include:
   - a plastic neck strap that prevents the facebow from coming out of the mouth.
   - a snap-away mechanism whereby the facebow easily disengages away from the head cap. Therefore if the facebow is pulled out of the mouth it will not remain attached to the head cap and so will not spring back into the patient's face.
   - modifications to the facebow, which can include turning the ends of the facebow over on themselves so they present a bigger and blunter surface area (Fig. 5.6(a)). An alternative method is to have an inner facebow whisker that locks into position (Fig. 5.6(b)).[3]

5.2 EXTRAORAL ANCHORAGE (EOA)

This is designed to prevent unwanted mesial movement of teeth as a consequence of their reaction to the active components of a fixed or removable appliance. As a general rule, the headgear must be worn 8–10 hours out of every 24 and the force applied is 250 g per side. However, if anchorage is to be preserved, it is important that the clinician has an understanding of the forces acting within the appliance and the headgear. Whether an anchor tooth will move mesially during treatment (loss of anchorage) depends on

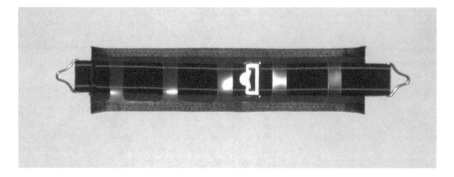

Fig. 5.5 In this case the cervical pull headgear is made of an elasticated material, which applies the force to the facebow.

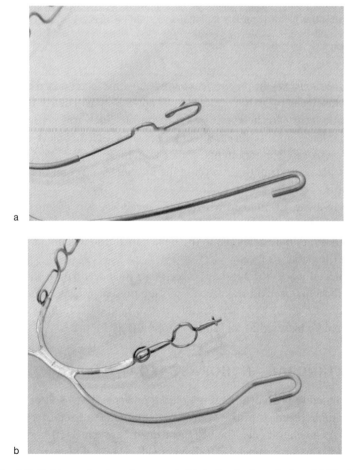

a

b

Fig. 5.6 Safety mechanisms incorporated into the facebow design. (a) The inner facebow has the end of the wire turned over itself. (b) An auxillary wire locks the facebow into place.

the forces acting and the root surface area of the anchor tooth. Generally the force required to move a single-rooted tooth using tipping forces is 25–40 g. To move the same tooth bodily requires a force of approximately 100 g. For multirooted teeth, such as first permanent molars, these forces will therefore be higher. It is because of the biological variation in the total root surface areas of different teeth that only generalizations can be made as to the forces required to move them, and hence the forces required to counteract such movement in the form of extraoral anchorage. Only by considering the root surface areas of the teeth can the forces and tooth movements be understood. Consider, for example, the loss of anchorage that can occur when excessive forces are applied to the teeth being moved. If this force leads to occlusion of the blood vessels on the pressure side of the periodontal ligament, normal surface resorption of the bony socket cannot occur and tooth movement will not occur. The periodontal ligament is said to undergo 'avascular necrosis' under such conditions and is said to look 'glassy' or 'hyaline' under the microscope. This is otherwise known as 'hyalinization'. At a distance from this area of excessive force, somewhere in the surrounding cancellous bone, the blood vessels will not be occluded. Since the force in these tissues will be below capillary blood pressure (approximately 30 mm/Hg), osteoclasts will begin resorbing the bone towards the pressure side of the ligament and eventually, when the periodontal ligament is reached, the tooth will begin to move. This resorption, beginning at some distance from the ligament, is known as 'undermining resorption'. In such instances there is a lag of around 2 weeks before the planned tooth movement begins to occur. Not only does this delay treatment, but during this lag phase the high force is dissipated amongst all the anchor teeth. It is therefore possible that the force acting on each individual anchor tooth is at the optimal level for the anchor tooth/teeth to move (see Chapter 1, Fig. 1.10). The frontal resorption taking place in the case of each anchor tooth will lead to their early unwanted mesial movement with a resultant loss of anchorage. Although extraoral anchorage will help prevent this movement, the clinician should only apply the correct forces to attain the desired tooth movements. However, even when the correct forces are applied, loss of anchorage can also easily occur. A common reason for this is that insufficient teeth are, or can be, utilized for anchorage (i.e. insufficient root surface). In addition, there is the ever-present additional effect of physiological mesial drift.[5]

Headgear used to reinforce anchorage is usually applied to the upper first permanent molars. This can be to tubes on the bands cemented to the first permanent molars in the case of fixed appliances (Fig. 5.7(a)), or to tubes soldered to the Adams' cribs on the upper first permanent molars in the case of removable appliances (Fig. 5.7(b)). The direction of pull of the headgear is just above the level of the occlusal plane for EOA on both fixed and removable appliances. This is because the anchor teeth are to remain stationary.

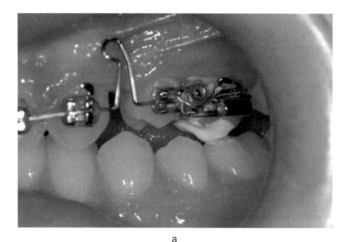

a

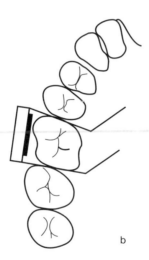

b

Fig. 5.7 The facebows fit either (a) into the tubes on molar bands or (b) into the tubes soldered on to the cribs of removable appliances.

Also anything other than an upward pull will dislodge an upper removable appliance.

5.3   EXTRAORAL TRACTION

Unlike extraoral anchorage the aim with extraoral traction (EOT) is to distalize teeth, usually the upper first permanent molar. In order to achieve this the force is generally 500 g per side and the headgear it is worn for at least

14–16 hours in every 24-hour period. The more hours per day the patient wears the headgear the more quickly the teeth move and treatment progresses. Occasionally, patients are prepared to wear it 24 hours per day, in which case it is possible to move the upper first permanent molars more than half a unit (half a premolar width) in 6–8 weeks. More often than not the opposite is the true, with it being difficult to motivate patients to wear their headgear for a sufficient number of hours to effect tooth movement. To overcome this problem and to monitor wear, timing devices have been developed that fit into the headgear and record the number of hours of wear. However, they are expensive to fit and have their limitations; inventive patients stretch the headgear when it is not being worn so that the recording device indicates more hours of wear than is actually taking place. A simple means of motivating patients, however, is the headgear chart or calendar which when compared with the actual number of hours worn is seldom totally accurate is still associated with an increased number of hours wear.[6]

When using EOT it is essential to consider the design of the headgear with respect to the movement achieved in all three spatial planes, i.e. anteroposterior, vertical, and transverse (Figs 5.8(a–c)). By utilizing the point of application of the headgear and the length of the inner and outer bows it is possible to vary the direction of pull in all three dimensions.[7] By varying the inner bow, it is possible to expand, contract, or maintain the position of the teeth in the transverse dimension (Fig. 5.9); the maxillary dentition has an increase in arch width from the anterior to posterior (see Chapter 6, Fig. 6.51).

An adjunctive appliance is a molar distalizing upper removable appliance, sometimes referred to as a nudger (see Chapter 3), or a bilateral screw appliance, sometimes referred to as a Y-plate. The use of a removable appliance is particularly useful if the molars need to be distalized more on one side of the mouth than on the other. Finally, the use of osseointegrated implants, and possibly onplants, would do away with the need for headgear and the problems of compliance altogether.[8]

Unlike EOA, the direction of the forces applied using EOT can be more variable. This is because it may be desirable to try to intrude or extrude the upper first permanent molars as part of the treatment. The types of movement that can occur, and the manner in which the headgear must be constructed to affect these movements, are related to the centre of resistance of the upper first permanent molar.

5.3.1   Centre of resistance and molar movements

As with all teeth, the application of a load to a tooth will cause the tooth to behave as though there is a centre of resistance.[7,9] The load of EOT applied to the tooth can act in one of several ways:

- *Bodily movement*—Here the tooth is moved along the Curve of Spee and there is no unwanted distal or mesial tipping (Fig. 5.10(a)).

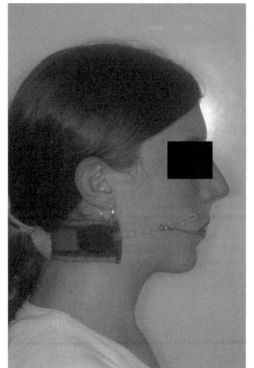

a

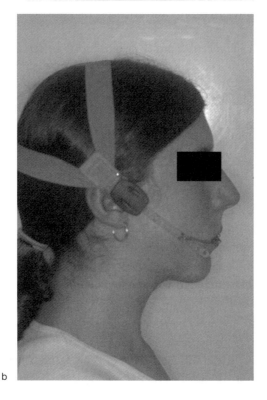

b

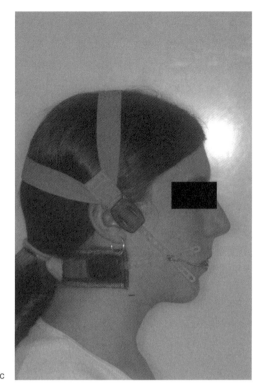

c

Fig. 5.8 Three types of headgear showing how the direction of pull may be adapted to the specific malocclusion. (a) Here the pull is directed in a cervical direction; this is ideal for cases requiring extrusion of the first molars.
(b) A higher occipital pull will intrude the first molars. (c) A combination will control movement along the curve of Spee, having no vertical influence on the molar position.

- *Bodily movement but with extrusion*—This is typical of the type of treatment required for low maxillary/mandibular plane angle cases (Fig. 5.10(b)).
- *Bodily movement but with intrusion*—This is typical of the type of treatment required for high maxillary/mandibular plane angle cases (Fig. 5.10(c)).
- *Distal movement of the crown*—This is typical of the type of treatment required on a maxillary second permanent molar when the tooth has tilted mesially following early loss of first permanent molars.

5.3.2   Headgear to modify growth directions

Having considered the application of headgear to a single tooth, the principle of a centre of resistance can be applied to the developing maxillary dentition. In this instance, headgear, if applied to an appliance with complete incisal and occlusal coverage and directed through the maxillary centre of

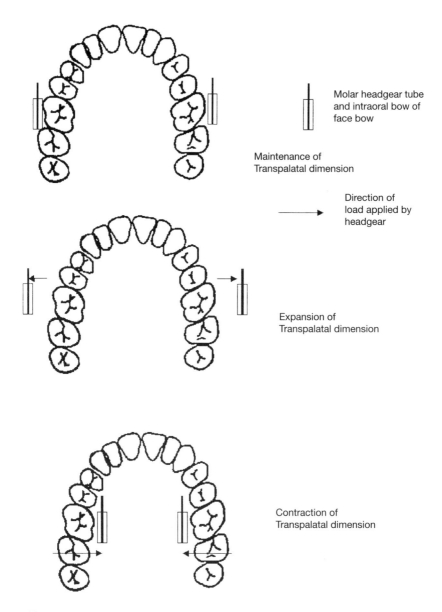

Molar headgear tube
and intraoral bow of
face bow

Maintenance of
Transpalatal dimension

Direction of
load applied by
headgear

Expansion of
Transpalatal dimension

Contraction of
Transpalatal dimension

Fig. 5.9 Adjusting the inner bow of the facebow allows the molars to be expanded, contracted, or maintained in the correct relationship.

resistance, could assist in controlling maxillary excess. This appliance, solely for intrusion, is referred to as an 'intrusion splint'.[10] The classic application of the headgear is between the first and second maxillary premolars and there is a need for a rigid inner bow, which can also be incorporated into other appliances, especially functional ones.[11,12] This type of treatment is identified for those patients with high maxillary mandibular plane angles

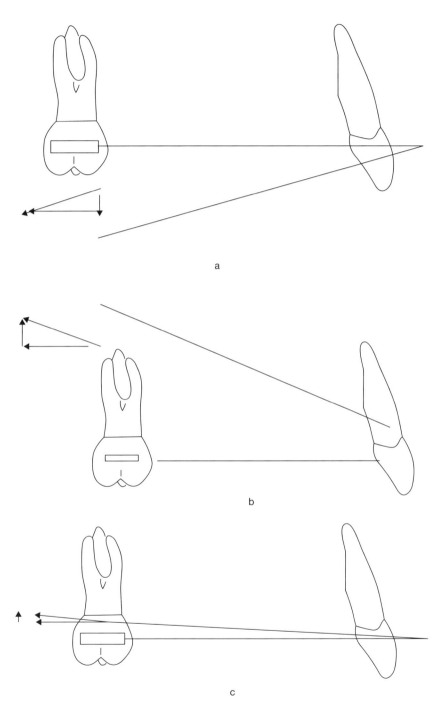

Fig. 5.10 Diagrams to illustrate the interaction of the facebow and the effects on the molar tooth for (a) extrusion, (b) intrusion, (c) no change in position along the curve of Spee.

and a high lip line who show excessive amounts of gingivae on smiling (Chapter 6, Fig. 6.38).

The controversy connected with this treatment is similar to that for functional appliances, and centres around the following questions:

1. Can the loading be applied to such an extent and duration that the whole maxillary dentition can be restrained to a clinically significant level?
2. Would the changes occur irrespective of treatment?
3. Is the headgear holding up the dentition whilst the soft tissues are developing around it?[13]
4. Following treatment does the growth pattern reinstate itself?

5.4   HEADGEAR FOR THE TREATMENT OF CLASS III INCISOR RELATIONSHIPS

The aim of treatment for Class III incisor relationship is to eliminate any anterior displacements of the mandible and to induce a degree of dento-alveolar compensation that will mask the underlying skeletal discrepancy. This implies not only proclination of the upper labial segment but also retroclination of the lower labial segment. This latter tooth movement can be achieved with fixed appliances, round arch mechanics preventing the expression of torque and can be supplemented by.

(1) headgear fitted to the lower arch (Fig. 5.11);
(2) a facemask (Fig. 5.12).

The hours of wear are similar to other headgears, but the forces have to be carefully monitored where they are applied directly to the labial dentition.

5.4.1   Headgear to the lower dentition

This is the Lee laboratory headgear (Fig. 5.11) with J hooks attached mesial to the mandibular canines on an archwire that is capable of supporting headgear forces (usually a 0.018-inch stainless-steel wire in a 0.022-inch bracket slot) but it can also be applied to a removable appliance with equal effect.[14] The intention is to apply a tipping force to the labial segment; there is often too little bone on the lingual aspect of the lower incisors for bodily movement.

5.4.2   Facemasks

These use the forehead and chin/pogonion area as the main attachment regions. Facemasks can be provided in two forms: customized facemasks[15] from impressions of the patient's chin and forehead; and prefabricated facemasks[16] available from several manufacturers (Fig. 5.12). Unlike the headgear to the mandibular dentition, facemasks are attached by elastics either to a removable appliance or to the fixed appliance; usually to the posterior

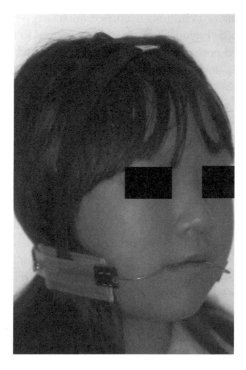

Fig. 5.11 An example of headgear fitted to the lower anterior labial segment to treat a Class III incisor relationship by retroclining the mandibular labial segment.

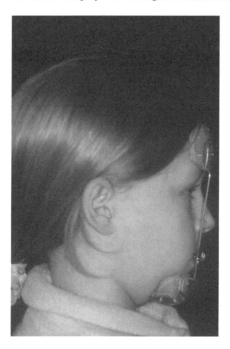

Fig. 5.12 A reverse 'facemask' for applying traction to the maxillary dentition for the correction of Class III malocclusions by proclination of the maxillary labial segment.

aspect of the maxillary dentition. If applied anteriorly, attachment is often to hooks in the canine region. The force is then applied to the extraoral face-mask structure, and pressure from the chin cap, whilst claiming to restrain mandibular growth, acts to retrocline the lower labial segment. There is evidence, similar to that for functional appliances, that the earlier the treatment commences (at about 9 years of age) the greater the effect, although the effect on mandibular growth was minimal.[17] However, the long-term effects appear to be minimal, especially with pre-existing growth patterns.[18]

5.5   SUMMARY OF MALOCCLUSIONS AND HEADGEARS USED

1. *Class I malocclusion EOA*—An Interlandi headgear worn 8–12 hours with an action along the Curve of Spee.
2. *Class II division 1 malocclusion with a normal maxillary/mandibular planes' angle*—EOT to distalize molars to correct the molar relationship to Class I; there should be no intrusive/extrusive vector of movement and the tooth should be moved bodily without tipping.
3. *Class II division 1 malocclusion with a high maxillary/mandibular planes' angle*—There should be a short outer bow with an occipital pull; the tooth should be moved both distally and intruded.
4. *Class II division 2 malocclusion with a low maxillary/mandibular planes' angle*—Such cases should have a cervical pull headgear to extrude the molar and so assist in correction of the overbite. The extrusion of the molar will increase the posterior face height, which is not stable due to the muscular sling of the medial pterygoid and masseter muscle.[19]
5. *Class III malocclusion with a normal maxillary/mandibular planes' angle*—Headgear may consist of either (1) a Lee laboratory straight-pull headgear attached to the lower archwire or (2) a reverse-pull face mask. It is important when using the latter not to extrude the posterior aspect of the maxillary dentition, which could have consequences on the vertical dimension.

It is important to realize that the influence headgear has on dental movements is fairly limited when compared to overall facial form and growth and development. In patients with 'long faces' with high maxillary mandibular plane angles and an increased lower face height, it is best to utilize mechanics that do not worsen this facial pattern. This would mean avoiding any form of vertical extrusion of the molars and would also limit the amount of possible palatal cusp extrusion.

5.6   LOADS APPLIED IN RELATION TO ROOT SURFACE AREA

It has been stated earlier that, by definition, headgear applies higher forces than can be applied by simple removable appliances (see Chapter 3). If headgear is applied to individual teeth it is possible to rapidly exceed the normal loading of the tooth by producing a pathological load. Teeth specifically at risk are those of the upper labial segment: if headgear is fitted to teeth in this segment, with a specific clinical goal, then loading must be reduced.[20]

5.7   SUMMARY

1. Components of headgear:
   - a head cap
   - a facebow or whisker
   - a means of applying force
   - safety mechanisms
2. Extraoral anchorage (EOA)
3. Extraoral traction (EOT):
   - centre of resistance and molar movements
   - headgear to modify growth directions
4. Headgear for the treatment of Class III incisor relationships:
   - headgear to the lower dentition
   - facemasks
5. Summary of malocclusions and headgears used.
6. Loads applied in relation to root surface area.

5.8   OBJECTIVES

1. Identify the two types of headgear applications, i.e. anchorage and traction.
2. Understand the types of tooth movement that can be induced.
3. Know the risks arising from the use of headgear and how to minimize them.

REFERENCES

1. Postlethwaite, K. M. (1990). Safety headgear products. *British Journal of Orthodontics*, **17**, 329–31.
2. Samuels, R. H. A. and Jones, M. L (1994). Orthodontic facebow injuries and safety equipment. *European Journal of Orthodontics*, **16**, 385–94.
3. Samuels, R. H. A. (1996). A review of orthodontic face-bow injuries and safety equipment. *American Journal of Orthodontics and Dentofacial Orthopedics*, **110**, 269–72.
4. British Orthodontic Society (2001). Advice sheet: facebows. BOS, London
5. Picton, D. C. and Moss, J. P. (1973). The part played by the trans-septal fibre system in experimental approximal drift of the cheek teeth of monkeys (*Macaca irus*). *Archives of Oral Biology*, **18**, 669–80.
6. Cureton, S. L., Regenniter, F. J., and Yancey, J. M. (1993). The role of a headgear calendar in headgear compliance. *American Journal of Orthodontics and Dentofacial Orthopedics*, **104**, 387–94.

7. Bowden, D. E. J. (1978). Theoretical considerations of headgear therapy: a literature review. *British Journal of Orthodontics*, **5**, 145–52.
8. Wehrbein, H., Merz, B. R., Diedrich, P., and Glatzmaier, J. (1996). The use of palatal implants for orthodontic anchorage. Design and clinical application of the Orthosystem. *Clinical Oral Implants Research*, **7**, 410–16.
9. Merrifield, L. L. and Cross, J. J. (1970). Directional forces. *American Journal of Orthodontics*, **57**, 435–64.
10. Orton, H. S., Slattery, D. A., and Orton, S. (1992). The treatment of severe 'gummy' Class II division 1 malocclusion using the maxillary intrusion splint. *European Journal of Orthodontics*, **14**, 216–23.
11. Clark, W. J. (1982). The twin block traction technique. *European Journal of Orthodontics*, **4**, 129–38.
12. Teuscher, U. (1986). An appraisal of growth and reaction to extraoral anchorage. Simulation of orthodontic–orthopedic results. *American Journal of Orthodontics*, **89**, 113–21.
13. Moss, J. P. and Picton, D. C. (1968). The problems of dental development among the children on a Greek island. *Dental Practitioner and Dental Record*, **18**, 442–8.
14. Orton, H. S., Sullivan, P. G., Battagel, J. M., and Orton S. (1983). The management of class III and class III tendency occlusions using headgear to the mandibular dentition. *British Journal of Orthodontics*, **10**, 2–12.
15. Battagel, J. M. and Orton, H. S. (1995). A comparative study of the effects of customized facemask therapy or headgear to the lower arch on the developing Class III face. *European Journal of Orthodontics*, **17**, 467–82.
16. Macdonald, K. E., Kapust, A. J., and Turley, P. K. (1999). Cephalometric changes after the correction of class III malocclusion with maxillary expansion/facemask therapy. *American Journal of Orthodontics and Dentofacial Orthopedics*, **116**, 13–24.
17. Yuksel, S., Ucem, T. T., and Keykubat, A. (2001). Early and late facemask therapy. *European Journal of Orthodontics*, **23**, 559–68.
18. Battagel, J. M. and Orton, H. S. (1993). Class III malocclusion: the post-retention findings following a non-extraction treatment approach. *European Journal of Orthodontics*, **15**, 45–55.
19. Bhatia, S. N., Yan, B., Behbehani, I., and Harris, M. (1985). Nature of relapse after surgical mandibular advancement. *British Journal of Orthodontics*, **12**, 58–69.
20. Marx, R. (1976), High pull Begg. *British Journal of Orthodontics*, **3**, 169–73.

6 Fixed appliances

CONTENTS

The principle behind the use of fixed appliances is one of three-dimensional control of tooth movement. The archwire and any auxiliaries, such as elastics and springs, apply forces to the tooth via the orthodontic bracket. It is the interaction of the archwire and the bracket slot which dictates the type of tooth movement that will occur, although other factors (such as the occlusion) will have an effect. Traditionally, the three dimensions of tooth movement are known as first-, second-, and third-order movements:

- *First-order movements* are those in the labiopalatal plane involving the whole or part of the crown of the tooth. Pure labiopalatal movement of the crown has its centre of rotation located at the root centroid (Fig. 6.1) and so can be considered a tipping movement. If the mesial or distal part of the tooth is moved in preference, the tooth will rotate along its long axis rather than tip labially or palatally.
- *Second-order movements* occur along the plane of the long axis of the tooth and include vertical movements of the whole, or part of the tooth. A tooth can therefore be extruded, intruded, or tipped in the mesiodistal direction by intruding/extruding the mesial or distal part in preference (Fig. 6.2).
- *Third-order movements* occur when the root is tipped in the labiopalatal direction in preference to the crown (Fig. 6.3). Here the centre of rotation is positioned within the bracket slot on the crown of the tooth, rather than at the centroid of the root as in first-order movements. Third-order movements are usually referred to as 'torqueing'.

It is the interaction of the archwire and the bracket slot to create these first-, second-, and third-order tooth movements that has led to the development of a number of appliance systems. Whatever the name of the

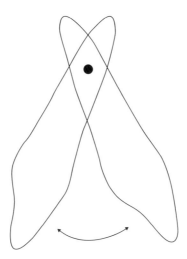

Fig. 6.1 First-order movements are labiolingual or buccolingual movements of the teeth within the dental arch and may involve rotation around the root centroid.

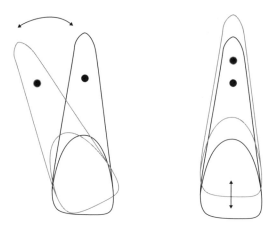

Fig. 6.2 Second-order tooth movements.

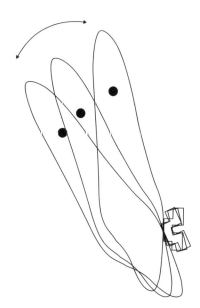

Fig. 6.3 Third-order movement of the root in a labiolingual or buccolingual direction with the centre of rotation at the archwire within the bracket slot.

system, they are based on two basic types: either the Edgewise appliance or the Begg appliance. The difference between these two systems centres on the bracket/archwire interaction. In the Edgewise appliance rectangular wires are used to gain three-dimensional control of the tooth by fitting into a rectangular cross-sectional slot in the face of the bracket (Fig. 6.4). In the Begg appliance, wires which are round in cross-section fit into a mesiodistally narrow, but an occlusogingivally long slot in the bracket (Fig. 6.5). The

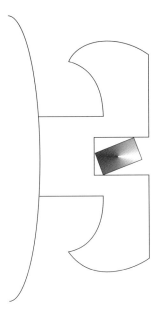

Fig. 6.4 A profile view of a preadjusted Edgewise appliance bracket with an archwire in place. Notice the rectangular cross-section of the archwire slot.

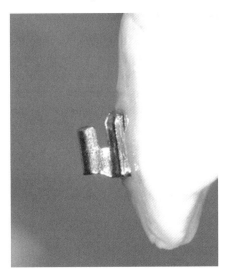

Fig. 6.5 A lateral view of a Begg bracket illustrating the vertical slot for the archwire.

round wires used in such a slot enable the tooth to tip both labiopalatally and mesiodistally. Three-dimensional control with this appliance is gained through the additional use of auxiliary springs (Fig. 6.6) to affect second- and third-order tooth movements.

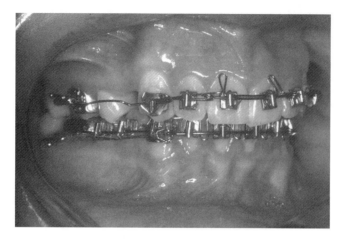

Fig. 6.6 Auxiliary springs on this Begg appliance to move the roots of the upper central incisors palatally on the round base archwire.

6.1 FIXED APPLIANCE COMPONENTS

The basic components of any fixed appliance include the following:
- *Brackets*—These are usually bonded directly to the labial surface of the incisor, canine, and premolar teeth in a predetermined position. It is the bracket design and dimensions which give rise to the numerous bracket systems currently available. These will be discussed later in this chapter.
- *Tubes*—These are either directly bonded to the buccal surface of the molar teeth or are carried on bands that are cemented to the molar teeth. These tubes, which are included in the appliance, carry the ends of the archwire on the most distal molar tooth. Additional tubes on upper molars may be used for fitting headgear.
- *Archwires*—These are available in many forms and can be purchased either on a reel or preformed into an arch shape. The variations in archwire composition and form are covered in detail in Chapter 7.
- *Other components*—These are bonding and banding agents, springs, hooks, metal ligatures, and elastomeric products such as separators, ties, elastic chains, and intraoral elastics.

Currently, most orthodontic treatment carried out with fixed appliances is performed using a modification of the Edgewise system known as the 'pre-adjusted Edgewise appliance' or the 'Straight-wire® appliance'. This system will be described first, not only because of its popularity, but because by understanding how this system works it is easier to appreciate the mode of action of other systems.

6.2   THE PREADJUSTED EDGEWISE OR STRAIGHT-WIRE® APPLIANCE

This was developed from the traditional Edgewise appliance by Andrews[1] from his observations of the study models of 120 patients he classified as non-orthodontic norms. By studying the teeth of normal occlusions he worked out his six keys to normal occlusion (see Chapter 2), he was then able to work backwards from the normal positions of the teeth to develop a bracket that was individualized for each tooth. In this way, an archwire bent only to a simple archform would move malpositioned teeth to their correct positions during treatment. Each tooth therefore has an individual bracket with a prescription for first-, second-, and third-order tooth movements built into it. Most of the previously developed bracket systems had been based on looking at malaligned teeth, and relied on the orthodontist bending wires and utilizing auxiliary wires and springs to move the teeth to their correct position. The brackets were essentially the same for each tooth. It is because the preadjusted system utilizes only a simple archform without additional wire bending that it became known as the Straight-wire® system.

6.2.1   The Straight-wire® bracket—design

The basic design of the Straight-wire® bracket is shown in Fig. 6.7. It consists of a horizontal slot, that is rectangular in cross-section, into which fits the archwire. Occlusally and gingivally to the slot, the bracket extends

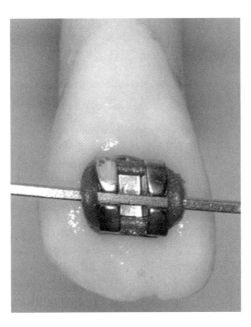

Fig. 6.7 A Straight-wire® bracket with a wire ligated into position.

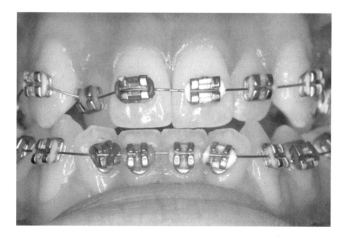

Fig. 6.8 Siamese brackets mean the archwire can be partially ligated into position when teeth are very malaligned.

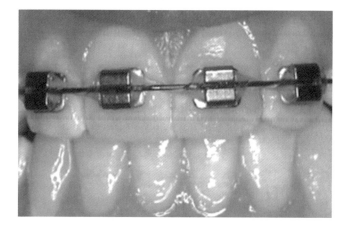

Fig. 6.9 Solid edgewise brackets (only two tie-wings per bracket).

to form the tie-wings, around which steel or elastomeric ligatures can be placed to hold the archwire in the slot during treatment. When there are four tie-wings, separated by the horizontal archwire slot and by a vertical slot, they are known as 'Siamese brackets'. The presence of four tie-wings is useful for very malpositioned teeth, which can be partially ligated to the archwire (Fig. 6.8). The vertical slot makes initial placement of the bracket on to the tooth, along its long axis, relatively straightforward (see Section 6.2.2). The alternative to a Siamese bracket is the solid bracket, but this is much less commonly used today (Fig. 6.9).

Joining the bracket slot and tie-wings to the bracket base is the stem. The stem is narrower occlusogingivally than the tie-wings that curve over it. This provides the necessary undercut for the steel or elastomeric ligatures. Ideally, the stem should also be narrower mesiodistally than the bracket

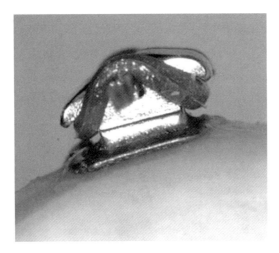

Fig. 6.10 The stem of the bracket is narrower than the base, which ensures the elastomeric module used to hold the archwire in place does not contact the enamel surface.

base, so that the ligatures, particularly elastomeric ligatures, rest against the bracket base and not the adjacent enamel surface (Fig. 6.10). This will minimize the chances of enamel decalcification during treatment.

Positioned between the bracket stem and enamel surface is the bracket base. In most instances, brackets are bonded directly to the enamel surface and the base provides the attachment with the bonding agent. Most bases therefore have some means of providing a mechanical interlock with the bonding agent. The mechanical interlock in the case of metal brackets may be in the form of one or more layers of gauze wire mesh which are welded/soldered to the bracket base (Fig. 6.11). Alternatively, the retentive

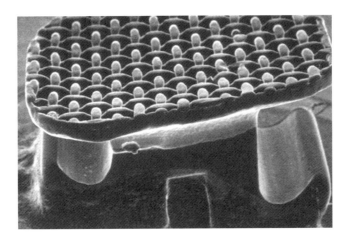

Fig. 6.11 A mesh-based metal bracket.

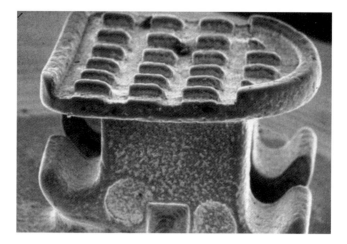

Fig. 6.12 A cast-metal bracket base.

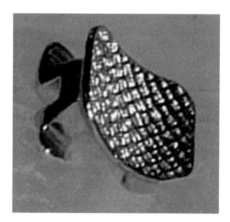

Fig. 6.13 Straight-wire® bracket bases are curved in order to fit the enamel surface accurately. They are known as 'compound contoured bases'.

mechanism can be integrally cast into the bracket base (Fig. 6.12). The mechanisms of bonding and the bracket-base designs of ceramic and plastic brackets, which can vary from those seen on metal brackets, will be dealt with in Chapter 7.

If Straight-wire® brackets, which are designed to facilitate first-, second-, and third-order movements, are to work effectively, not only must they bond to the enamel, but they must accurately fit the tooth surface. The bracket base is therefore curved both occlusogingivally and mesiodistally and is described as being 'compound-contoured' (Fig. 6.13). This ensures a close and accurate fit to the enamel surface of the particular tooth for which the bracket is designed, so that the prescription built into the bracket can be fully and correctly realized during treatment.

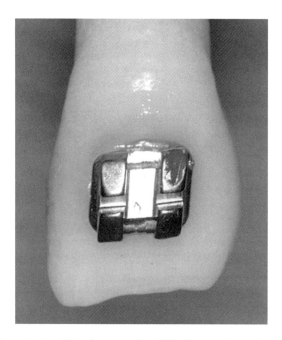

Fig. 6.14 Straight-wire® brackets are identifiable by a mark on the distogingival tie-wing.

Since each tooth in the arch has its own individual bracket, it is import-ant that the operator is able to identify and orientate each bracket. It is com-mon practice among manufacturers to place an identifying mark on the dis-togingival aspect of the face of the bracket. These marks are usually different on upper arch brackets from those on lower arch brackets. For example, the mark on upper brackets may be a dot, whilst those on lower brackets are a dash. Metal brackets usually have this mark cast into the face of the bracket (Fig. 6.14) and when new this is often painted a specific colour to denote the tooth. With practise it becomes relatively easy to tell which bracket is which. Further indications include:

• Incisor brackets have bracket bases that are less curved than canine and premolar brackets.
• Lower incisor brackets all appear the same and sometimes have a chamfered finish to the occlusal tie-wings to reduce occlusal interference with the upper incisor teeth.
• Upper lateral incisor brackets have a greater labiopalatal thickness than upper central incisor brackets.
• Premolar brackets have gingival tie-wings that are set further away from the bracket base to aid tying in the archwire.
• Second premolar brackets can be denoted from first premolar brackets by the mark they also carry on the mesiogingival part of the bracket. This might be a cross cast into the face of metal brackets.

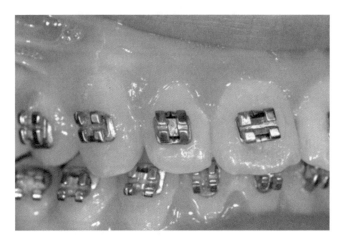

Fig. 6.15 Preadjusted Edgewise brackets demonstrating different degrees of angulation (mesiodistal tip) built into the brackets.

Like the traditional Edgewise bracket system before it, the brackets in the preadjusted Edgewise or Straight-wire® system utilize a rectangular slot into which progressively larger wires are placed as treatment progresses. The final archwire is usually rectangular in cross-section and the dimensions are so large that it will almost fully occupy the bracket slot. In this way, the individual prescription of each bracket, in all three spatial planes, will be fully expressed by the end of active treatment. The prescription varies from tooth to tooth in the following ways:

- *First order*—The labiopalatal thickness of the brackets varies from the bottom of the bracket slot to where the bracket base contacts the enamel surface. Therefore the length of the stem affects the first-order movement of the teeth, often referred to as 'in/out tooth movement'.
- *Second order*—Within the dental arch the long axis of each tooth displays a varying degree of mesiodistal tip. This 'angulation' is therefore also built into the slot of the bracket (Fig. 6.15).
- *Third order*—The long axis of each tooth also displays varying degrees of labiopalatal (buccopalatal) tip. This 'inclination' or 'torque', is also built into the slot of each bracket.

6.2.2   The Straight-wire® bracket—positioning

As already mentioned, in order for Straight-wire® brackets to create the desired tooth movements, it is essential they are placed in the correct position on the teeth. The centre of the bracket slot must be positioned on the labial enamel surface at a point known as the 'facial axis (FA) point'.[2] This point is to be found halfway between the incisal edge/cusp tip and the gingival margin (cementoenamel junction), along a line known as the 'long axis of the clinical crown' (LACC). As the name suggests, this is on the long

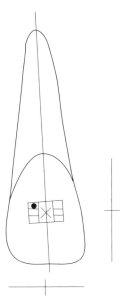

Fig. 6.16 FA point. Notice the centre of the bracket base is positioned halfway between the mesial and distal surfaces and halfway between the incisal edge and the gingival margin of the clinical crown.

axis of the crown of the tooth and midway between its mesial and distal surfaces. It is easily visualized on the labial surfaces of the canine and premolar teeth, where it is denoted by the central ridge. In the case of molar teeth, it is denoted by the mid-buccal groove in the upper arch and by the anterior buccal groove in the lower arch.

When positioning the Straight-wire® bracket the centre of the bracket slot should overlie the FA point, so that the mesial and distal sides of the bracket are parallel with and straddling the LACC. In this way the bracket is also usually placed equidistant from the mesial and distal surfaces of the tooth (Fig. 6.16). Bracket placement using this technique has been shown to be remarkably accurate, certainly when horizontal and vertical positioning of the bracket are studied. However, correct angulation and inclination of the bracket slot during placement are not so consistently attained.[3,4]

To make it easier to visualize where to place the brackets, especially for the inexperienced operator, it has been recommended that the LACC and the FA points are marked up on a duplicate set of study models using a pencil. These models can then be used as a guide at the chairside during bracket placement (Fig. 6.17). However, it is not recommended that the etched enamel surfaces of the patient's teeth are marked with a pencil, since the pencil marks may remain on the surface for some time after completion of treatment.[5] Even with many years of experience, it is quite common to get bracket placement incorrect on one or two teeth during the initial bond-up

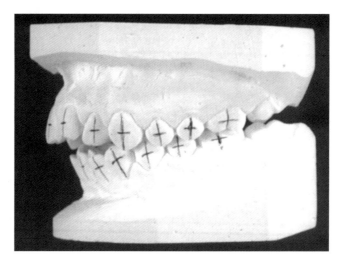

Fig. 6.17 On these study models the LACC and FA points have been marked with a pencil to act as a guide to bracket placement at the chairside.

appointment. Often this becomes apparent within a few months of starting treatment, and it is at this time that the bracket should be removed and repositioned to save the need for later wire bending and to reduce treatment time (Fig. 6.18). In some instances it is not possible to place the brackets in the idealized positions on the teeth at the beginning of treatment. Examples where this might be the case include teeth which are:
- partially erupted
- severely rotated
- abnormal in size or shape, e.g. a peg-shaped upper lateral incisor.

However, the bracket can be repositioned during treatment as the correct bonding position on the tooth becomes more accessible. Another instance where bracket positioning may vary is when the amount of visible crown of a tooth is different from the other teeth in the arch, even though the tooth may be at the correct occlusal level. This is commonly seen in the lower incisor region. For example, if one tooth appears to have a longer or shorter clinical crown length than the other three incisors, it may be necessary to position the bracket on this tooth either closer to the incisal edge or to the gingival margin, respectively (Fig. 6.18). If the crown lengths are all different, then the most normal length tooth can be used as a guide to bracket placement on the other three teeth. In this case, the normal tooth is bracketed first and the incisal edge to bracket slot distance can be measured and used on the other three incisors during bracketing. A measuring gauge can be used for this purpose (Fig. 6.19). A similar problem can arise on canine and premolar teeth. Here it is important to look at the adjacent teeth and in particular the opposite tooth in the same arch, to ensure the tooth appears neither intruded nor extruded. To maintain

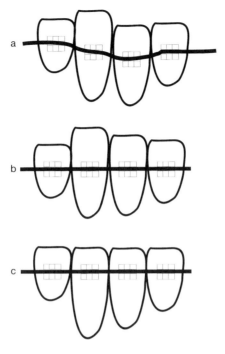

Fig. 6.18 If the brackets are positioned on the teeth at the FA point with no account taken of the length of the anatomical vs. clinical crown heights (a), then as the teeth level and align the incisal edges will be at different levels (b). To get the incisal edges to level up when one or more of the teeth have different clinical crown lengths (c), it is important to measure the centre of the bracket to incisal edge height during the bonding procedure.

symmetry, some operators prefer to place the brackets on each side of the arch, one at a time, beginning at the back of the arch. In other words, place the upper left second premolar first, followed by the upper right second premolar, and then proceed to the upper first premolar, left and right, and so on, around to the central incisors.

In the case of both molar and premolar teeth the brackets can be bonded directly to the enamel surface, although many orthodontists still use banded attachments, particularly on molars (Fig. 6.20). This is because brackets bonded to these teeth frequently fail,[6] either due to occlusal forces, or due to the difficulties in maintaining a dry field during the bonding procedure. Banded attachments are also necessary in the upper arch if headgear is required. They are also useful where the tooth is partially erupted and a bracket would have to be positioned, touching the gingival margin. Bonding in such circumstances may be unsuccessful.

In positioning a banded molar attachment it can be difficult to determine the correct position of the bracket slot on the buccal aspect of the tooth, because the band itself obscures most of the tooth. On molar teeth,

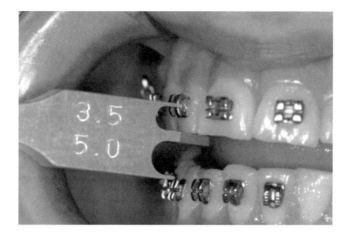

Fig. 6.19 A height measuring gauge in use.

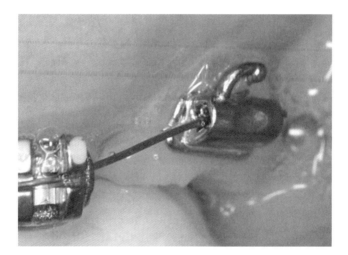

Fig. 6.20 A bonded molar tube.

mesiodistal positioning is straightforward, because the band is contoured to fit in the buccal groove, where the LACC is located. By ensuring the occlusal part of the bracket on the band is parallel with the cusp tips of the molar, the angulation of the bracket/tube slot relative to the long axis of the tooth will be correct (Fig. 6.21). However, the FA point can still be difficult to see, and getting the occlusogingival height of the slot to overlie the FA point can be a problem. In this instance, the operator can use a set of study models and mark the required level of the molar slot on the adjacent second pre-molar tooth on the models (Fig. 6.22), referring to this during bond/band placement.

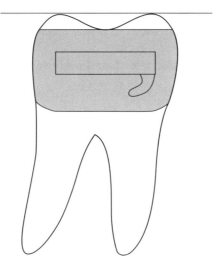

Fig. 6.21 When placing molar bands the tube should be parallel with the cusp tips.

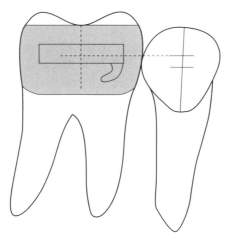

Fig. 6.22 Using study models, a pencil mark on the second premolar can help to identify the FA point during molar band placement.

6.2.3   The Straight-wire® bracket—common variations in design

Straight-wire® brackets can vary from one manufacturer to another in many respects. With very few exceptions, it is not recommended that the brackets of one design are used with those of another design on the same patient. This is not only because of possible differences in the in/out, angulations, and inclinations built into the brackets, but it can be difficult to place the brackets correctly and symmetrically when the brackets on one side of the mouth look different, in size and shape, to those on the other side of the mouth. Common variations in design include:

- bracket size
- number of tie-wings—Siamese (four tie-wings) vs. solid brackets (two tie-wings)
- ligature vs. ligatureless brackets
- prescriptions—in/out, angulation, and inclination
- archwire slot dimensions—0.018 inches (0.45 mm) vs. 0.022 inches (0.55 mm).

Variations in the material composition of brackets will be discussed in Chapter 7.

Bracket size

A number of conflicting ideals have to be considered when designing an orthodontic bracket with respect to its size. For most patients the ideal would be a bracket so small as to be invisible to others. However, for the orthodontist there are other considerations. The bracket must be of sufficient size to enable the tooth movements to be accurately controlled in all three spatial planes. Too narrow mesiodistally and it will be difficult to correct rotations of the teeth around the long axis. Conversely, if the brackets are too wide mesiodistally there will be insufficient wire between adjacent brackets for even relatively thin wires to be flexible enough to move the teeth effectively without the wire becoming distorted, or perhaps applying too much force to the teeth[7] (see Chapter 1). Another consideration in orthodontic tooth movement, and which is affected by the mesiodistal width of the bracket slot, is friction between the bracket and the archwire. However, the evidence concerning the level of friction between narrow vs. wide brackets when a tooth is sliding along an archwire is somewhat equivocal.[8–10]

If the brackets are too narrow occlusogingivally, the tie-wings may be so small that it will be impossible to place more than one ligature on the tooth at any one time. If the bracket is too large in this dimension it may cause occlusal interference, leading to wear of the opposing tooth (Fig. 6.23), especially if it is a ceramic bracket[11] and thereby delay tooth movement. Brackets that are too narrow labiopalatally may restrict ligature placement. It may also lead to the ligatures lying close to, or even directly on the enamel surface, encouraging enamel decalcification. Too thick labiopalatally, and the patient may suffer discomfort on the inside of the lips and cheeks.

Number of tie-wings

Most brackets in use today have four tie-wings and are known as 'Siamese brackets'. The alternative types are two or even three tie-wings. The advantage of having more than two tie-wings is that an archwire can be partially ligated to the bracket slot. This is particularly useful early on in

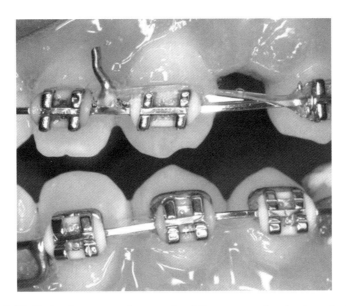

Fig. 6.23 Notice the wear on the cusp tip of the upper canine due to occlusion with the lower arch metal bracket.

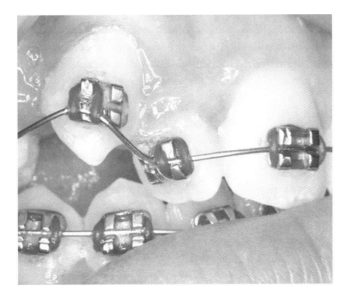

Fig. 6.24 Siamese brackets means teeth can be partially ligated to the archwire.

treatment (Fig. 6.24). The rationale behind having three tie-wings is that partial ligation is still a possibility and yet the bracket is relatively narrow mesiodistally compared with a four tie-wing bracket. This will help reduce interbracket span,[12] which has been discussed under bracket size.

Ligature vs. ligatureless brackets

During orthodontic treatment the teeth can either be moved with or along the archwire. In the case of the latter, there will inevitably be friction between the wire and the bracket slot, something that has been the subject of a great deal of investigation. The amount of friction is thought to be related to the:

• bracket material
• archwire material
• surface roughness of the bracket slot and the archwire
• mesiodistal width of the bracket
• size of the archwire
• type of ligature used to hold the archwire in the bracket slot.

The principle behind ligatureless brackets, otherwise known as 'self-ligating brackets', is that the mechanism used to hold the archwire in the bracket slot should provide a tube through which the archwire runs. Conventional steel ligatures and elastomeric ties often apply a force that will push the wire firmly into the base of the slot, which will increase the friction between the bracket and archwire. A bracket that doesn't use such ligatures or ties will not demonstrate this binding or friction to the same degree. Examples of such ligatureless brackets include: the Speed bracket,[13] the Activa bracket,[14] and, most recently, the Damon bracket[15] (Fig. 6.25). Another advantage of ligatureless brackets is improved cross-infection control, since there are no individual ligatures to be stored or handled, particularly the potentially sharp ends to steel ligatures.

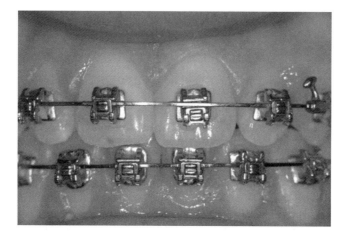

Fig. 6.25 Ligatureless Damon II brackets. The slider is open on the upper left central incisor and closed on all the other teeth.

Prescriptions

Although many systems with variations in bracket prescriptions are sold, the basic principle is still that of the Straight-wire® system. Individual orthodontists have refined the original bracket prescriptions determined by Andrews. Of the more popular and well-known prescriptions are those of Roth and of McLaughlin, Bennett, and Trevisi (MBT). In each case there are variations to both the second- and third-order prescription of one or more brackets. Indeed, although Andrews developed the original Straight-wire® brackets for non-extraction cases with essentially a Class I or very mild Class II skeletal relationship, he later developed brackets for extraction cases and for variations in skeletal pattern,[16] as well as to deal with different degrees of crowding and anchorage requirements. In the extraction series of brackets, of which there were the minimum, medium and maximum extraction series, differing degrees of additional tip and counter-rotation devices were introduced into the brackets to prevent teeth tipping and rotation into adjacent extraction sites (Table 6.1).

The terms 'minimum', 'medium', 'maximum' in Table 6.1 refer to the amount of movement required, in millimetres, by the adjacent teeth following extractions for the relief of crowding. Minimum series brackets were used when only 2 mm of movement was required, medium series were designed for 3–4 mm of movement, and maximum for 5 mm or more of movement. Andrews also produced upper and lower incisor brackets with varying degrees of incisal torque. For a Class I skeletal pattern the S series was used, for Class II skeletal patterns the A series was used, and for Class III the C series. The tip and the in/out values were the same in each case, but the torque values were different (Table 6.2).

It was as a result of all these Andrews' variations on the Straight-wire® theme, that Roth developed his own bracket prescription, with the aim being to produce just one set of brackets for all malocclusions. These brackets were designed to overcorrect the positions of the teeth, since settling is expected to occur at the completion of treatment. This overcorrection included:
• more torque in the upper incisor region;
• less torque for the upper canines;

Table 6.1 Additional degrees of tip- and counter-rotation built into the original Andrew's prescription according to the need to move the teeth adjacent to an extraction site

Extraction series	Tip	Rotation	Translation
Minimum	2°	2°	For 2 mm
Medium	3°	4°	For 3–4 mm
Maximum	4°	6°	For >5 mm

Table 6.2 The torque values of the upper and lower incisor brackets for each of the series A, S, and C. Note how the values vary according to the skeletal pattern (ANB angle)

Bracket series	Incisor tooth	Lateral	Central
A Series	Upper	−2°	2°
ANB <5°	Lower	4°	4°
S Series	Upper	3°	7°
ANB 0–5°	Lower	−1°	−1°
C Series	Upper	8°	12°
ANB <5°	Lower	−6°	−6°

- more mesial crown tip (angulation) of the upper canines;
- more rotation to the mesial, around the long axis, for the upper canines and premolars;
- the upper premolars and molars have 0° of tip;
- greater distal rotation around the long axis of the upper molars.

However, for specific cases even Roth had variants of his own bracket prescription. For example, for Class II division II incisor relationships that may require more torque in the upper incisor region[17] 'Super torque' brackets were recommended.

The prescription in the MBT system differs form both the Andrews' and Roth prescriptions. These differences include:

- Even greater torque provided in the upper incisor region.
- Reduced tip (mesial angulation) of the upper arch teeth, which thereby reduces the mesial movement of these teeth and hence the anchorage demands in the upper arch.
- Greater lingual crown torque obtained for the lower incisors. This helps to reduce the proclination commonly seen during levelling and aligning. It also helps to create/maintain a Class I incisor relationship in combination with the increased torque described for the upper incisors.
- Greater buccal root torque obtained for the upper molars to prevent their palatal cusps from hanging down.
- Reduced lingual crown torque obtained in the lower premolars and molars. This is to prevent, amongst other effects, the tendency for the crowns of, in particular, the lower second molar from rolling lingually.

Once again there are variations in the MBT prescription for specific cases, notably for the upper second premolars. Not infrequently these teeth may have a small crown and so an MBT bracket is available with an increased in/out (second order) thickness of 0.5 mm.

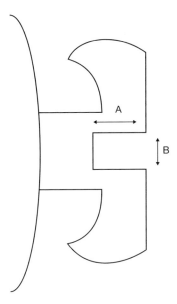

Fig. 6.26 The dimensions of a 0.022-inch edgewise bracket.

The permutations in prescription of the Straight-wire® appliance are vast and largely based on the clinical experience of those advocating the use of any particular system. It is worth reiterating that the principles of the Straight-wire® system are the same whatever the subtle changes in bracket prescription. However, patients do not have identical teeth and skeletal relationships and so an appliance made to an average prescription will often require modification.[18] This can either be in the form of altered bracket prescription, bracket placement, or the orthodontist may have to perform localized or generalized wire bending.

Archwire slot dimensions

The cross-sectional dimensions of the bracket slot are often described in Imperial units of thousands of an inch, and there are two sizes to choose from: 0.018 × 0.025 inches (0.45 × 0.63 mm) and the more commonly used 0.022 × 0.028 inches (0.55 × 0.70 mm). These dimensions refer to the height (B) and the depth (A) of the bracket slot, respectively (Fig. 6.26). The length of the slot will depend upon the mesiodistal width of the bracket, and, to confuse matters, this dimension is often described in metric units. In some cases the corners of the bracket slot are rounded to reduce the effects of binding against the archwire.

6.2.4 The Straight-wire® appliance—treatment phases

Following placement of the Straight-wire® appliance there are usually six treatment phases, dependent on the starting malocclusion. Typically these phases are:

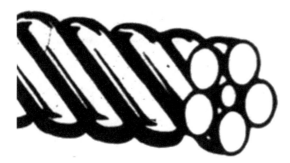

Fig. 6.27 Cross-section of a multistrand stainless-steel wire.

- initial alignment
- overbite correction
- overjet correction
- space closure
- finishing
- retention.

At the end of treatment Andrews' six keys should have been achieved, although it is not always possible to achieve all six, even in the hands of experienced clinicians.[19] Each of these phases will now be discussed in turn.

Initial alignment

Once the brackets and tubes have been correctly positioned on each of the teeth, initial alignment can begin. This involves placing an archwire, which will flexible enough to be tied into most, and hopefully all, of the bracket slots. It is important the wire does not undergo permanent deformation when it is tied into position using either elastomeric modules or steel ligatures. In this way, a light force will be applied to each of the teeth in order to initiate and sustain tooth movement (see Chapter 1) in all three spatial planes. With the 0.022-inch (0.55 mm) system the initial wire is usually one of three types and dimensions:

- multistrand stainless-steel wire. This is usually 0.015 (0.38 mm) or 0.0175 (0.44 mm) inches in cross-section (Fig. 6.27).
- nickel–titanium. This is usually superelastic 0.012- (0.3 mm), 0.014- (0.35 mm), or 0.016- (0.4 mm) inch wire, which is also round in cross-section.
- thermally active nickel–titanium. Here the initial wire can be round, square, or rectangular in cross-section. Initial wires made from thermally active nickel–titanium are usually of a larger dimension than initial wires made from superelastic nickel–titanium. The reasons for this will be discussed in Chapter 7. Examples of the initial wire sizes are 0.018 inches round, 0.016 × 0.016 inches square (0.4 × 0.4 mm), and 0.016 × 0.022 inches rectangular. (0.4 × 0.55 mm)

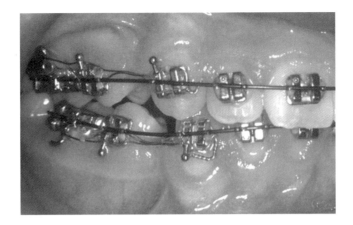

Fig. 6.28 Lacebacks in position beneath the archwire.

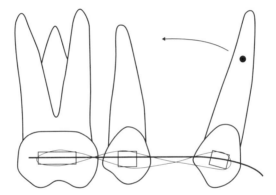

Fig. 6.29 The laceback will reportedly prevent mesial tipping of the canine crown and instead will encourage the root to move distally. Data however does not confirm this.

In addition to placing the archwires, it is common practice to place lace backs from the first permanent molar to the canine in all four quadrants (Fig. 6.28). The purpose of the lace backs is twofold:

1. To protect the archwire from masticatory forces which might otherwise distort it and/or cause it to disengage from the brackets and tubes. This is particularly so if a premolar tooth has been extracted as part of the treatment, leaving the wire unsupported at the extraction site.

2. To reportedly prevent mesial tipping of the crown of a distally angulated canine, which will instead, encourage distal movement of the canine root (Fig. 6.29).

However, it should be remembered that lace backs can increase plaque retention (see Chapter 9). Lace backs can remain in position until the phases of overjet reduction and space closure are reached, when larger dimension steel wires will be in place that require less protection. Also,

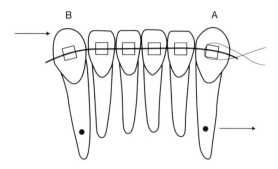

Fig. 6.30 By using a laceback on just one side (A), the crown of the distally angulated canine on this side is prevented from moving mesially. The absence of a laceback on the other side (B) enables the crown of the also distally angulated canine to tip mesially and thereby help move the centreline towards the opposite side.

by this time, the angulation built into the canine bracket will have been expressed by the larger dimension wire and no further mesial movement of the canine crown, or distal movement of the root, will take place.

Sometimes a lace back is only placed on one side of the arch. This may be because only one canine is distally angulated, or teeth have not been extracted on this side of the arch. However, even when both canines are distally angulated, by using a lace back to restrict mesial crown movement of only one canine, the lace back can be used to help correct the centreline (Fig. 6.30). The centreline will move towards the side with the lace back.

The precise tooth movements that will occur during initial alignment will also depend upon a number of other factors, including those listed below.

• *The position of the adjacent teeth in the same arch*—Teeth will initially tend to move to an average position within the arch due to reciprocal forces from the archwire acting on adjacent teeth. Therefore very proclined teeth will become less proclined, whilst adjacent retroclined teeth will become more proclined (Fig. 6.31). Traditionally, the initial wires used in the Straight-wire® system have been round in cross-section, e.g. 0.012-inch (0.3 mm) nickel–titanium alloy in a 0.022-inch (0.55 mm) bracket. Therefore the wire is a very loose fit in the bracket and the forces applied by the wire will tend to tip the teeth around the root centroid, certainly in a labiopalatal direction. With the use of larger dimension, thermally active, nickel–titanium wires for initial alignment, torqueing movements may also occur early on in treatment. Once again, very proclined teeth will become less proclined, whilst adjacent retroclined teeth will become more proclined. Whatever the initial aligning wire, partially erupted teeth may be extruded, whilst the adjacent fully erupted teeth will be intruded. This can, in some cases, cause a canting of the occlusal plane. Where a tooth is rotated, reciprocal movement of the adjacent teeth may also occur (Fig. 6.32).

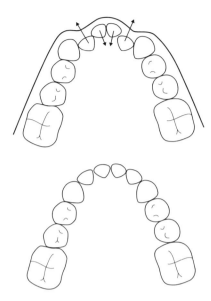

Fig. 6.31 The incisors in this case will take an average position within the arch during initial alignment. Notice how the central incisors move lingually and the lateral incisors move labially.

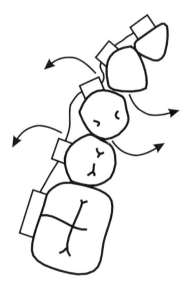

Fig. 6.32 When derotating a tooth, reciprocal movement will occur in the adjacent teeth.

- *The number of adjacent teeth and the size of their root surface* areas—This equates to the anchorage balance between the tooth/teeth to be moved and the adjacent tooth or teeth (see Chapter 3, Anchorage). If the most mal-positioned tooth has the greatest surface area then the adjacent teeth are likely to move towards the malposed tooth rather than the other way around. It is because of this that such teeth are sometimes ignored early on in treatment, either to let them align spontaneously, or so that all the adjacent teeth can be incorporated together on to a larger dimension arch wire, thereby increasing their anchorage value. In this way the malposed tooth can be aligned later without inadvertently moving the adjacent teeth in an unwanted direction

• *The interaction of the archwire and bracket slot*—Excessive binding (friction) of the wire in the bracket slot may prevent the teeth from sliding along the archwire. Instead of the wire moving through the brackets, the tooth/teeth will move with the wire as it tries to return to its original shape. Indeed, it is common for incisor teeth to procline during initial alignment due to this effect. Binding can occur either due to the malposition of the tooth/teeth, or due to the effects discussed under the heading 'Ligature vs. ligatureless brackets', earlier.

• *Spacing/crowding*—The averaging of tooth positions mentioned earlier will only occur in an idealized system, where teeth can slide freely along an archwire and have the space in which to do so. Where there is crowding, this averaging can only take place if the adjacent teeth move around the arch to allow the most malpositioned teeth to move into the arch (Fig. 6.31). As a consequence, crowded teeth may move towards any space that has been created by extractions.

• *Occlusal interference*—An occlusal interference from an opposing tooth may prevent initial alignment. In such instances it is either necessary to wait for the opposing tooth to move or for the vertical overlap (overbite) to be reduced. The overbite can either reduce as initial alignment takes place in the vertical plane, or transiently perhaps by using a biteplane, or even propping the bite by using glass poly(alkenoate) cement or acrylic blocks on two or more posterior teeth (Fig. 6.33).

Overbite reduction

Although the phases of fixed appliance therapy are often described as distinct phases, in reality they merge with one another. Overbite reduction will often therefore begin during the initial alignment phase. The exception to this will be when the canines are distally angulated. In this instance the overbite will actually increase in the early stages of treatment and it is not until the canine angulation is corrected that the overbite will begin to reduce (Fig. 6.34). When teeth are moved in one direction, only to be moved back again at a later date, it is known as 'round tripping'. Sometimes, in order to prevent such round tripping, the incisor teeth are not bonded during the early stages of treatment when the canines are very distally angulated. They are bonded later when the canines are approaching their correct angulation (Fig. 6.35).

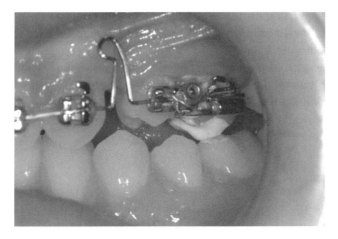

Fig. 6.33 Glass polyalkenoate cement placed on the upper molars to prop the bite and remove occlusal interferences.

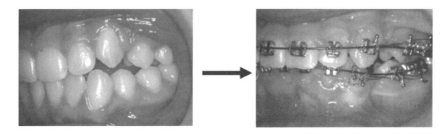

Fig. 6.34 The distally angulated lower canine in combination with the preadjusted Edgewise bracket has led to the archwire moving occlusally in the incisor region, with a consequent extrusion of these teeth and a worsening of the overbite from the pretreatment position to the midtreatment position.

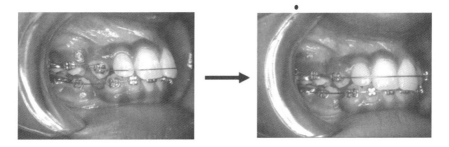

Fig. 6.35 In this case the incisor were not bonded initially. See how incisal the archwire is on the upper incisors. As the canines align, with the root apex moving distally, the archwire on the incisors moves to a more gingival position and the incisor brackets can now be placed.

Overbite reduction usually begins in earnest when stainless-steel wires are used. As initial alignment progresses, the archwires are changed to those of a larger cross-section. Whether round, square, or rectangular nickel–titanium wires were used at the start, these are replaced with progressively larger (often nickel–titanium) wires, until stainless-steel wires can be fitted relatively easily. These latter wires may also initially be round in cross-section, for example 0.018 inches (0.45 mm) and then 0.020 inches (0.5 mm), but it is usual to progress into larger cross-sectional rectangular wires up to what is usually termed the 'final working archwire' (see Section 6.2.6).

If overbite reduction is slow, a number of other steps can be taken, including those listed below.

• *Bending a reverse Curve of Spee in the lower archwire*—Care must be taken when using a close-fitting rectangular archwire, this is because the reverse Curve of Spee will introduce unwanted labial crown torque to the lower incisors (Fig. 6.36) and buccal crown torque into the buccal segment teeth. It may be necessary to bend the archwire to remove this torque whilst maintaining the reverse Curve of Spee. Another unwanted side-effect of labial crown torque in the lower incisor region is that the roots of these teeth may be forced against the lingual cortical plate of bone. This will not only slow overbite reduction but may induce apical root resorption in these teeth. It is possible to purchase rectangular nickel–titanium alloy wires with the reverse curve already bent into the archwire—these are known as 'rocking horse wires' or 'counterforce wires' (Fig. 6.37). However, with these latter wires it is not possible to remove the unwanted torque and so they should not be left in place for long periods.

• *Bending an increased Curve of Spee into the upper archwire*—It is important when assessing the patient not to assume it is always the lower incisor position that needs to be altered when reducing an overbite. Often the upper incisors need to be intruded, particularly when the patient displays a great

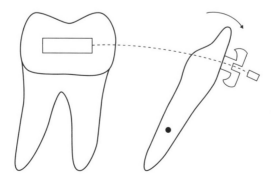

Fig. 6.36 Proclination of the lower incisors as a result of placing a reverse Curve of Spee in the lower archwire.

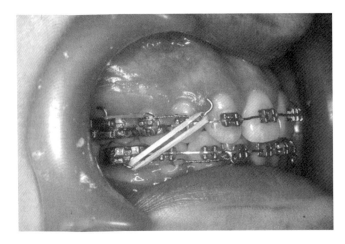

Fig. 6.39 Class II intermaxillary traction will aid overbite reduction by extruding the lower molars.

Using Class II intermaxillary elastics—This can help overbite reduction by ruding the lower first permanent molars (Fig. 6.39). An unwanted effect be extrusion of the upper incisors.

Providing an anterior biteplane—This can either be in the form of an per removable appliance, which may be used in conjunction with or prior he treatment with the fixed appliance, or by the use of bonded palatal achments.

rjet reduction

lowing initial alignment and overbite reduction, if the malocclusion was ginally a Class II division 1, there will still be an overjet to reduce at this ge. The upper canines and incisors will be in contact and space will be sent distal to these teeth. Using the upper molars and premolars as chorage, the upper labial segment teeth will be moved palatally. From oks bent, soldered, crimped, or screwed (Fig. 6.40) to the archwire ween the upper lateral incisors and the canines, either elastomeric chain, stomeric rings on a steel ligature, or nickel–titanium springs are used to ply a force to the upper labial segment teeth back to hooks on the first lars. The archwire therefore moves with the upper labial segment teeth d slides through the brackets and tubes of the posterior anchor teeth. This known as 'sliding mechanics' for this reason. For this sliding to take place e wire should be stainless steel; when using a 0.022-inch (0.55 mm) acket slot size, the minimum size of this stainless-steel wire should be)18-inch (0.45 mm) round wire. A wire made from another material ch as nickel–titanium alloy or a wire of smaller dimension than)18 inches (0.45 mm) will not be sufficiently stiff to prevent dumping. umping' is where the teeth either side of a space tip into the space rather

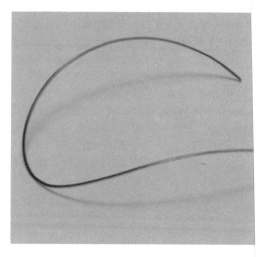

Fig. 6.37 A counterforce or rocking horse nickel–titanium pronounced Curve of Spee.

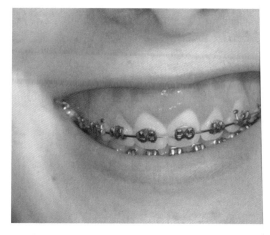

Fig. 6.38 This patient displays an excessive amount of upper smiling.

deal of the upper incisors and associated gingivae on Care must again be taken with the unwanted torque t duced into the archwire.

- *Using localized intrusion bends*—These are placed segment teeth are intruded relative to the buccal segme

- *Placing bands/bonded tubes on the second permanent mo* to reduce the overbite by extruding the premolars relativ incisors.

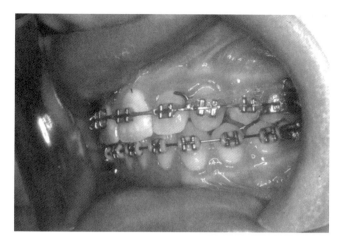

Fig. 6.40 Hooks on the archwire between the lateral incisor and canine can be used to close space and reduce an overjet.

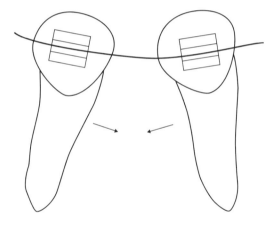

Fig. 6.41 If the archwire is not stiff enough then space closure can result in teeth tipping towards one another rather than moving bodily. This is commonly known as 'dumping into an extraction space'.

than move bodily (Fig. 6.41). Overjet reduction is commonly carried out on a rectangular stainless-steel wire (e.g. 0.019×0.025 inches (0.48×0.63 mm)); this will not only prevent any such dumping, but will also control the upper incisors, minimizing palatal tipping of their crowns. Although the use of a large-dimension, stainless-steel wire will prevent the teeth either side of a space from tipping into it on a macroscopic scale, there will be some tipping on a microscopic scale. The reason for this is the looseness of the fit of the archwire in the bracket slot. Consider Fig. 6.42 where the tooth is being moved along the archwire. As it does so, the tooth and its bracket tip in the direction of movement until the corners of the bracket engage the archwire. At this point the bracket will bind against the wire due to

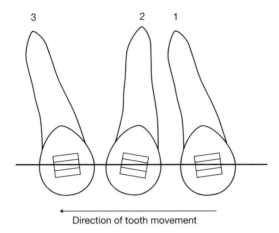

3   2   1

← Direction of tooth movement

Fig. 6.42 The tooth on the right (position 1) is being moved along a stiff archwire. As it does so it will tip (position 2) by an amount determined by the looseness of the fit of the archwire in the bracket slot (mesiodistally). Eventually it will no longer be able to tip due to binding of the wire in the bracket slot, instead the root will move distally to reach position 3. This is known as 'walking along the archwire' and commonly occurs.

friction and will be unable to move freely. A force couple will be exerted on the tooth, which will encourage the apex of the tooth to move in the same direction of the crown. Eventually the bracket will be able to move along the wire once more, until it binds again. In this way the tooth moves in a series of tipping and uprighting movements, and is said to 'walk along the wire'. In general, the narrower the mesiodistal width of the bracket, the more pronounced this tipping and uprighting will be, and the slower the tooth movement.

Sometimes the movement of the archwire through the posterior attachments isn't as free sliding as it should be, resulting in slow movement. If this is the case, sliding may be improved by reducing the cross-sectional dimensions and polishing the archwire posteriorly where it passes through the premolar and molar brackets/tubes, or by using loose-fitting ligatures on the premolar brackets. However, a downside of these actions can be the induction of increased mesiodistal tipping and possible unwanted rotations, respectively. If overjet reduction is still slow, then a looped archwire can be bent up (Fig. 6.43). This looped wire is activated by pulling the free end through the attachment or the most posterior tooth, usually through the tube on the first permanent molar. The activation is then maintained by tying the archwire to the first molar attachment. Although this eliminates unwanted friction within the system, looped archwires are difficult to bend and care has to be taken not to introduce other unwanted tooth movements, such as arch expansion. If the loops are overactivated then too much force will be applied, which can lead to loss of anchorage or root resorption (see

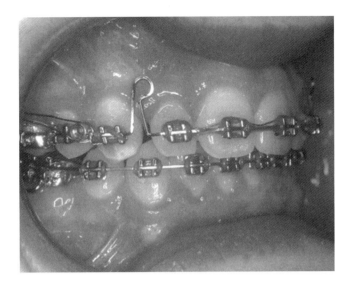

Fig. 6.43 A looped archwire used to reduce an overjet.

Chapter 9). If the upper incisor teeth are very proclined at this stage then overjet reduction can begin on a round stainless-steel archwire, with the incisors tipping palatally. However, if the upper incisors need to be moved bodily in a palatal direction then a rectangular stainless-steel wire should be used. In a 0.022-inch (0.55 mm) bracket slot this usually means a 0.019 × 0.025-inch (0.48 × 0.63 mm) steel archwire (see Section 6.2.6).

It is important the overbite is fully reduced at this stage in order to facilitate overjet reduction. If it isn't, then the upper labial segment teeth will be prevented from moving palatally. This in turn will increase the likelihood of the anchor teeth moving mesially, resulting in a loss of anchorage.

Space closure

Once the overjet has been reduced in a Class II division 1 incisor relationship, or alignment and overbite reduction have been achieved in a Class I or Class II division II incisor relationship, there may be residual space within the arches that will need to be closed. This will entail a continuation of the sliding mechanics initiated during overjet reduction. In reality, overjet reduction and space closure are not usually distinct phases, but merge into one. It is important during space closure to keep in mind the final incisor and molar relationships that need to be attained. Although the final incisor relationship will be Class I, the molar relationship will be Class I if the malocclusion was treated without premolar loss, or if one premolar was extracted in each quadrant. It will be Class II if one premolar was extracted in each upper arch quadrant only. Intermaxillary elastics can aid space closure. Class II elastics, worn from hooks on the lower first molars to the hooks on the upper archwire between the canine and lateral incisors, can

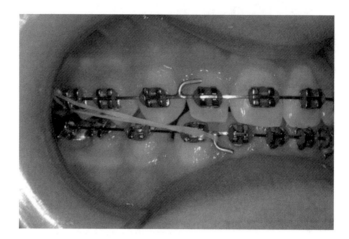

Fig. 6.44 Class III intermaxillary elastics.

help to move the lower molars mesially and the upper labial segment distally (see Fig. 6.39). During space closure in the lower arch, as well as the posterior teeth moving mesially the lower incisors will be tipped lingually. This movement of the lower incisors not only makes overjet reduction more difficult, since the upper incisors will need to be moved more palatally, but will result in the lower incisors relapsing to a more labial position at the end of treatment. Therefore Class II intermaxillary elastics can be useful in helping to maintain the labiolingual position of the lower incisors during space closure. Conversely, if the lower incisors have become inadvertently proclined during initial alignment, or the upper incisors are being retroclined during upper arch space closure creating a Class III incisor relationship, Class III intermaxillary elastics can be used. This runs from an archwire hook between the lower lateral incisor and canine, up to the hook on the upper first permanent molar (Fig. 6.44). It is also possible to have Class II elastics on one side of the mouth and Class III elastics on the other if the centrelines are not coincident and require correction. In addition, the patient can be asked to wear an anterior cross-elastic (Fig. 6.45). Whereas a patient should be asked to wear intermaxillary elastics full time, including during eating, for maximum effect, and to change the elastics every day, anterior cross-elastics obviously cannot be worn during mealtimes.

Finishing

At the completion of overjet reduction and space closure it is possible that treatment may still not be complete. As discussed previously, in Section 6.2.3 on bracket prescriptions, it is unlikely that the Straight-wire® appliance, made to suit the average patient, will always finish to a perfect result. This may be the case even when the orthodontist has placed the brackets in the correct positions on the teeth at the start of treatment. In such

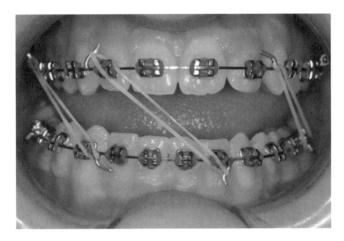

Fig. 6.45 An anterior cross-elastic in combination with Class II elastics on one side and Class III on the other.

instances, it may be necessary to reposition some of the brackets and place a smaller dimension nickel–titanium archwire once again. Alternatively, bends can be placed into the steel archwire to affect the necessary movement. These bends, known as 'artistic positioning bends', can be placed into the final rectangular stainless-steel wires, or into smaller dimension round stainless-steel wires when first- or second-order movements are required. If a tooth or teeth require third-order torqueing movement, this can be bent into the final rectangular stainless-steel wire. Occasionally, larger cross-section titanium–molybdenum alloy wires (see Chapter 7) are used to apply such torque instead.

At the completion of active treatment, the occlusion should not only have reached the desired aesthetic result, but should also function correctly. During lateral excursions of the mandible, the occlusion should demonstrate either canine guidance or group function on the working side and there should be no non-working side interferences. Such idealized functional occlusal results are not always found to be present at the completion of treatment.[20] Finishing for function may therefore be required. For example, it might be necessary to extrude the canines to achieve canine guidance and to apply buccal root torque to the upper molars and premolars if their palatal cusps are causing non-working side interferences.

Retention

Once active treatment has been completed, the fixed appliances can be removed and the patient begins the period of retention. The rationale behind the need for retention, the most appropriate retainers, and the length of time they need to be worn does not currently have a sound evidence base.[21-24]. Retention, following tooth movement, is thought to be necessary

in order to maintain the corrected occlusion during the period of reorganization of the supporting dentoalveolus. In particular, reorganization of the
periodontal ligament and associated gingivae, and the formation of mature
cancellous bone from the immature woven bone formed during tooth movement. Relapse of tooth positions following orthodontic treatment can be
seen in both the short and the long term. Short-term relapse is also known
as 'orthodontic relapse', whilst longer term relapse, seen some considerable
time after cessation of retention, is thought to be part of the normal process
of maturation that would occur even if orthodontic treatment had not been
carried out.

There are essentially two types or orthodontic retainer: removable or fixed.
Removable retainers can be made from stainless-steel wire and cold-cure
acrylic like a conventional removable appliance, a well-known example of
which is the Hawley retainer. An alternative design is to have the retainer
made from polypropylene, which is pressure-formed to fit the new position
of the teeth (Fig. 6.46). However, because of the close overall fit of these
retainers, and the ability of an upper retainer in particular, to act as a reser-
voir in which food and drink can accumulate, it is not advisable for these to
be worn full time.

Fixed orthodontic retainers are also of two basic types: flexible and inflexible. Flexible retainers usually comprise multistrand steel wire but they can
be made from woven Kevlar. The advantage of a flexible bonded retainer is
that the teeth can still move to a very small degree during function. Inflexible retainers usually comprise a steel bar, with or without bond pads at
each end. These retainers suffer from the same problems as acid-etch
retained bridges, which are fixed at both ends. Namely, if, during function,
the tooth at one end of the fixture moves more than the tooth at the other
end, the retainer is likely to debond. Flexible retainers are bonded to each

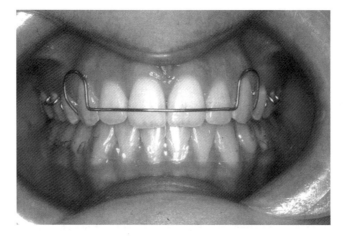

Fig. 6.46 An upper Hawley and lower vacuum-formed retainer in place.

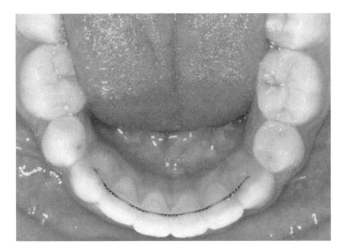

Fig. 6.47 A flexible bonded retainer bonded to each tooth.

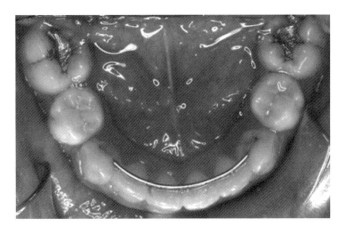

Fig. 6.48 An inflexible bonded retainer which is only bonded to the lower canines and not the incisors.

individual tooth that is to be retained (Fig. 6.47). Inflexible retainers are bonded only to the teeth at the ends of the retainer (Fig. 6.48). Whatever type of bonded retainer is used, the dilemma is knowing when it can be removed without relapse occurring. As with any retention regimen, the only way of guaranteeing the teeth remain in their post-treatment position is to retain forever. With removable retainers this may mean wearing the retainer for 1–2 nights per week at least until facial growth ceases, or forever as the only real guarantee the teeth will remain in perfect alignment. However, this is not without its problems, e.g. prolonged appliance maintenance: repair or replacement.

6.2.5   Factors that can affect the stability of tooth positions following treatment

Orthodontic relapse can be seen both in the short and long term. Long-term changes, years after treatment has ceased, are usually due to continued facial growth, which can occur well into adulthood and possibly forever, albeit at a very reduced rate.[25,26] Changes in the occlusion as a result of this facial growth would have occurred whether or not orthodontic treatment had been performed, and are beyond the control of the orthodontist unless the patient wears a retainer forever. Short-term relapse however, usually known as 'orthodontic relapse', can be minimized by the orthodontist. A number of factors are thought to be implicated in orthodontic relapse, which are discussed below.

Changing the intercanine width; changing the intermolar width

Both intercanine and intermolar widths are thought to alter with age, particularly in the lower arch. Whilst intermolar width may increase with age in males, it tends to decrease in females. It is therefore important not to exacerbate this by expanding either width during orthodontic treatment, although it is known that maintenance of intercanine width in itself doesn't guarantee stability.[27,28]

Proclining the lower incisors

Teeth are thought to be in a position of soft tissue stability, being between the tongue on one side and the lips and cheeks on the other. As a result, moving teeth from this position of soft tissue balance can lead to relapse. The initial position of the lower incisors is thought to be the best guide to the position of post-treatment stability.[29,30] Exceptions to this include retroclined lower incisors as a result of a digit-sucking habit, or trapping in the palate in some Class II division 1 incisor relationships.[31] Care must be taken when using Class II intermaxillary elastics, even with rectangular wires, as their continued use can lead to an unwanted degree of proclination of the lower incisors.

Alteration of archform

This is thought to increase the likelihood of relapse,[32] therefore archwires should, wherever possible, be bent to conform to the original archform of the patient rather than to a preformed shape. Archwires made from nickel–titanium alloy are usually preformed and are not altered by the orthodontist. However, it is important to use stainless-steel archwires in the latter stages of fixed appliance therapy, so that the arch dimensions and archform of the patient seen at the beginning of treatment can be maintained or re-established. Study models taken at the commencement of treatment are therefore an essential reference against which these archwires can be altered. Archform is related to the intercanine and intermolar widths discussed earlier.

Creation of a fully interdigitated anteroposterior buccal segment relationship

It is known that a fully interdigitated, anteroposterior buccal segment relationship, whether it is Class I, II or III, is associated with improved post-treatment stability, as measured by tooth alignment. Part way between any of these relationships proves to be less stable in the longer term.[33]

The periodontium

Teeth that have been derotated during treatment have a high tendency to rotational relapse, either as a result of stretching of the collagen fibres within the periodontal ligament,[34,35] or as a result of stretching the gingival tissues as a whole.[36] The correction of rotations can occur early on in treatment with fixed appliances, and, provided the standard of oral hygiene is good, consideration should be given to carrying out pericision[37] on initially, very rotated teeth. Here, the supragingival, principal fibres of the periodontium are severed to allow for release of any tension in the soft tissues. Pericision has been shown to reduce the degree of rotational relapse many years' post-retention.[38]

6.2.6 Archwire sequencing

There is no definitive archwire sequence that has to be used during the phases of fixed appliance therapy. Orthodontists often have their own routine archwire sequences. However, the basic principle is the same in each case, namely to begin with a wire that provides a light force and which can be tied into all the brackets, without undergoing permanent deformation and without being readily fractured or dislodged by the patient. As the teeth begin to align and the bracket slots line up, wires with a larger cross-sectional dimension can be used. These fill more of the bracket slot and in this way the full bracket prescription will eventually be expressed. The final working archwires, in which sliding mechanics are used, should be made from stainless steel.

With the advent of the newer wire technologies the choices for the orthodontist are often bewildering. The use of these newer wires may require fewer archwire changes to reach the final working wire, e.g. 0.019 × 0.025-inch (0.48 × 0.63 mm) rectangular stainless steel in a 0.022-inch (0.55 mm) bracket slot. Examples of typical archwire sequences are given in Table 6.3. This list of sequences is not exhaustive and will vary according to personal preference and the specific features of the malocclusion, e.g. initial degree of irregularity, depth of overbite, inclination of the upper incisors. In all cases, when stainless-steel wires are used, both the shape and size of the archform should conform to that of the patient at the start of

Table 6.3 Typical archwire sequencing according to the phase of treatment and the types of wires being used

Treatment phases	Traditional wire sequence; only stainless-steel wires	Nickel–titanium wires followed by stainless steel	Thermally active nickel–titanium wires followed by stainless steel
Appliance placement: Initial alignment	0.015- (0.38 mm) or 0.0175-inch (0.44 mm) multistrand steel	0.012- (0.3 mm), 0.014- (0.35 mm), 0.016-inch (0.4 mm) nickel–titanium	0.016- (0.44 mm) or 0.018-inch (0.45 mm) thermally active nickel–titanium
Continued alignment: Overbite reduction	0.016-inch (0.4 mm) stainless steel	0.016- (0.44 mm) or 0.018-inch (0.45 mm) nickel–titanium	0.020 × 0.020-inch (0.5 × 0.5 mm) thermally active nickel–titanium
Continued alignment: Overbite reduction	0.018-inch (0.45 mm) stainless steel, or 0.016 × 0.022-inch (0.4 × 0.55 mm) stainless steel	0.019 × 0.025-inch (0.48 × 0.55 mm)– nickel titanium, or 0.020-inch (0.5 mm) stainless steel	—
Continued alignment: Overbite reduction	0.020-inch (0.5 mm) stainless steel, or 0.016 × 0.022-inch (0.4 × 0.55 mm) stainless steel	—	—
Space closure	0.019 × 0.025-inch (0.48 × 0.63 mm) stainless steel	0.019 × 0.025-inch (0.48 × 0.55 mm) stainless steel	0.019 × 0.025-inch (0.48 × 0.55 mm) stainless steel
Finishing	0.014- (0.35 mm) or 0.016-inch (0.4 mm) stainless steel, or braided rectangular steel 0.019 × 0.025 inches (0.48 × 0.55 mm)	0.014- (0.38 mm) or 0.016-inch (0.44mm) stainless steel 0.019 × 0.025-inch (0.48 × 0.55 mm) TMA	0.016 × 0.022-inch (0.48 × 0.55 mm) or 0.017- (0.43 mm), 0.019- (0.48 mm), or 0.0215 × 0.025-inch (0.54 × 0.63 mm) titanium–niobium

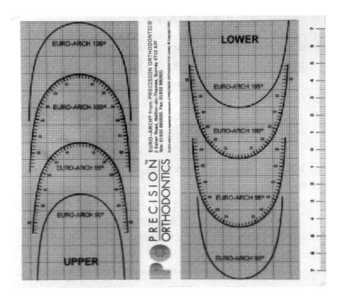

Fig. 6.49 A symmetry chart.

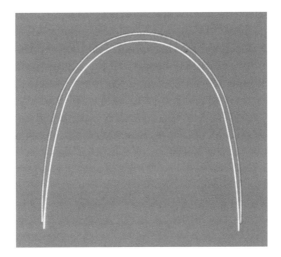

Fig. 6.50 Coordinated upper and lower archwires.

treatment. It is therefore important to refer back to the original study models each time a new steel archwire is placed. A symmetry chart (Fig. 6.49) is used to check that the archform displays symmetry and a glass slab is useful to check that the wire is flat, unless of course an increased Curve of Spee or a reverse Curve of Spee is being intentionally bent into the archwire. Finally, when upper and lower steel arches are being placed the arches should be checked to see if they are coordinated, such that the upper archwire will fit outside the lower (Fig. 6.50).

6.3 THE EDGEWISE APPLIANCE

This was developed by Edward Angle[39] in 1928 and was in common usage up until the early 1980s. Like Straight-wire® brackets, Edgewise brackets have a rectangular slot 0.018 inches (0.45 mm) or 0.022 inches (0.55 mm) within their face into which fits the archwire. In their simplest form the brackets for each tooth are all the same size and shape, as is the archwire slot position within the face. The only variation is that brackets bonded to incisor teeth have flat bases, while those bonded to canines and premolars have curved bonding bases. This enables the base to more closely fit the buccal enamel surface of the teeth. When the brackets are bonded to the teeth the operator ensures that each bracket is placed on the labial/buccal surface, with the bracket slot at right angles to the long axis of the tooth. The bracket is placed equidistant from the mesial and distal surfaces of the tooth, but there is some variation in positioning occlusogingivally. For example, in the upper arch the bracket slot to incisal edge distance of the central incisor is 0.5 mm greater than that of the lateral incisor, but 0.5 mm less than that of the canine. During bracket placement it was common practice to use a measuring gauge to assist the orthodontist in getting these bracket slot to incisal edge/cusp tip distances correct (see Fig. 6.19). It was because the brackets were placed in approximately the same position on each tooth (except for some variation in occlusogingival positioning) that the archwires needed to be bent by the orthodontist, in all three dimensions, first-, second-, and third-order, to achieve the desired tooth movements. Examples of the first-order bends that typically had to be placed into the archwires are shown in Fig. 6.51. Whereas space closure with the Straight-wire® appliance is often achieved using sliding mechanics, the bends placed into conventional Edgewise wires meant space closuring was not usually possible

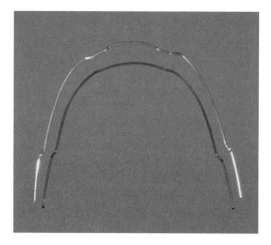

Fig. 6.51 First-order bends in an upper and a lower edgewise archwire.

with this method. Instead closing loops also had to be bent into the wires (see Fig. 6.43). All this wire bending, throughout treatment, required much more clinical time, and the final occlusal results were often inconsistent compared to those obtained with the Straight-wire® appliance. Hardly surprising then that the Straight-wire® appliance, or preadjusted Edgewise system, has replaced the conventional Edgewise appliance.

6.4 THE BEGG APPLIANCE

This appliance was developed by P. R. Begg[40] from the ribbon arch appliance of Edward Angle. The principles behind the mechanics of this appliance are light forces and simple tipping movements of the teeth. This was made possible by using round wires within a bracket that is relatively narrow mesiodistally, but which has a long archwire slot, occlusogingivally (0.020 × 0.045 inches) (0.5 × 1.13 mm) (Fig. 6.52). This long slot permits the use of more than one archwire, when required. At the start of treatment, bands are placed on the first permanent molars, and brackets are only bonded on to the canines and incisors. The initial archwires are made of 0.016-inch (0.4 mm) stainless steel. Alignment of the teeth can be achieved either by increasing its flexibility with the use of multiple loops, or by using a very flexible multistrand steel wire beneath the 0.016-inch (0.4 mm) base archwire (Fig. 6.53). As the teeth align, only the plain base archwire, in 0.016-inch (0.4 mm) stainless steel, is left in place. At the same time, the patient wears intermaxillary elastics. Class II elastics are used in Class I and II incisor relationships, whereas Class III elastics are used in Class III incisor relationships.

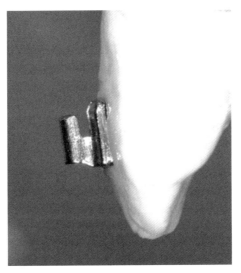

Fig. 6.52 A Begg bracket in profile view. Notice the long bracket slot which opens gingivally.

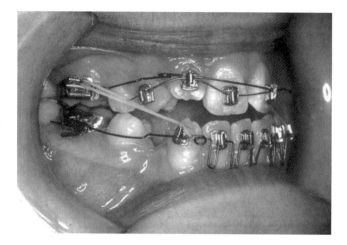

Fig. 6.53 This case at the bond-up appointment in the lower arch has a multilooped lower archwire for increased flexibility in the lower labial segment. In the upper arch there is a flexible multistrand upper archwire in place at the same time as a stiffer base archwire.

Typically, treatment using the Begg appliance is divided into three distinct stages. The objectives and treatment for each of these stages are as follows:
1. **Stage I**:
   (a) *Objectives*:
      • Align the labial segments and close spacing.
      • Reduce the overbite (overcorrect).
      • Reduce the overjet (overcorrect).
      • Overcorrect the labial segment rotations.
      • Overcorrect the molar relationship and any rotations.
      • Correct posterior crossbites.
   (b) *Treatment*:
      • Bond the canines and incisors.
      • Band the first permanent molars.
      • Place multilooped 0.016-inch (0.4 mm) stainless-steel archwires, or a plain 0.016-inch (0.4 mm) stainless-steel base archwire, with a multistrand auxiliary wire when the teeth are very malaligned. Anchor bends are bent into the 0.016-inch (0.4 mm) stainless-steel archwire from the start.
      • Begin intermaxillary elastic wear from the start of treatment.
      • When the incisors and canines are aligned, use just the plain 0.016-inch (0.4 mm) steel base archwire and continue with anchor bends to aid overbite reduction.
When all the stage I objectives have been achieved, treatment can progress to stage II.

2. **Stage II**:
   (a) *Objectives*:
      - Maintain all the stage I objectives.
      - Close all the extraction spaces.
   (b) *Treatment*:
      - Begin space closure using intramaxillary traction.

Once the stage II objectives have been reached, treatment can progress to stage III.

3. **Stage III**:
   (a) *Objectives*:
      - Overcorrect the angulations and inclinations of the teeth.
      - Maintain the overcorrection of rotations.
      - Maintain space closure.
   (b) *Treatment*:
      - Bond the premolars and use prestage III 0.016-inch (0.4 mm) wires to align them.
      - Replace the prestage III wires with 0.018-inch (0.45 mm) lower and 0.020-inch (0.5 mm) upper stainless-steel wires. Use hook pins to hold the wire in the slot and to reduce mesiodistal tipping.
      - A torqueing auxiliary, in 0.014-inch (0.35 mm) stainless steel, may be used to torque the upper incisors to the correct inclination (Fig. 6.54). The continued use of Class II elastics, in a Class II case, will prevent this torqueing auxiliary from proclining the upper incisors and instead will encourage the roots of these teeth to move palatally. However, these elastics may encourage the lower incisors to procline. To reinforce the anchorage of the lower arch and to prevent this proclination, a reverse torqueing auxiliary,

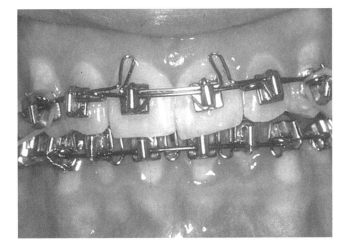

Fig. 6.54 A torqueing auxiliary in place in the upper arch and a reverse torqueing auxiliary in the lower arch.

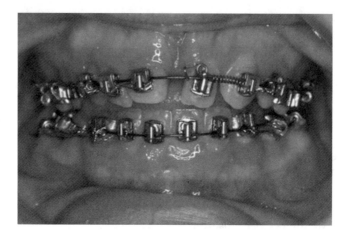

Fig. 6.55 An uprighting spring used to alter the angulation of the upper left incisor tooth.

known as a 'cow's udder', might be used. Uprighting springs may be used in either arch to correct the angulations of the teeth, or to act as brakes and increase the anchorage value of a particular tooth or teeth (Fig. 6.55).

This is obviously a simplified look at Begg mechanics, but nevertheless the principles are: light forces, simple tipping movements of the teeth, and the extensive use of intermaxillary elastics, whereby the teeth in one arch are moved reciprocally against the teeth in the opposing arch. In this way, by carefully managing the anchorage, it is unusual for headgear to be used during treatment with the Begg appliance.

6.5   THE TIP-EDGE APPLIANCE

The Tip-Edge appliance uses similar treatment principles to those seen with the Begg technique, namely light forces and tipping movements, followed by uprighting of the teeth using auxiliary springs. However, the Tip-Edge bracket is very different in design from that of the Begg bracket. Although narrow like the Begg bracket, it has a rectangular archwire slot in its face like an Edgewise bracket. What is unique about the Tip-Edge bracket and what permits the teeth to tip mesiodistally up to 25° like a Begg bracket, is that wedges have been removed from either end of the archwire slot (Fig. 6.56). This wedge removal also means that the rectangular archwire slot has two cross-sectional dimensions, dependent upon the angulation of the tooth. When at the correct angulation the archwire slot is of a conventional dimension, namely 0.022 × 0.028 inches (0.55 × 0.7 mm), but the slot is larger when the tooth is tipped, measuring 0.028 × 0.028 inches (0.7 × 0.7 mm). This larger slot is available when the teeth are malaligned and so the initial 0.016-inch (0.4 mm) steel archwire may fit into the arch-

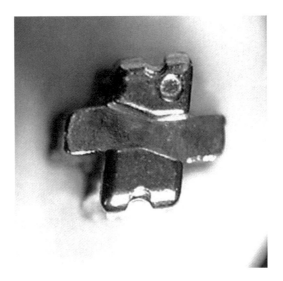

Fig. 6.56 Front view of a Tip Edge bracket.

wire slot on most of the teeth at the initial visit. A lighter nickel–titanium wire can be used at the same time in the case of very malposed teeth. Once larger 0.020-inch (0.5 mm) and eventually 0.0215×0.028-inch (0.54×0.7 mm) stainless-steel wires are in place, uprighting springs known as Side-Winder springs can be used to achieve the correct tooth angulations. As this uprighting occurs, the slot dimensions in contact with the archwire change from the larger 0.028×0.028 inches (0.7×0.7 mm) to the smaller 0.022×0.028 inches. The close approximation of the latter slot size to the final 0.0215×0.028-inch (0.54×0.7 mm) rectangular archwire means that as the latter slot size comes into play, so the third-order tooth movements are expressed by the wire. This final use of a rectangular archwire in a pretorqued rectangular slot gives the treatment finishing advantages of the Straight-wire® appliance, something that is not seen with the Begg appliance.

6.6 LINGUAL APPLIANCES

Lingual fixed appliances have been available since the 1970s and were developed in order to provide 'invisible fixed braces.' Those currently available are preadjusted Edgewise appliances, and so the treatment principles are the same as those of the Straight-wire® appliance. Therefore, following bracket placement, light wires are used for initial alignment, followed by progression to larger wires for overbite correction, overjet correction, space closure, and finally finishing. It is important to realize that such preadjusted lingual appliances are not just conventional preadjusted Edgewise brackets bonded to the lingual, rather than the labial, surfaces of the teeth. The brackets have bases

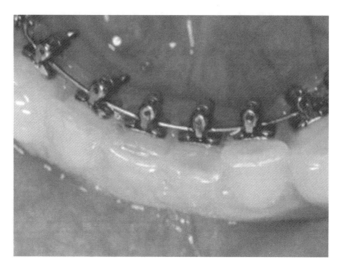

Fig. 6.57 Lingual preadjusted Edgewise brackets in position. These are self-ligating brackets. Notice the very narrow interbracket distance.

designed to fit the contours of the lingual surfaces of the teeth and the arch-wire slots have individualized prescriptions for each tooth. Like conventional brackets, lingual brackets have been made both ligatureless and as ones requiring ligatures (Fig. 6.57). Unlike conventional brackets, they have been made with either a lingual or an occlusally facing archwire slot.

As with the Straight-wire® appliance on the labial surfaces of the teeth, accurate bracket positioning at the start of treatment is essential if the pre-programmed advantages of the system are to be realized. Direct bonding the brackets to the lingual surface of the teeth can be very difficult and as a result indirect bonding is recommended. Here the brackets are placed in their correct positions on study model teeth in the laboratory. A transfer tray is then made on this model, over the brackets, so that when the tray is removed from the model only the bonding bases of the brackets are exposed. Using this tray, the brackets are then bonded to the teeth in the mouth with the orthodontist being confident they are in their correct positions. The tray is then removed leaving the brackets on the teeth.[41]

Due to the small interbracket distance on the lingual aspect of the teeth, not only must lingual appliance brackets be narrow mesiodistally, but also the largest archwires used with this appliance are either 0.016 inches (0.4 mm) round or 0.016 × 0.016 inches (0.4 × 0.4 mm) square in cross-section. A typical archwire sequence might be 0.012-inch (0.3 mm) nickel–titanium, 0.016-inch (0.4 mm) nickel–titanium, followed by 0.016 × 0.016-inch (0.4 × 0.4 mm) nickel–titanium, and then the same dimension wire but in stainless steel. With the advent of thermally active nickel–titanium wires, larger dimension wires (e.g. 0.016 × 0.022 inches (0.4 × 0.55 mm)) can be used, even though the interbracket span is reduced. Also,

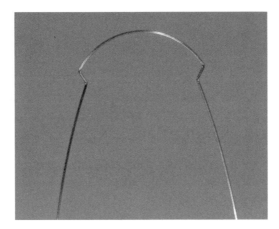

Fig. 6.58 A Lingual archform.

they can be used from the beginning of treatment, necessitating fewer arch-wire changes.[42] Preformed archwires are available for lingual appliances, but the archform is very different from the conventional labial appliance (Fig. 6.58).

Lingual appliances have a number of reported advantages over the more conventional labial fixed appliances,[43] namely:
- Aesthetics are improved.
- The labial surfaces of the teeth remain unaffected by the bonding and debonding processes.
- The risk of noticeable enamel decalcification is reduced.
- The ability of the orthodontist to see the labial surfaces of the teeth means that the final tooth positions can be more accurately assessed.

However, lingual appliances are not in widespread use by orthodontists worldwide, possible reasons for this include:
- Access is restricted.
- It is difficult to obtain moisture control during bonding.
- It is difficult to achieve accurate bracket placement during bonding.
- Indirect bonding is recommended due to problems in bracket placement.
- The high variability of lingual tooth morphology can affect bracket prescriptions.
- The small interbracket span means smaller dimension wires must be used, which are less efficient in controlling final tooth positions.
- The narrow brackets means that rotational control of tooth movement is not as effective as that seen with the wider, labially placed brackets.
- Lingual archwires have first-order bends (e.g. canine offsets), which can preclude sliding mechanics.
- Specially designed instruments with longer handles are often required.
- If the overbite is deep then the patient will occlude on the upper brackets, which can be uncomfortable.[44]

- The patient may complain of a sore tongue due to the position of the brackets.[44]
- Treatment time can be longer for both the individual appointments and overall.

6.7   FIXED APPLIANCES WITH REMOVABLE AND FUNCTIONAL APPLIANCES

So far, removable, functional, and fixed appliances have largely been discussed in isolation, but there are instances when it is useful to use more than one appliance at the same time.

Different appliances can be used in opposing arches or within the same arch, and at the same time. For example, an upper removable appliance with an anterior biteplane can be very effective where there is a deep overbite to reduce. If a lower fixed appliance is also fitted this will not only align the lower arch teeth but will also assist in overbite reduction. Once the overbite has been fully reduced, the lower fixed appliance will maintain this correction, the upper removable appliance can be discarded, and upper fixed appliance therapy might begin.

Fixed appliances can also be used in conjunction with functional appliances. For example, if a functional appliance is to be used in a Class II division 2 incisor relationship, the upper incisors must be proclined, either before starting treatment with the functional appliance, or at the same time as the functional. Proclination prior to using the functional appliance can be accomplished using a removable appliance, a fixed appliance, or a combination of the two. Proclination during functional appliance therapy can be accomplished with the aid of a fixed appliance. This appliance can be used on all the upper arch teeth, or only some of them, in which case it is known as a 'sectional fixed appliance' (see Chapter 4, Section 4.6.2).

6.8   SUMMARY OF FIXED APPLIANCES

1. The three dimensions of tooth movement are: first-, second- and third-order movements.
2. Fixed appliance components comprise: brackets, tubes archwires, and others (e.g. elastics).
3. The Straight-wire® appliance is a preadjusted Edgewise appliance. Each tooth has an individual prescripted bracket. Accurate bracket positioning on the tooth is therefore essential.
4. Common variations in Straight-wire® bracket design:
    - bracket size
    - number of tie-wings—Siamese vs. solid brackets
    - ligature vs. ligatureless brackets

- prescriptions—in/out, angulation, and inclination
- archwire slot dimensions—0.018 inches (0.45 mm) vs. 0.022 inches (0.55 mm).

5. The Straight-wire® appliance—usually six phases of treatment with this appliance:
   - initial alignment
   - overbite correction
   - overjet correction
   - space closure
   - finishing
   - retention.

6. Factors that affect the stability of tooth positions following treatment:
   - changing the intercanine width
   - changing the intermolar width
   - proclining the lower incisors
   - alteration of archform
   - creation of a fully interdigitated anteroposterior buccal segment relationship
   - the periodontium.

7. Archwire sequencing:
   - the basic principle used to be: begin treatment with wires that are narrow and round in cross-section, before progressing to larger dimension wires. With the introduction of new alloys, larger dimension wires are being used from the beginning.

8. Appliances:
   - the Edgewise appliance
   - the Begg appliance
   - the Tip-Edge appliance
   - lingual appliances
   - fixed appliances with removable and functional appliances.

6.9   OBJECTIVES

1. Describe the three dimensions of tooth movement.
2. List the basic components of a fixed appliance.
3. Describe the principle behind the Straight-wire® appliance.
4. Describe common variations in Straight-wire® bracket design.
5. List the six common stages of treatment with the Straight-wire® appliance.
6. List the factors influencing final treatment stability.
7. Describe some common archwire sequences and the principle behind the use of different wires.
8. Briefly describe alternative fixed appliance techniques.

FURTHER READING

Kesling, P. C. (1992). *Tip-Edge® guide and the differential Straight-arch® technique*. TP Orthodontics Inc., La Porte, Indiana

Romano, R. (1998). *Lingual orthodontics*. B. C. Decker Inc, Hamilton, Ontario.

REFERENCES

1. Andrews, L. F. (1972). The six keys to normal occlusion. *American Journal of Orthodontics*, **62**, 296–309.
2. Andrews, L. F. (1989). *Straight-wire: the concept and appliance*. L. A. Wells, San Diego.
3. Fowler, P. V. (1990). Variations in the perception of ideal bracket location and its implications for the pre-adjusted edgewise appliance. *British Journal of Orthodontics*, **17**, 305–10.
4. Taylor, N. G. and Cook, P. A. (1992). The reliability of positioning pre-adjusted brackets: an *in vitro* study. *British Journal of Orthodontics*, **19**, 25–34.
5. Springate, S. D. (1992). Indelible bond location marks: an avoidable aesthetic hazard. *British Journal of Orthodontics*, **19**, 139–41.
6. Mizrahi, E. (1983). Orthodontic bands and directly bonded brackets: a review of clinical failure rate. *Journal of Dentistry* **1**, 231–6.
7. Schudy, G. F. and Schudy, F. F. (1989). Intrabracket space and interbracket distance: critical factors in clinical orthodontics. *American Journal of Orthodontics and Dentofacial Orthopedics*, **96**, 281–94.
8 Frank, C. A. and Nikolai, R. J. (1980). Frictional resistances between orthodontic bracket and arch wire. *American Journal of Orthodontics*, **78**, 593–609.
9. Tidy, D. C. (1989). Frictional forces in fixed appliances. *American Journal of Orthodontics and Dentofacial Orthopedics*, **96**, 249–54.
10. Kapila, S., Angolkar, P. V., Duncanson, M. G., and Nanda, R. S. (1990). Evaluation of friction between edgewise stainless steel brackets and orthodontic wires of four alloys. *American Journal of Orthodontics and Dentofacial Orthopedics*, **98**, 117–26.
11. Viazis, A. D, DeLong, R., Bevis, R. R., Rudney, J. D., and Pintado, M. R. (1990). Enamel abrasion from ceramic brackets. *American Journal of Orthodontics and Dentofacial Orthopedics*, **98**, 103–9.
12. Viazis A. D. (1995). Bioefficient therapy. *Journal of Clinical Orthodontics*, **29**, 552–68.
13. Hanson, G. H. (1986). JCO Interviews—Dr. G. Herbert Hanson on the SPEED bracket. *Journal of Clinical Orthodontics*, **20**, 183–9.
14. Harradine, N. W. T. and Birnie, D. J. (1996). The clinical use of the Activa self-ligating bracket. *American Journal of Orthodontics and Dentofacial Orthopedics*, **109**, 319–28.
15. Damon, D. H. (1998). The Damon low-friction bracket: a biologically compatible straight-wire system. *Journal of Clinical Orthodontics*, **11**, 670–80.
16. Andrews, L. F. (1976). The straight-wire appliance. Extraction brackets and 'Classification of Treatment'. *Journal of Clinical Orthodontics*, **10**, 360–79.
17. Roth, R. H. (1987). The Straight-wire appliance—17 years later. *Journal of Clinical Orthodontics*, **21**, 632–42.
18. Creekmore, T. and Kunik, R. L (1993). Straight wire: the next generation. *American Journal of Orthodontics and Dentofacial Orthopedics*, **104**, 8–20.
19. Kattner, P. F. and Schneider B. J. (1993). Comparison of Roth appliance and standard edgewise appliance treatment results. *American Journal of Orthodontics and Dentofacial Orthopaedics*, **103**, 24–32.

20. Clark, J. R. and Evans, R. D. (1998). Functional occlusal relationships in a group of post-orthodontic patients: preliminary findings. *European Journal of Orthodontics*, **20**, 103–10.

21. White, L. W. (1999). Retention strategies: a pilgrim's progress. *Journal of Clinical Orthodontics*, **33**, 336–68.

22. Blake, M. and Garvey, M. T. (1998). Rationale for retention following orthodontic treatment. *Journal of the Canadian Dental Association*, **64**, 640–3.

23. Blake, M. and Bibby, K. (1998). Retention and stability: a review of the literature. *American Journal of Orthodontics and Dentofacial Orthopedics*, **114**, 299–306.

24. Melrose, C. and Millett, D. T. (1998). Toward a perspective on orthodontic retention? *American Journal of Orthodontics and Dentofacial Orthopedics*, **113**, 507–14.

25. Behrents, R. G. (1985). *Growth in the ageing craniofacial skeleton*. Monograph 17, *Craniofacial growth series*. Center for Human Growth and Development, University of Michigan. Ann Arbor, Michigan.

26. Behrents, R. G. (1985). *Atlas of growth in the aging craniofacial skeleton*. Monograph 18, *Craniofacial growth series*. Center for Human Growth and Development, University of Michigan. Ann Arbor, Michigan.

27. Little, R. M., Wallen, T. R., and Riedel, R. A. (1981). Stability and relapse of mandibular anterior alignment: first premolar extraction cases treated by traditional edgewise orthodontics. *American Journal of Orthodontics*, **80**, 349–65.

28. Little, R. M., Riedel, R. A., and A[o]rtun, J. (1988). An evaluation of changes in mandibular anterior alignment from 10 to 20 years post-retention. *American Journal of Orthodontics and Dentofacial Orthopedics*, **93**, 423–8.

29. Shields, T. E., Little, R. M., and Chapko, M. K. (1985). Stability and relapse of mandibular anterior alignment: a cephalometric appraisal of first premolar extraction cases treated by traditional edgewise orthodontics. *American Journal of Orthodontics*, **87**, 27–38.

30. Houston, W. J. B. and Edler, R. (1990). Long-term stability of the lower labial segment relative to the A-Pog line. *European Journal of Orthodontics*, **12**, 302–10.

31. Mills, J. R. E. (1968). The stability of the lower labial segment: a cephalometric survey. *Dental Record*, **18**, 293–306.

32. De La Cruz, A., Sampson, P., Little, R. M., A[o]rtun, J., and Shapiro, P. A. (1995). Long-term changes in arch form after orthodontic treatment and retention. *American Journal of Orthodontics and Dentofacial Orthopedics*, **107**, 518–30.

33. Kahl-Nieke, B., Fischbach, H., and Schwarze, C. W. (1995). Post-retention crowding and incisor irregularity: a long-term follow-up evaluation of stability and relapse. *British Journal of Orthodontics*, **22**, 249–57.

34. Reitan, K. (1958). Tissue rearrangement during retention of orthodontically rotated teeth. *Angle Orthodontist*, **29**, 105–13.

35. Edwards, J. G. (1968). A study of the periodontium during orthodontic rotation of teeth. *American Journal of Orthodontics*, **54**, 441–61.

36. Redlich, M., Rahamim, E., Gaft, A., and Shochan, S. (1996). The response of supraalveolar gingival collagen to orthodontic rotation movement in dogs. *American Journal of Orthodontics and Dentofacial Orthopedics*, **110**, 247–55.

37. Edwards, J. G. (1970). A surgical procedure to eliminate rotational relapse. *American Journal of Orthodontics*, **57**, 35–46.

38. Edwards, J. G. (1988). A long-term prospective evaluation of circumferential supracrestal fiberotomy in alleviating orthodontic relapse. *American Journal of Orthodontics and Dentofacial Orthopedics*, **93**, 380–7.

39. Angle, E. H. (1928). The latest and best in orthodontic mechanisms. *Dental Cosmos*, **70**, 1143–58.

40. Begg, P. R. (1965). *Begg orthodontic theory and technique*. W. B. Saunders, Philadelphia.

41. Hickman, J. (1993). Predictable indirect bonding. *Journal of Clinical Orthodontics*, **27**, 215–17.

42. Wiechmann, D. (2000). Lingual orthodontics (Part 4): economic lingual treatment (ECO-lingual therapy). *Journal of Orofacial Orthopedics*, **61**, 359–70.

43. Creekmore, T. (1989). Lingual orthodontics—its renaissance. *American Journal of Orthodontics and Dentofacial Orthopedics*, **2**, 120–37.

44. Miyawaki, S. Yasuhara, M., and Koh, Y. (1999). Discomfort caused by bonded lingual orthodontic appliances in adult patients as examined by retrospective questionnaire. *American Journal of Orthodontics and Dentofacial Orthopedics*, **115**, 83–8.

7 Materials

CONTENTS

7.1 REMOVABLE/FUNCTIONAL APPLIANCE MATERIALS

This section is intended to provide information on the materials specifically used in both removable and functional appliances. It will not cover the adjunctive materials used in the construction of these appliances such as alginate, plaster, stone, and separating media. Essentially, there are two types of material used in removable and functional appliances: acrylic and wires.

7.1.1 Acrylic

The polymer used to fabricate removable and functional appliances is based on methyl methacrylate. Methyl methacrylate monomer, which is a liquid at room temperature, can undergo polymerization to form the solid polymer, poly(methyl methacrylate). The polymerization reaction is known as 'free-radical addition polymerization'. For this to take place, free radicals, which have an unpaired electron, must be generated from a chemical initiator, usually a peroxide, e.g. dibenzoyl peroxide. The initiator has to be activated by one of the following:

- *Electromagnetic radiation*—e.g. ultraviolet or visible light usually in the range of 364–367 nm or 440–480 nm, respectively.[1] The radiation acts upon a photosensitized free-radical initiator, such as camphorquinone, which is an α-1,2 diketone and an amine reducing agent (such as dimethyl *p*-toluidine).[2,3] The excited ketone may then abstract a hydrogen atom from the amine, thereby creating a free radical that will lead to the polymerization of a monomer.
- *Heat*—dibenzoyl peroxide will decompose at temperatures between 50 and 100 °C to provide free radicals.
- *Chemicals*—e.g. tertiary aromatic amine, thiols, tri-*n*-borane derivatives[4] can activate dibenzoyl peroxide to provide free radicals.

The polymerization reaction is illustrated in Fig. 7.1. Upon reacting with a free radical (R·) the methyl methacrylate monomer becomes a free radical, which is then able to react with more of the monomer, and so on, to produce poly(methyl methacrylate):

Heat-cured acrylic

Activation with heat, not surprisingly, produces what is known as 'heat-cured acrylic'. This material contains very little residual monomer. As a result it is strong and durable, and is usually reserved for those instances

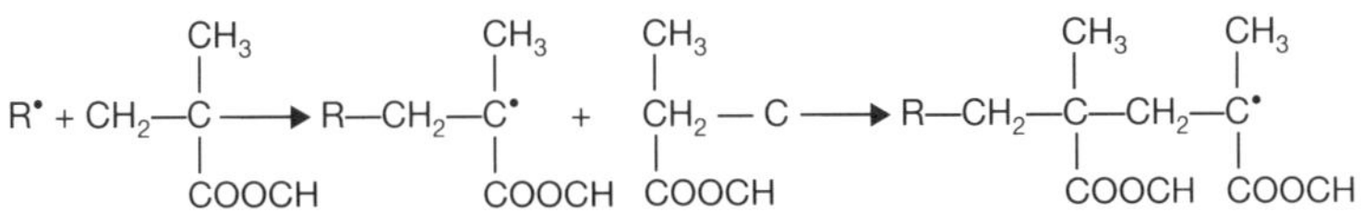

Fig. 7.1 Free-radical addition polymerization.

where the appliance has to last a long time. It is thus used for denture bases and for those functional orthodontic appliances that have to be made in thin sections.

In the formation of appliances from heat-cured acrylic, methyl methacrylate (monomer liquid) is mixed with poly(methyl methacrylate) (polymer powder) to the consistency of wet sand. The powder also contains the initiator, dibenzoyl peroxide. Within a very short time the wet-sand consistency changes as the powder absorbs the monomer and the particles swell and stick together to produce a dough. This is then packed into a plaster mould and heated to a temperature of approximately 72 °C for 16 hours under a pressure of about 17 MPa. Within this mould will be the wirework of the final appliance. Polymerization of the monomer is accompanied by a considerable shrinkage, generally around 21%. Mixing the monomer and polymer, rather than using just monomer, not only makes the material easier to handle, but the polymerization shrinkage is reduced to around 7%. Packing and holding the acrylic under pressure during the polymerization process also reduces the formation of voids. Producing orthodontic appliances using heat-cured acrylic is a time-consuming and therefore expensive technique. Not only do large plaster moulds have to be made, but the acrylic has to cure for many hours. The technician then has the difficult task of unpacking the appliance from the mould without damaging it in the process.

Light-cured acrylic
Light-cured acrylic is rarely used for removable or functional appliances, but it is commercially available.

Cold-cured acrylic
Acrylic activation for the production of removable and functional appliances is most commonly achieved with the use of a suitable chemical. Because it requires no external heat source, it has become known as 'cold-cured acrylic'. Like heat-cured acrylic, monomer and polymer are mixed together to reduce the degree of polymerization shrinkage. However, the monomer liquid in this case contains an activator, such as a tertiary aromatic amine, e.g. dimethyl-*p*-toluidine. A stabilizer, such as hydroquinone, is also included to prevent premature and unwanted polymerization of the monomer prior to use. Unlike the heat-cured technique, where monomer and polymer are mixed together in a glass jar and then packed into a plaster mould once it has reached the dough stage, in the cold-cured technique the two are integrated directly on a damp working model. The polymer powder is gently and evenly poured over the plaster model, where the wire components of the final appliance are already in place. Liquid monomer is then dripped on to the dry powder, so that it again takes on the consistency of wet sand. In this way, it flows around the metal components but remains sufficiently viscous

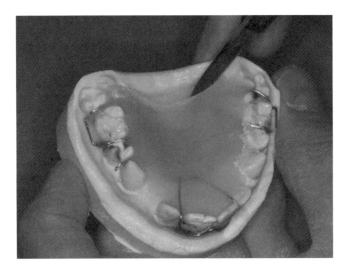

Fig. 7.2 Cold-cure acrylic being shaped during fabrication of a removable appliance.

to stay on the model, allowing the technician to mould and cut it where necessary (Fig. 7.2). Powder and liquid are repeatedly poured on to the model until the desired thickness is achieved. Once the material has been shaped, the model, with its wire components and acrylic, is placed in a hydroflask to cure for 10 minutes. This flask contains warm water, at a temperature of approximately 45 °C, and by using compressed air the pressure within the hydroflask is raised to approximately 130 kPa. The heat accelerates the chemical reaction and the pressure reduces the formation of voids within the acrylic, which would otherwise occur due to vaporization of the monomer during the curing process. Functional appliances are also easily made using this technique: the acrylic being dripped on to articulated models which have the wirework of the appliance already in place.

7.1.2 Wires

Wires used in removable and functional appliances have three basic functions:
- to retain the appliance in the mouth, e.g. Adams' cribs;
- to move a tooth or teeth, e.g. a palatal finger spring;
- to retain a tooth position and prevent movement, e.g. a soft stop.

To meet these three basic functions a wire should have the following ideal properties. It should be:
- formable by the technician during construction of the appliance;
- sufficiently stiff to resist deformation by the patient during use, e.g. during removal, placement, and mastication;
- able to provide forces at an acceptable physiological level capable of producing tooth movement where required;

- safe and non-toxic;
- corrosion resistant;
- solderable;
- weldable;
- cheap and readily available;
- free from changes during storage (i.e. it should have a long shelf-life).

Stainless-steel wires

The most suitable wires for this purpose and the ones that possess most of the above ideal properties are made from stainless steel. Stainless steel is an alloy comprising principally iron (with less than 0.2% carbon) together with chromium and nickel. The stainless-steel alloys used for orthodontic wires are often described as 18:8 stainless steels, referring to the percentage content of chromium and nickel, respectively. Both metals affect the crystal structure of the alloy as well as imparting corrosion resistance.

Not only can stainless-steel wires with slightly different alloy compositions be purchased, but they are also available with differing mechanical properties. Steel wires are fabricated from ingots that are rolled to progressively smaller dimensions before finally being drawn through small metal dies to produce a wire of the desired dimensions. In removable and functional appliance construction the wire dimensions are usually: 0.5 mm (0.020 inches), 0.6 mm (0.024 inches), 0.7 mm (0.028 inches), 0.8 mm (0.032 inches), 0.9 mm (0.036 inches), and 1.2 mm (0.048 inches).

Stainless steel, like all metals and alloys, has a crystalline structure, which results in the formation of grains. As wires are pulled through progressively smaller dies the grains become elongated and give a fibrous structure to the wire. In order to understand how this fibrous structure can affect the mechanical properties, it is important to understand what happens when a wire undergoes plastic deformation. If the crystalline structure of the wire was perfectly regular, then in order for the wire to deform plastically, it would be necessary to move one layer of atoms over another. This would take a very large amount of energy indeed. However, there are irregularities within the crystal structure known as 'dislocations' (Fig. 7.3). When plastic deformation occurs it is these dislocations that move; a process that requires much less energy. Dislocations can be likened to rucks within a carpet. To move a large carpet that has been perfectly laid, on say a concrete floor, would be difficult. However, if there was a ruck in the carpet, moving this ruck would gradually lead to movement of the carpet, and with much less effort. However, just like dislocations, if there were two rucks in the carpet and at different angles to each other, each ruck would impede the movement of the other, unless even more energy was applied. The movement of a dislocation is not only affected by other dislocations, but they are unable to pass across grain boundaries. During the manufacturing process, when the wire is pulled through smaller and smaller dies, or during the fabrication of

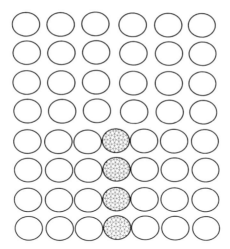

Fig. 7.3 Dislocation within a crystal structure. Notice the extra column of atoms which can be likened to a ruck within a carpet.

components of a removable or functional appliance, the density of these dislocations increases, and the material is said to be 'cold-worked'. Cold-working leads to the tangling of dislocations and the phenomenon known as 'work-hardening'. The effects this has on the physical properties of the wire will be discussed below

Work-hardening

This can be relieved by a process known as 'annealing', in which the wire is heated to a temperature below that which will alter the grain structure (i.e. below the recrystallization temperature of approximately 950 °C), but which is sufficiently great to enable the number of dislocations to be reduced. Overheating can lead to the problem of weld decay, which is discussed later. Too much work-hardening will eventually lead to the wire breaking, either when being formed to create a removable appliance component, or during clinical use of this component in the mouth. For this reason, wires are available from the manufacturer with differing hardness values. If a great deal of wire bending is required to fabricate a removable appliance component, a softer material can be selected. There is currently no uniformity in the description of hardness—examples of descriptors used by manufacturers include soft, half-hard, and hard; others include soft, hard, hard plus, spring hard, spring hard plus, and extra spring hard.

The corrosion resistance of stainless steel is largely due to the presence of chromium in the alloy, which creates a passive layer of chromium oxide at exposed surfaces. Although good news in terms of corrosion resistance, the presence of chromium has two disadvantages in orthodontic wires:

1. The passive layer of chromium oxide must be removed before soldering. This is achieved by using a flux, the most effective of which are the fluoride-containing fluxes such as potassium fluoride. Care must be exercised when using such fluxes as they can produce toxic fluorides on heating.

2. If the steel is heated above 500 °C for a protracted period, for instance during soldering or annealing, the chromium precipitates out of the alloy to form chromium carbide. This in turn has two effects. First, the amount of chromium available to form the passive layer is reduced (a minimum 12% being required) and so the steel is more prone to corrosion. Second, precipitation of the carbide occurs at the grain or crystal boundaries within the steel, making it more brittle and therefore liable to fracture in use. This phenomenon, known as 'weld decay', can be reduced by heating the wire to a temperature above 500 °C for only a very short time during the soldering process. For this reason, a low melting-point silver solder (600–750 °C) is used to solder stainless steel. Incorporating small quantities of titanium or niobium into the steel can reduce the formation of chromium carbide. These metals form carbides in preference to chromium, and the steels containing them are known as 'stabilized stainless steels'.

Physical properties of stainless-steel wires

At this point it is worth considering some of the mechanical properties of stainless-steel wires. The easiest way of understanding these properties is to consider the stress/strain characteristics of stainless-steel wire loaded in tension, as shown in Fig. 7.4. The y-axis label is stress, which is the force applied per unit area of the wire (N/m^2). The x-axis label is strain, which is the change in length relative to the original length of wire and so is expressed as a percentage.

*   *Elastic or Young's modulus*—This property depends on the chemical composition and so will be the same for all wires of the same composition. This modulus (E) can be determined from the slope of the stress–strain graph where the wire undergoes linear elastic deformation between zero and the elastic limit.
*   *Proportional limit*—Up to this point the wire shows linear elasticity.
*   *Elastic limit*—The elastic limit occurs just beyond the proportional limit and so linear elasticity is not observed between the two points. However, when the stress is removed the wire returns to its original shape, without any plastic deformation (permanent set). It is between zero and the elastic limit that the useful spring properties of a wire can be used to move a tooth.
*   *Yield strength*—This is the point at which a wire no longer behaves elastically when a load is applied, but begins to undergo plastic deformation. Experimentally, this point is very difficult to identify and '0.1% proof stress' is an alternative term used for comparison between wires. This is

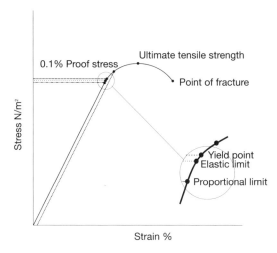

Fig. 7.4 Stress–strain curve for stainless-steel wire.

the load at which 0.1% strain occurs. It is between the yield point and the ultimate tensile strength that the wire can be formed into shape, for example to bend up springs and Adams' cribs.

- *Ultimate tensile strength*—Beyond this point, even if the wire is no longer stressed, it will continue to demonstrate a change in strain.
- *Point of fracture*—Beyond the ultimate tensile stress the wire continues to demonstrate strain and rapidly reaches the point of failure.
- *Work-hardening*—Although work-hardening has already been discussed, it is worth noting the effects it will have in relation to the stress–strain curve. If a wire is strained beyond the elastic limit, it will undergo plastic deformation and inevitably some work-hardening. If it is strained to the 0.1% proof stress and then unloaded the stress will return to zero, but there will be some permanent set in the wire. If it is subsequently reloaded, the work-hardening that has taken place will have the effect of raising the yield strength and the elastic limit. It will also increase the value of the ultimate tensile strength. However, the distance on the stress–strain curve between the yield strength and ultimate tensile stress will be reduced. There is therefore less opportunity to plastically deform the wire to create a desired shape, such as a spring or crib, without the wire breaking in the process. The wire is now less ductile. It is for this reason that wires are available in various hardnesses and are purchased according to the amount of work-hardening they are likely to be subjected to during the construction of an appliance.

Cobalt–chromium wire

Cobalt–chromium is very occasionally used in the construction of removable and functional appliances. Like steel wires they are available in various grades, with the grades denoted by a colour, e.g. blue, yellow, green, and red. However, unlike steel wires, cobalt–chromium wires are designed to be heat-treated in the laboratory. They are bent to the desired shape when soft and then hardened by heat treatment. The soft blue grade is used where a great deal of wire bending is proposed, while the harder red grade can be used where less wire bending is planned. In practice, most laboratories would stock only the softer blue grade and then heat-treat this as required. In the heat-treatment process the wire is heated to a temperature above 480 °C for 7–12 minutes[5] and then rapidly cooled. This leads to the formation of a fine grain or crystal structure in which the alloy composition or phases may vary within the grains. This precipitation of different phases within the crystal structure can impede the movement of dislocations and is known as 'precipitation hardening'. It leads to an increase in the yield and ultimate tensile strengths of the wire, but with little effect on the stiffness. Cobalt–chromium rectangular wire can be fabricated in the soft state to form a Hawley bow and then heat-treated to provide a bow of sufficient stiffness to act as a retainer.

7.2 FIXED APPLIANCE MATERIALS

Essentially, there are five components to fixed appliances:
- archwires
- bracket/bands
- bonding/banding agents
- elastomerics
- auxiliary components, e.g. nickel–titanium springs, hooks, ligatures.

These will be dealt with in turn.

7.2.1 Archwires

Several types of archwire materials are available to the orthodontist:
- stainless steel
- nickel–titanium
- titanium–molybdenum alloy
- titanium–niobium
- cobalt–chromium
- aesthetic archwires.

These will be dealt with below.

Stainless steel

As with stainless-steel wires for removable appliances, stainless-steel archwires are available in various guises. The variables include:
- *Composition*—There are subtle differences in the composition of some of the steels used in orthodontic archwires, but usually in the lesser constituents.

- *Degree of work-hardening*—As with removable appliances it is possible to buy wires with differing hardnesses described as hard, spring hard, and extra spring hard. One manufacturer uses a completely different set of descriptors, e.g. regular, special, special plus, and extra special plus. This variability of descriptors can lead to confusion and make comparison of wires between manufacturers difficult.
- *Packaged form*—Steel wires are available in straight lengths or on the coil, and so have to be bent into the desired arch shape. Also available are pre-formed archforms.
- *Archforms*—Three basic archforms are available:
  (1) Bonwill–Hawley—here the wire from canine to canine is curved. Distal to the canines the wire is straight (Fig. 7.5).
  (2) Catenary curve—this is the shape demonstrated when a chain is allowed to hang between two points. Obviously the precise shape will depend on the length of the chain and the distance between the points from which it is suspended (Fig. 7.6). The catenary curve approximates the shape of the dental arch from first molar to first molar.
  (3) Trifocal ellipse or Brader archform[6]—This is more egg-shaped and although similar to the catenary curve from the first molar anteriorly, unlike the catenary curve it tapers inwards, distal to the first molar (Fig. 7.7).
  These archforms are also often available in different overall sizes. However, it is important to realize that in each case preformed arches are only the starting point. The archwire should be made to conform to the patient's original archform, particularly in the Straight-wire® technique.

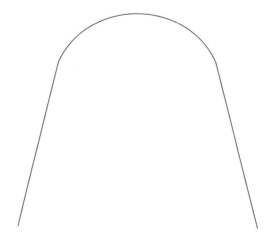

Fig. 7.5 Bonwill–Hawley archform.

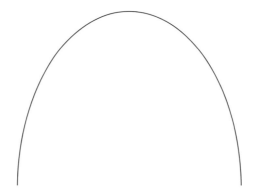

Fig. 7.6 A catenary curve.

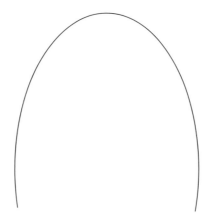

Fig. 7.7 A trifocal ellipse or Brader archform.

- *Cross-sectional shape*—Archwires for use in the Straight-wire® technique are available in round, square, and rectangular cross-section. In the case of the square and rectangular wires they are also available with slightly rounded corners in an attempt to reduce the frictional resistance of the bracket moving along the archwire.
- *Cross-sectional dimensions*—Even though metric measurements are used when discussing the overall size of an orthodontic bracket, the archwires and the slot within the bracket, into which the wire fits, are still described in Imperial units. For wires that are circular in cross-section (round wires) the diameter of the wire can vary as follows:

  Round wires: 0.008 (0.2 mm), 0.010 (0.25 mm), 0.012 (0.3 mm), 0.014 (0.35 mm), 0.016 (0.4 mm), 0.018 (0.45 mm), and 0.020 inches (0.5 mm);

  Square wires: 0.016 × 0.016 inches (0.4 × 0.4 mm), 0.018 × 0.018 inches (0.45 × 0.45 mm), and 0.020 × 0.020 inches (0.5 × 0.5 mm);

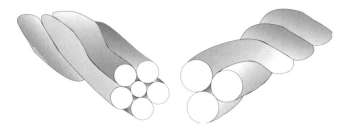

Fig. 7.8 Multistrand wires.

Rectangular wires: available in various sizes, e.g. 0.016 × 0.022 inches (0.4 × 0.55 mm), 0.017 × 0.025 inches (0.45 × 0.63 mm), 0.018 × 0.025 inches (0.45 × 0.63 mm), 0.019 × 0.025 inches (0.48 × 0.63 mm), 0.021 × 0.025 inches (0.53 × 0.63 mm).

- *Numbers of strands to the wire*—Most of the modern wires in use today are made from one strand. However, prior to the advent of very flexible nickel–titanium wires, multiple stainless-steel wires were often wrapped together to form a multistrand or braided archwire. These wires consist of three or more wires of similar dimensions twisted together, or three or more wires of similar dimension twisted around a central core of wire (Fig. 7.8). In a 0.022-inch (0.55 mm) slot Straight-wire® system a common initial aligning archwire was a 0.0175-inch (0.44 mm) multistrand wire made from three 0.008-inch (0.2 mm) wires twisted together. Such wires are said to demonstrate the elastic deformability of the individual small wires and the flexural rigidity of the sum of all the wires.[7]

Nickel–titanium alloy

Nickel–titanium archwires have been in use in orthodontics since the 1970s, with the original Nitinol (3M) wire having been developed by the Naval Ordinance Laboratories in the USA.[8–11] Hence the name Nitinol, an acronym of **ni**ckel–**ti**tanium **n**aval **o**rdinance **l**aboratory.

Essentially, there are three types of commercially available nickel–titanium wires:[12]
- martensitic stable (conventional alloy)
- austenitic active (pseudoelastic)
- martensitic active (thermoelastic).

These will be dealt with in turn.

Martensitic stable

Nickel–titanium wires are composed of approximately 50% nickel and 50% titanium. The original nickel–titanium wires used in orthodontics, of which Nitinol was an example, were cold-drawn through dies during manufacture and subsequently demonstrated linear elastic behaviour, like stainless steel. It is described as having a 'martensitic crystal structure', a term that has

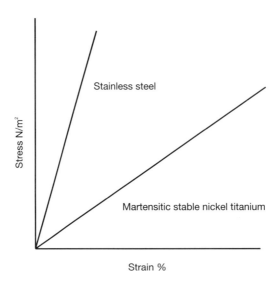

Fig. 7.9 Idealized stress–strain graph showing the relative stiffness of stainless steel and nickel–titanium alloy. Stainless steel is approximately 5–6 times stiffer.

been historically associated with a particular phase, or crystal structure, of an iron alloy. However, unlike stainless steel the elastic modulus (stiffness) is much lower, so that for any given activation (deflection) the force applied by a martensitic stable nickel titanium wire is between one fifth and one sixth of that applied by an equivalent dimension stainless-steel wire[13] (Fig. 7.9). In addition, the strain that can be applied to the wire before it reaches its yield strength is much greater than for stainless steel. This means that a nickel–titanium wire can move a tooth with a lighter force and for a longer period than a stainless-steel wire of equivalent size.

Austenitic active

This type of nickel–titanium wire has not been cold-worked to the same degree as the martensitic stable form and as a result demonstrates 'pseudoelastic' or 'superelastic' behaviour. This type of behaviour is best explained by considering the stress–strain curve in Fig. 7.10. This curve is very much an idealized version of the behaviour of the wire in the mouth. Before it is placed under load, by tying the wire into the brackets, it is said to have an austenitic structure. As the wire is placed under stress (loaded), being pushed into the bracket slot on a malaligned tooth, it initially demonstrates linear elastic behaviour: i.e. from points a to b, the plot follows a straight line in a similar fashion to that seen with the other alloys so far discussed. As the orthodontist continues to push the wire into the bracket, the wire then begins to undergo a change in its crystal structure towards the martensitic phase. During this time the stress within the wire remains the same, which gives the plateau effect seen on the stress–strain graph— i.e. from points b to c. The changes in the crystal structure that take place

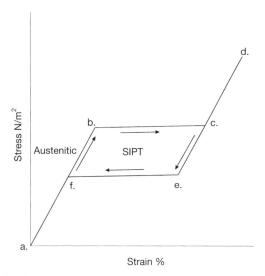

Fig. 7.10 Idealized stress–strain curve for austenitic stable nickel–titanium wire showing the plateaus that occur during stress-induced phase transformations (SIPT).

are known as 'stress-induced phase transformations'. Eventually the alloy reaches the martensitic phase throughout and begins to demonstrate linear elastic behaviour once more—i.e. points c to d. If the wire is now fully displaced into the bracket slot and has been tied in place, a force will be applied to the tooth and it will begin to move. As it does so, the stress within the wire will reduce—i.e. points d to e. With continued tooth movement, the stress within the wire will begin to plateau once again as the alloy transforms back to the austenitic phase—i.e. points e to f. For the orthodontist, the most important part of the stress–strain curve is this unloading plateau from points e to f, since this will mean a light continuous force is applied to the tooth, even though it is moving and the deflection (strain) of the wire is reducing. Eventually the stress-induced phase transformation will have been reversed and the austenitic structure will have returned. With continued unloading, linear elastic behaviour will once again be demonstrated by the wire—i.e. points f to a. The reason the wire is called pseudoelastic is that, despite having this unusual non-linear elastic behaviour, it behaves elastically, returning to its original shape with little appreciable plastic deformation.

It has been demonstrated that by heat-treating austenitic active nickel–titanium wires, the stress (loading) at which the phase transformations take place can be altered.[14–16] The unloading-force plateau can therefore be altered to give differing force values to wires of the same cross-sectional dimensions. The orthodontist must therefore choose which wire to use not only according to the alloy and the cross-sectional dimensions, but also by the heat treatment to which it has been subjected during manufacture.

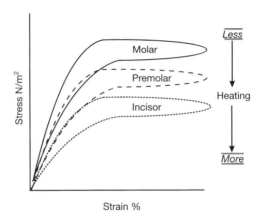

Fig. 7.11 Stress–strain graph showing the effect that heat treatment can have on nickel–titanium wire.

Furthermore, it is also possible to purchase a single archwire that has different force values in different parts of the same wire. One single archwire can therefore have different unloading values in the labial segment, the premolar segments, and the molar segments, e.g. Bioforce Sentalloy (GAC International Inc. New York, USA) (Fig. 7.11).

Another interesting phenomenon is also demonstrated by some austenitic active wires as a result of the change in modulus of elasticity with differing degrees of strain.[17] It is possible to increase the unloading force of the wire by untying it from a bracket, allowing the wire to return to its original shape and then pushing it back into the bracket and retying it. This is because the unloading plateau seen on the stress–strain graph is generally higher for small initial deflections of the wire compared to greater initial deflections. Whether this effect is intentionally utilized by orthodontists is doubtful, but it may inadvertently be used each time the elastic ties are routinely replaced at recall appointments.

Martensitic active

This type of nickel–titanium wire not only undergoes the stress induced phase transformation of its crystal structure, as seen with the austenitic active (pseudoelastic or superelastic) wire, but also demonstrates a change in crystal structure with a change in temperature. More importantly, when classifying a wire as martensitic active, this change in crystal structure occurs at around mouth temperature. These wires are frequently referred to as thermally active, heat activated or thermoelastic nickel–titanium wires. The temperature at which the phase change occurs is not a point temperature but a temperature range, referred to as the temperature transition range (TTR). Below the TTR the wire is in the martensitic phase with a low modulus of elasticity and it can be deformed (strained) very easily. Therefore

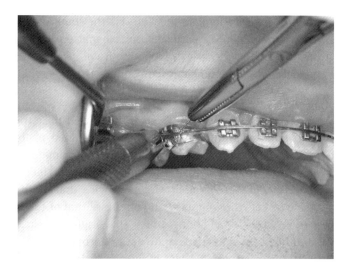

Fig. 7.12 By cooling down the heat-activated wire it is easy to tie it into the brackets.

when the wire is cooled below the TTR it is easy to ligate it to a misplaced tooth (Fig. 7.12). As the wire temperature rises towards mouth temperature, the wire begins its transition from the martensitic to the austenitic phase and the modulus of elasticity increases. The wire then returns to its original shape, increasing the loading on the tooth and encouraging it to move. This return to shape with a change in temperature is known as the 'shape memory effect' and was first observed over 70 years ago with a gold–cadmium alloy[18] and with nickel–titanium alloys in the 1960s.[10]

The TTR is not unique to the thermoelastic wires, being demonstrated by all the nickel–titanium alloys having almost equal parts of nickel and titanium. The TTRs for these wires range from −200 up to 110 °C[19] and can be altered from one extreme to the other with only minor changes in the principal constituents of the alloy, e.g. 3 or 4%. It is known that changes of only 150 parts per million can change the TTR by 1 °C.[20] With such small changes in composition having such profound effects on the properties, it is easy to see the difficulty in producing a clinically useful thermoelastic alloy with a TTR at around mouth temperature. Although the usefulness of thermoelastic wires in orthodontics has been recognized for over 20 years,[21] it has only been in the past few years that they have been commercially available to the orthodontist. It is now possible to purchase wires with predetermined TTRs of 27 °C, 35 °C, and 41 °C. The 27 °C wire has a TTR below mouth temperature and so behaves as an austenitic active (pseudoelastic or superelastic) wire. The 35-°C wire has a TTR around mouth temperature and is therefore martensitic active (thermally active, heat activated, or thermoelastic). It is cooled to facilitate insertion into the brackets of the malaligned teeth and then undergoes a phase transformation to the austenitic form and applies a force to the teeth via the shape memory effect. The 41 °C wire will remain in the easily deformable martensitic form, unless the patient has hot food or drink, in which case it will lead to intermittent loading of the teeth when the ambient temperature rises above 41 °C.

Titanium–molybdenum alloy

This alloy is otherwise known as TMA™ or β-titanium. Unlike the original martensitic stable nickel–titanium wires, which contained approximately 50% nickel and 50% titanium, this alloy contained approximately 78% titanium, 11.5% molybdenum, 6% zirconium and 4.5% tin.[12] The modulus of elasticity, or stiffness, of TMA is approximately twice that of the original martensitic stable nickel–titanium alloy and one-third that of the equivalent size stainless-steel wire. In addition, unlike the original nickel–titanium wires, TMA could be bent into shape quite easily (formable) and could also be welded. But its uses are limited by its high coefficient of friction when compared with nickel–titanium and stainless-steel wires, which is important since space closure with the Straight-wire® appliance largely entails sliding mechanics. The supposed advantages of formability and weldability are also of limited value in most instances. However, TMA sectional wires have been described for use in applying traction to unerupted upper canine teeth[22] and are occasionally used as finishing wires.

Titanium–niobium alloy

This alloy has recently been introduced as another finishing wire in a similar manner to TMA wires. It is reported to have a modulus of elasticity approximately 50% of stainless steel and is similar, if not slightly greater, than that of TMA.[23] Like TMA it is also weldable.

Cobalt–chromium alloy

Cobalt–chromium alloy has largely been discussed above. This wire, known in its commercial form as Elgiloy™, is composed of approximately 40% cobalt, 20% chromium, 16% iron, 15% nickel, 7% molybdenum and 2% manganese. It is used infrequently as an archwire with present-day fixed appliances, but was extensively used when looped archwires were in common use (such as in the Rickett's technique, a modification of the Standard Edgewise appliance). Complex looped archwires were bent up with the wire in its soft state and then heat-treated to increase the yield and ultimate tensile strengths of the wire, but with little change in the overall stiffness.[24] There are four different types of Elgiloy™ available: blue, yellow, green, and red. Although Elgiloy™ may have a soft feel to the orthodontist in its preheat-treatment state, it should be remembered that it has the approximate stiffness of the equivalent size stainless-steel wire both before and after heat treatment, Such heat treatment can be achieved by heating in an oven, or by passing an electrical current through the wire. A colour-changing paste can be applied to the wire that indicates when the heat treatment is complete.

Aesthetic archwires

Aesthetic wires can be considered to be of two basic types: coated metal wires and non-metallic materials.

Coated metal wires have been around for many years and can be either coated stainless steel or nickel–titanium. The coating can be a white epoxy resin or a Teflon coating that initially appears quite good in the mouth, but the problems with such coatings are essentially twofold. First, the coating inevitably occupies some space and so the wire beneath the coating cannot be as large as might be desired by the orthodontist. Second, the coating wears off in a relatively short time.

Non-metallic materials have appeared in various presentations. Some have never progressed beyond the experimental stage for use in orthodontics, e.g. poly(acetyl).[25] Others, such as Optiflex (Ormco, USA), which consists of a laser-drawn silica core coated in nylon, have been marketed for use during initial alignment. Yet other more promising materials are currently being developed and are based on, for example, unidirectional glass fibres coated with a polymeric matrix, making them composite-based materials.[26]

Choice of archwire

For the orthodontist the choice of archwire is no longer dependent purely upon the cross-sectional shape and dimensions of the wire, as was the case when only stainless-steel archwires were available for fixed appliances. Today the choices are much greater and often more bewildering. The orthodontist is now able to select wires with very different moduli of elasticity, which can often be altered by various heat treatments prior to use, as well as stress and heat during treatment.

7.2.2 Brackets

Orthodontic brackets are made from one of three types of materials:
• metals—e.g. stainless steel, cobalt–chromium, titanium, gold;
• polymers—e.g. polycarbonate, poly(urethane);
• ceramics—e.g. monocrystalline aluminium oxide, polycrystalline aluminium oxide, zirconium oxide.
These will be considered in turn.

Metal brackets

The design of metal brackets has been covered in Chapter 6, Section 6.2.1. They are most commonly made from various grades of stainless steel and are:
• milled from a piece of metal;
• cast using a technique similar to the lost-wax technique; or
• metal injection moulded (MIM). Here, powdered metal is forced into a mould and heated, which causes the powder particles to fuse together to create the desired bracket. This fusion is otherwise known as 'sintering'.
Other metal brackets include:

- stainless steel plated with gold or coated with titanium nitride;
- cobalt–chromium;
- titanium.

Gold-plated brackets are used for their aesthetic effect. A similar appearance can be achieved by coating stainless steel with titanium nitride. In recent years cobalt–chromium brackets have been marketed as an alternative to stainless steel for use in patients with a nickel allergy. Fortunately, such cases of true intraoral nickel allergy are extremely rare.[27] In fact, cobalt–chromium brackets are not nickel-free but marketed as 'low nickel'. If a true intraoral allergy does exist, then the lowest permissible level of nickel in a bracket will be unknown, bringing into question the value of a low-nickel bracket.[28,29] If a patient does have a true intraoral nickel allergy then pure titanium brackets, which are nickel-free, could be used. However, no nickel would mean that most archwires (steel, nickel–titanium, etc.) would be unusable.

Whatever the material, metal brackets rely principally on mechanical retention to the tooth. The bracket base is roughened and this provides the mechanical interlock with the bonding agent, which is flowed on to its surface during the bonding process. To aid this retention, the bracket base can take various forms:

- *Mesh*—one-, two-, or three-ply stainless mesh is brazed to the bracket base. This mesh base is also sometimes sandblasted by the manufacturer to further increase the opportunity for mechanical retention (Fig. 7.13).
- *Slots and grooves*—these are cast or milled into the bracket base (Fig. 7.14)
- *Laser etched*—a roughened surface is created by laser etching.
- *Sintered metal/ceramic powder*—the powder, when sintered to the bracket base, provides a rough surface for a mechanical interlock with the bonding agent.

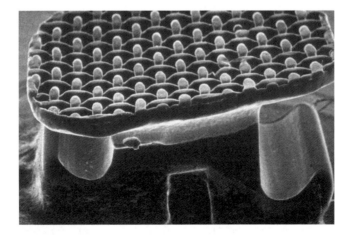

Fig. 7.13 Scanning electron micrograph of a mesh-based steel bracket.

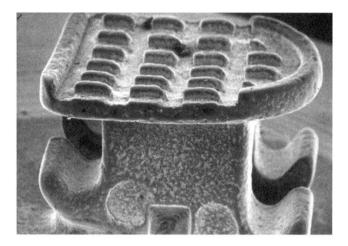

Fig. 7.14 Scanning electron micrograph of a cast bracket base.

Plastic brackets

Plastic brackets are usually made from polycarbonate or polyurethane and are either transparent or white in colour, this being dependent to some extent on the presence or absence of glass filler particles.

The main reason for their use is that they demonstrate good aesthetics. However, they do suffer from a number of disadvantages. The early plastic brackets discoloured in time and needed to be replaced during treatment. In addition, a low abrasion resistance led to surface loss during toothbrushing, which in turn would weaken the bracket and could lead to the eventual loss of one or more tie-wings. The final problem with such brackets is associated with the viscoelastic properties of polycarbonate. Thus, not only does polycarbonate demonstrate elastic behaviour, with a fairly low modulus of elasticity, but with time it also demonstrates creep. Therefore, torqueing forces applied to the bracket with a rectangular wire will not only cause the bracket to flex and the slot to widen at the face of the bracket in the short term (elastic behaviour), but with time it will also lead to gradual permanent deformation of the bracket and its slot (creep). In an attempt to overcome these problems, manufacturers have incorporated glass filler particles into the bracket and provided metal slot inserts. Of these two modifications, the metal slot insert does improve torque transfer to the tooth by reducing the immediate flexing of the bracket slot under the influence of a rectangular archwire.[30] However, creep is still likely to occur, even in the presence of this metal insert.

Polycarbonate brackets are available either with a relatively smooth bonding base or with a base that has a system of integral slots to facilitate mechanical attachment via the bonding agent. Smooth bases require coating with a primer prior to placement of the bonding agent. This is usually methyl methacrylate or a low molecular weight dimethacrylate. Such primers have the effect of chemically roughening the bracket base.

Polyurethane bracket bases have an integral system of slots for mechanical retention of the bonding agent.

Ceramic brackets

The second type of aesthetic bracket is the ceramic bracket, which first became available in the late 1980s. At the present time they are made from aluminium oxide (alumina). Brackets based on zirconium oxide, a tougher material, were introduced but did not find favour due to their relatively poor aesthetics compared with those made from alumina. There are two types of alumina brackets: monocrystalline or polycrystalline.

• *Monocrystalline brackets*—These are milled from a single crystal of alumina (sapphire). The crystal is grown by heating aluminium oxide to above 2100 °C and seeding the molten material, followed by slow cooling. Brackets are then milled from this single crystal. The milling process can create surface imperfections as well as internal stresses and so a final heat treatment is performed to remove them. This is important because such imperfections and stresses would otherwise have detrimental effects on the mechanical properties of the final bracket. Crack propagation can be initiated at surface imperfections, reducing both the tensile and compressive strengths of the bracket and increasing the likelihood of failure during use. The finished bracket is translucent and colourless (Fig. 7.15).

• *Polycrystalline brackets*—These are formed by blending aluminium oxide particles with a binder, followed by moulding to the desired bracket shape. The moulded material is then heated to approximately 1800 °C, which leads to burnout of the binder and fusion of the alumina particles. Once roughly formed in this way, the bracket is machined to the correct dimensions before it is heat treated to remove surface imperfections and to relieve stresses created during machining.[31] The final bracket is less translucent than the monocrystalline bracket and is white in colour (Fig. 7.16). This is because the polycrystalline alumina has grain boundaries that reflect light. The larger the alumina grains used in bracket fabrication the more translucent the bracket, but the less resistant the bracket is to crack propagation. Most polycrystalline brackets are made from aluminium oxide particles measuring 0.3 µm diameter, which fuse to create grains 20–30 µm in diameter. Although ceramic brackets demonstrate good aesthetics, they suffer from several potential disadvantages:

1. *Wear of opposing teeth*—Due to their hardness they can cause wear of opposing teeth, and it is for this reason they are used infrequently on lower arch teeth.[32,33]

2. *Risk of enamel fracture at debond*—It has been found that there is an increased risk of enamel fracture when debonding ceramic brackets. This will be discussed further in Section 7.2.8.

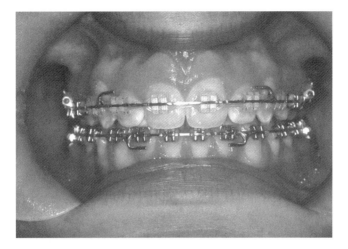

Fig. 7.15 Monocrystalline ceramic brackets in the upper arch.

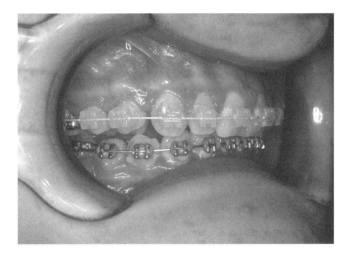

Fig. 7.16 Polycrystalline ceramic brackets in the upper arch.

3.   *Bracket fracture*—Due to the brittle nature of ceramic brackets it is not unusual for one or more tie-wings to fracture in service.[34] This is not only inconvenient, slowing treatment progress and perhaps requiring bracket replacement, but there is always the potential risk of the patient inhaling or swallowing the radiolucent bracket fragments.

4.   *Friction during sliding mechanics*—Friction between the archwire and bracket during sliding mechanics is undesirable. *In vitro* experiments have produced conflicting results as to whether ceramic brackets have a higher coefficient of friction than steel brackets. It has been suggested that ceramic brackets produce greater levels of friction than equivalent dimension steel brackets by some workers,[35] and contradictory lower levels by others.[25] It is

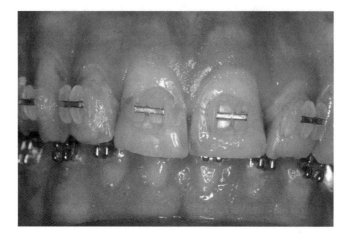

Fig. 7.17 Polycrystalline ceramic brackets with metal slot inserts to reduce friction.

probable that there is little difference between ceramic and steel brackets and that there are other factors, such as wire material and wire size, which are of greater importance.[30] However, some manufacturers have endeavoured to allay fears that the frictional coefficients of ceramic brackets might be higher than steel by incorporating steel slot inserts into their ceramic brackets (Fig. 7.17).

5.   *Cost*—Generally the cost of ceramic brackets is much higher than stainless-steel brackets.

7.2.3   Bands

Orthodontic bands were originally the only method of attaching brackets and tubes to the teeth. With the advent of direct bonding their use is now more restricted, being used mainly on posterior teeth, notably the molars, and particularly when headgear is to be attached to the upper first molars. They are also used when bonding might be difficult: such as on partially erupted teeth; where the enamel is defective, e.g. in cases of amelogenesis imperfecta; or when a bonded attachment repeatedly fails due to heavy occlusal forces. Bands are made from stainless steel and the bracket or tube is welded directly to it (Fig. 7.18). They are usually shaped to fit the contours of the tooth and are available in various sizes. The inner surface of the band is sometimes sandblasted, or laser- or micro-etched. Such surface treatment has been found to reduce the number of bands that become uncemented during treatment, particularly when cemented in place using glass polyalkenoate cement.[37]

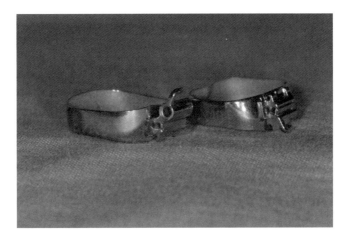

Fig. 7.18 Orthodontic bands with prewelded attachments.

7.2.4 Banding and bonding

There is some overlap in the use of materials for banding and bonding in orthodontics, although the enamel preparation will differ depending upon whether the material is to be used for banding or bonding. For simplicity the materials will be dealt with together, but reference will be made to their common usage, banding, bonding, or both.

Banding

Before band placement it is important to ensure the enamel surface is clean. It has been common practice to polish the enamel with a slurry of pumice, or a proprietary polishing paste, in a rubber cup using a slow-speed handpiece. There is, however, no evidence to suggest that this procedure improves the retention of the cemented band to the tooth. Therefore it could be argued that if the tooth is unclean and requires polishing prior to band placement, then the standard of toothbrushing is obviously insufficient for orthodontic appliance therapy to be contemplated.

Once the enamel is clean, the band can be cemented in place using one of a number of materials. Previously they were cemented using a material such as zinc phosphate cement, which largely acted as a gap filler between the band and the enamel surface. Today the materials used will often adhere to the enamel surface, the inner surface of the steel band, or to both and they are largely based on the glass polyalkenoate cements and their derivatives. With these materials the enamel surface should be clean, but there is no need for it to be dry since the materials are commonly water based. The inside of the band should also be clean.

Bonding

Prior to bond placement it has been common practice to prepare the enamel surface, with the type of preparation being dependent on the bonding agent to be used. The two broad types of materials in common usage are the acrylates, most notably the diacrylates, and the glass polyalkenoate cements and their derivatives. The possible stages of enamel pretreatment are:

- *Pumicing*—In all cases it has been customary to polish the enamel with a slurry of pumice in a rubber cup using a slow-speed handpiece in order to remove plaque and any pellicle that might interfere with subsequent enamel pretreatment and bonding. This step has been found to be unnecessary both with the diacrylates and the resin-modified glass polyalkenoate cements[38,39] If pumicing is being performed just to remove plaque, then it is questionable whether orthodontic treatment should be undertaken on a patient with such poor oral hygiene.

- *Enamel acid etching/conditioning*—Bonding to the enamel surface using the diacrylates relies on micromechanical retention. The enamel surface is therefore roughened to provide this mechanical retention by acid-etching using a solution or gel of 37% *o*-phosphoric acid for 15–30 seconds per tooth. The enamel surface is then washed with water and dried with oil-free compressed air until it is frosty white in appearance (Fig. 7.19). Etching of the tooth surface is possible due to the prismatic nature of enamel, and usually occurs preferentially at either the prism cores or prism boundaries.[40] The honeycomb pattern produced consists of pores 5–6 µm in diameter, etched to a depth of 50–60 µm into which the diacrylate can penetrate.[41] The diacrylate tags within the enamel surface provide the mechanical interlock. Subsequently, five types of etch pattern were recognized, namely: at the prism cores, prism boundaries, combinations of both these two, a pitted enamel surface unrelated to the prisms, and finally a flat smooth surface.[42,43] More recently, the boundary between the diacrylate tags and the etched enamel surface has been described as being less distinct than was first thought. Instead, an interfacial resin-enamel interdiffusion zone has been demonstrated, which may provide adhesion between the enamel and diacrylate that is more than just mechanical.[44]

When the glass polyalkenoate cements and their derivatives are used for direct bonding many different types of acid etchants have been suggested and tested, but the results of what are often laboratory tests are inconclusive. The etchants/conditioners tested include solutions of 37% *o*-phosphoric acid, 10% poly(acrylic) acid, and 10% maleic acid. Successful bonding *in vivo* is certainly possible without the need for acid etching/conditioning, as demonstrated by Silverman *et al.*[45] All teeth were bonded, including the first and second molars, using a resin-modified glass polyalkenoate cement and the observed bond failure rate was very low, being only 3.2% over an 8-month period. What is important, when using the glass polyalkenoate

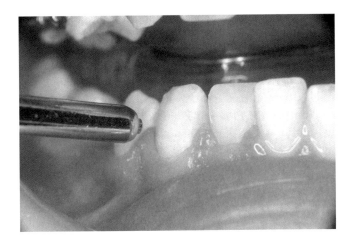

Fig. 7.19 Frosty white enamel after etching, washing, and drying.

cements and their derivatives for bonding, is that the enamel should be damp and must not be thoroughly dried prior to bond placement.

• *Washing and drying*—Following enamel etching with 37% *o*-phosphoric acid and prior to using the diacrylate resins, it is necessary to thoroughly wash the enamel surface with water. The Council on Dental Materials, Instruments and Equipment (1982) state that as a rule 10–15 seconds of rinsing with copious amounts of water per quadrant of the mouth is clinically acceptable. If an acid gel is used, washing for twice this time is recommended.[46] In reality, washing is usually performed for a much shorter time than this, otherwise moisture control is difficult. Contamination of etched enamel with saliva can reduce the effectiveness of the etch for subsequent bonding; if it does occur then the enamel should be etched for a further 10 seconds.[47] After rinsing it is necessary to thoroughly dry the enamel prior to bonding with diacrylate bonding agents. If an acid conditioner is used prior to the use of glass polyalkenoate cement or one of its derivatives, the enamel should still be washed, but must not be thoroughly dried prior to bonding.

• *Sealants and primers*—A low-viscosity sealant or primer may be placed on to an etched enamel surface prior to the use of a diacrylate bonding agent. This is to ensure the etched enamel surface is thoroughly wetted prior to using a higher viscosity, filled diacrylate bonding agent (see Section 7.2.5, Diacrylates). Unfortunately, the terms 'sealant' and 'primer' are often used synonymously. However, a sealant can usually be cured on the enamel surface independently from the filled diacrylate. On the other hand, primers are not usually cured independently from the filled resin, but may contain reactive components necessary for polymerization of the filled diacrylate that is to follow. Some primers contain HEMA (hydroxyethyl methacrylate), which is hydrophilic and therefore can be used when the etched enamel surface has been contaminated with moisture or even saliva.

• *Self-etching primers*—Recently, an enamel pretreatment for use prior to bonding with a light-cured diacrylate has become available, whereby the enamel is etched and primed in one step. No rinsing is required after etching. Called 'Transbond™ Plus Self Etching Primer' (3M Unitek) it contains an aqueous solution of methacrylated phosphoric acid esters. It is brushed on to the enamel surface for 3 seconds and then the solvent is evaporated by directing a gentle airburst at the tooth away from the gingivae. In this way an enamel etch pattern similar to that seen with the more conventional acid-etch technique is said to be produced. Self-etching primer is currently recommended for use with a visible light-cured diacrylate adhesive.

7.2.5 Banding and bonding materials

The materials used for banding and bonding are:
• diacrylates
• cyanoacrylates
• glass polyalkenoate cement
• glass polyphosphonate cement
• resin-modified glass polyalkenoate cement
• compomers (polyacid modified resin composites).
These will be dealt with in turn:

Diacrylates

Diacrylate bonding agents are used to bond brackets and tubes to teeth. They are often referred to as 'composite resins' and are most commonly based on the aromatic dimethacrylate monomer bis-glycidyl methacrylate (bis-GMA) or Bowen's resin.[48]

This monomer, like methyl methacrylate (see Section 7.1.1), undergoes free-radical addition polymerization. Its larger molecular structure, with side chains capable of undergoing cross-linking, means that it demonstrates both a lower polymerization shrinkage and coefficient of thermal expansion than methyl methacrylate-based adhesives. However, the large molecular structure also means that it is very viscous. In order to make it clinically usable it is diluted with lower viscosity dimethacrylate monomers, such as diethylene glycol dimethacrylate (DEGDMA) or triethylene glycol dimethacrylate (TEGDMA). In recent years other dimethacrylate monomers, such as urethane dimethacrylate (UDMA), have been used to substitute for all or some of the bis-GMA.

Having a lower viscosity, less of the other diluent monomers are required in urethane dimethacrylate-based adhesives, and they are said to be particularly useful for use in light-cured products.[49] Also present within the dimethacrylate are filler particles consisting of glass beads or rods, aluminium silicate, barium, strontium, and borosilicate glasses. The filler content of commercially available dimethacrylate (diacrylate) bonding agents can vary greatly and may form in the order of 15–80% by weight of the material. The term 'composite' applies only to those resin-based materials that contain at least 50% of filler by mass. Fillers reduce the polymerization shrinkage and coefficient of thermal expansion of the material as well as improving abrasion resistance. Whether these factors are important in the thin section found beneath orthodontic brackets is unclear. Indeed, orthodontic bonding using unfilled dimethacrylate alone may be possible. Nevertheless, most diacrylates used in orthodontic bonding today are filled because other factors, such as improved viscosity and ease of handling, are also important to the orthodontist. The filler particles are often silane-coated to promote adhesion to the dimethacrylate resin. The most commonly used silane is γ-methacryloxypropyltrimethoxysilane. Properties such as the Young's modulus, tensile and compressive strengths, and wear resistance are all increased when the filler particles are able to bond to the resin matrix.[50]

The setting mechanisms of the acrylics, of which the dimethacrylates are but one type, have already been discussed (see Section 7.1.1). In orthodontic bonding they are either chemically cured or light-cured, although dual-cured materials have been suggested for orthodontic use:

• *Chemically cured*—These materials are available in two forms, namely: Twin paste and 'No-mix'. In the Twin paste form the activator is within one paste and the initiator is within the other. Mixing the pastes causes the activator to react with the initiator to produce the necessary free radicals for addition polymerization to take place and for the material to set. In the 'No-mix' system the operator paints the initiator peroxide, which is within a fluid carrier, on to both the etched enamel surface and the bracket base. Following this, filled dimethacrylate resin containing the activator is applied to the bracket base. Once the bracket is applied to the tooth surface, rapid polymerization takes place as the thin sandwich of 'initiator/activator containing resin/initiator' is subsequently created. The use of such a 'No-mix' curing mechanism is only possible where the dimethacrylate is required in thin section, such as in orthodontic bonding. In thick section, polymerization would either be too slow, or may be incomplete within the bulk of the adhesive.

• *Light-cured*—The use of light-cured dimethacrylates for bonding metal orthodontic brackets was first described by Tavas and Watts.[51] Light-curing of bonding agents beneath metal brackets is made possible by transillumination through the enamel, whereas with ceramic brackets light will also pass through the bracket. Both metal and ceramic brackets are available with the dimethacrylate already on the bracket base, so-called Adhesive Pre Coat brackets (APC—3M Unitek). The light sources available to cure such adhesives include halogen, plasma arc lamps, and LED (light-emitting diode) lamps. Whatever the source it is important that the light has a wavelength of approximately 440–480 nm for photoinitiation to take place.

• *Dual-cured*—Combined chemically and light-cured bonding agents, known as 'dual cure', have also been tested as possible orthodontic bonding agents. The suggested advantages of their use include more accurate bracket positioning, easier removal of excess, and an assurance that complete polymerization will take place in thick section.[52] They are not commonly used in orthodontics, particularly since the bondline thickness of the adhesive in orthodontics is not usually a problem.

Cyanoacrylates

These adhesives were first developed by Jeremias[53] of Eastman Kodak. Like other acrylates, cyanoacrylate monomer can be polymerized by free-radical addition, although it more usually undergoes anionic addition. It is this latter mechanism that has given the cyanoacrylates very attractive properties as adhesives, since they can be initiated by weak bases such as water. Cyanoacrylates can therefore cure very rapidly when in contact with only the smallest amounts of moisture, as is present on most surfaces. Unfortunately, they have not been demonstrated to be useful orthodontic bonding agents.[54-56] This is probably due to their limited moisture resistance on metal substrates. Water ingress along metal oxide coatings, such as the passive layer found on a stainless-steel orthodontic bracket, will lead to hydrolytic degradation of the cyanoacrylate monomer and eventual failure of the bond.[57,58]

Glass polyalkenoate cements

These cements were first introduced in 1972 and are otherwise known as 'glass ionomer cements'. Their principal use in orthodontics is as a band cement, although they have been used with limited success to directly bond brackets to teeth. They have two main components:
• liquid—an aqueous solution of an organic acid, such as poly(acrylic), poly(maleic) acid; and
• powder—consists of ion-leachable glasses, namely calcium alumino-fluorosilicate glasses.

On mixing the powder and the liquid there is an acid–base reaction between the organic acid and the basic glass powder. Calcium and aluminium ions are released from the surface of the glass, with the former being released more quickly than the latter. Calcium polyacrylate chains form and the cement demonstrates changes in consistency. At this point it is said to enter the gelation stage. As setting continues, the aluminium ions also become incorporated into the gel and begin to form a cross-linked calcium–aluminium carboxylate gel. The cement then gradually becomes hydrated and enters what is known as the maturation phase. In the mixing

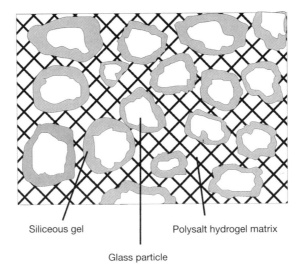

Siliceous gel   Polysalt hydrogel matrix

Glass particle

Fig. 7.20 Diagram of set glass polyalkenoate cement.

of these cements there is an excess of powder and so the acid–base reaction creates a final heterogeneous set material of glass particles coated in a siliceous gel, all surrounded by a polysalt hydrogel matrix (Fig. 7.20).

Zinc phosphate cements were the mainstay orthodontic band cements for many years, but the newer glass polyalkenoate cements have a number of advantages over the formerly used cements. These include: adhesion both to enamel and to stainless steel, a lower solubility once set, and the theoretical ability to show sustained fluoride release. However, the first-generation glass polyalkenoates were particularly susceptible to moisture contamination, a problem that has been largely overcome with the second-generation glass polyalkenoates. In the latter, the liquid may be water or an aqueous solution of tartaric acid, and the powder a blend of aluminosilicate glass and a powdered polyacid. These cements certainly show increased fluoride release soon after band placement, but this falls rapidly with time. Fluoride will be released if the cement begins to dissolve, particularly in an acidic environment, as perhaps might occur at a potentially carious site. Such a site can be beneath an orthodontic band. Certainly decalcification rates beneath bands have been reported to be lower with glass polyalkenoate cements than with the older zinc phosphate cements.[59]

Glass polyphosphonate cement

These cements have been available for use in restorative dentistry for some time and have recently been tried clinically as orthodontic band cements. They have been found to be as effective at retaining the bands, but with a less unpleasant taste, than the glass polyalkenoate cements.[60]

Resin-modified glass polyalkenoate cement

First available in the early 1990s, these cements differ from the glass polyalkenoate cements in that they also possess a resin component, namely HEMA (hydroxyethyl methacrylate). This can form up to 10% of the cement and can be chemically or light activated. Resin-modified glass polyalkenoate cements are supplied as a powder and a liquid and demonstrate the acid–base reaction described for the glass polyalkenoate cements; also, the HEMA undergoes polymerization to form polyHEMA. In orthodontics they have been used mainly as an alternative to the diacrylates as bonding agents, although, like the glass polyalkenoates. they can also be used as band cements. When used for direct bonding, reported clinical bond failure rates have been found to be comparable with those seen using diacrylate bonding agents. This appears to be so whether the enamel has been pre-treated using poly(acrylic acid) conditioner or not.[45,61] Where very high bond failure rates have been reported for resin-modified glass polyalkenoate cements, the enamel has been dried excessively prior to bond placement.[62] It is important that the enamel remains moist prior to bond placement regardless of whether it has been etched or conditioned beforehand.

Compomers (polyacid-modified resin composites)

These differ from resin-modified glass polyalkenoate cements principally in the size of the resin component, which is in the order of 30 50%.[63] Compomers are supplied as single-component materials within a syringe or a compule. They are light-cured, with the resin component undergoing free-radical addition polymerization following photoinitiation. Although the remainder of the compomer is similar in composition to a glass polyalkenoate cement, the acid–base reaction can only take place in the presence of water. Water is not actively mixed with the cement during placement, but must diffuse into the polymeric matrix from the saliva once the material is in place beneath the bracket. Therefore the extent of the acid–base reaction will of necessity be fairly limited. The clinical bond failure rates of brackets bonded using compomer have been found to be comparable to those seen with diacrylate bonding agents. However, because the filler particles release fluoride once water has diffused into the set material, the compomer may have the additional advantage of reducing the risk of in-treatment decalcification.[64]

7.2.6   Elastomeric products

The elastomeric products used in orthodontics include separators, ligatures, bands, and chains and are usually made from latex or polyurethane. An elastomer can be considered to be a material that can be stretched many times its original length without breaking, and that will return to its original size when it is released. Elastomers are high molecular weight amorphous polymers consisting of linear molecules that are convoluted and in random motion within the bulk of the material. An amorphous polymer being one whose polymer chains are not arranged as ordered crystals. These polymer chains can uncoil and slide past each other, although there may be some degree of cross-linking between the chains that will limit the sliding movement. The greater the degree of cross-linking, the higher the elastic modulus (stiffness) of the material. If a tensile force is applied to an elastomer, the long chains begin to unfold and take up a more ordered alignment. If the material is sufficiently strained, the molecules will become so ordered that the elastomer will begin to crystallize and eventually the covalent bonds within the chains and cross-links will begin to break. This is known as 'strain-induced crystallization'. If the force is removed before this point is reached, the material will return to its original shape without any plastic deformation. Should the primary bonds break, exceeding the elastic limit of the material, some permanent deformation will occur and it will not return to its original shape.

The behaviour of elastomers is, however, not this straightforward, because they also exhibit a property known as 'viscoelasticity'. If the material is cooled, the motion of the molecules within the material is reduced and it behaves like a glassy solid. Above a certain temperature, known as the 'glass transition temperature' (T_g), the material behaves more like a rubber. As the temperature continues to rise even further, the motion between the molecules can increase to such an extent that the material will behave more like a viscous liquid (Fig. 7.21). The glass transition temperature is dependent on a number of factors, such as the principal molecular structure of the elastomer, any side-chain molecules, or any cross-linking, all of which can increase the T_g. On the other hand, the presence of plasticizers (i.e. lower molecular weight materials that are able to penetrate between the large molecular chains of the elastomer) has the effect of lowering the T_g. In orthodontics, the T_g of some of the elastomeric materials so far discussed should be below room temperature if they are to be rubbery for use in the mouth.

Elastomers also demonstrate other unusual properties, namely:

• *Creep*—This is the time-dependent permanent deformation that occurs when the material is subjected to a constant load.

• *Stress-relaxation*—As the name suggests, this is the decrease in stress that occurs with time when an elastomer is subjected to constant strain. An example in orthodontics would be when an elastic tie is holding an archwire in a bracket slot. Some stress-relaxation will also inevitably occur in powerchain stretched between teeth, or from a tooth such as the first molar to a hook on the archwire between the lateral incisor and canine. This is because tooth movement is relatively slow and can almost be considered as keeping the elastomeric powerchain under constant strain (see 'Elastomeric chain' below).

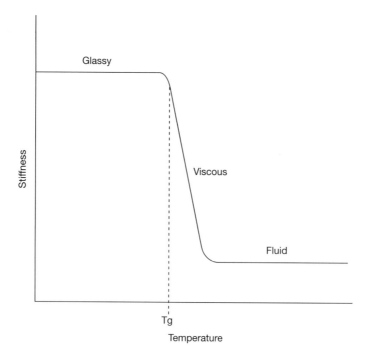

Fig. 7.21 Viscoelasticity of an elastomer.

• *Hysteresis*—This is the loss of mechanical energy seen between the loading and unloading curves for an elastomer on a stress–strain curve. Therefore the force applied by an elastomeric chain or thread used to move tooth will be less than the force applied to stretch the elastic in the first instance.

• *Hysteresis loss*—With repeated loading and unloading, energy will be repeatedly lost at each cycle (Fig. 7.22). This might occur when a patient is wearing intermaxillary elastics, where the elastic bands will undergo loading and unloading as the patient repeatedly opens and closes their mouth during the day.

The following list includes examples of elastomerics used in orthodontics, these are either die-stamped or injection-moulded to create the desired shape during manufacture:

• *Separators*—These are placed at the interstices, usually between molar and or premolar teeth, in order to move adjacent teeth apart. This happens over a relatively short period of a week, so that an orthodontic band carrying a bracket, or more often a tube, can be cemented around the tooth. A not uncommon problem with elastic separators is that they move subgingivally and can be both difficult to see and to remove (Fig. 7.23). Visibility is improved by colouring the separators blue. Some are also radiopaque.

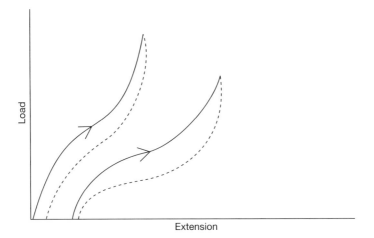

Fig. 7.22 Hysteresis loss.

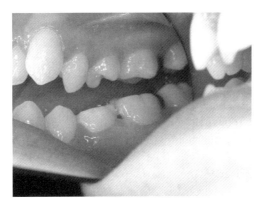

Fig. 7.23 Blue elastic separators on a lower molar tooth. Notice how the mesial elastic has slipped subgingivally.

- *Elastomeric ties*—These are used to retain the archwire in the bracket slot. Some are available with fluoride-releasing abilities, and, although they are less elastic and more prone to discolouration and swelling in intraoral use than conventional elastomeric ties, their use can dramatically reduce the incidence of enamel decalcification.[65] Elastomeric ties are routinely changed every 4–6 weeks during treatment and so this fluoride-releasing effect can be sustained throughout treatment. Elastomeric ties are available in multiple colours in an attempt to improve patient motivation towards their orthodontic treatment (Fig. 7.24). More recently, elastomeric ties have been produced with a water-insoluble coating in an attempt to reduce friction as the archwire slides between the bracket base and the elastomeric tie.

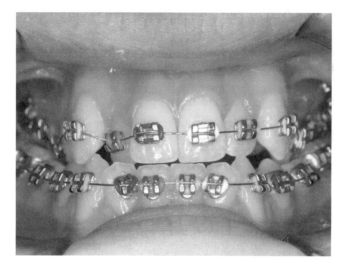

Fig. 7.24 Coloured elastomeric modules used to hold the archwires in place.

- *Elastomeric chain*—This consists of a number of elastomeric ties in series and is used to move or hold adjacent teeth together (Fig. 7.25). However, like any elastomer they undergo stress-relaxation and within a relatively short time will lose much of their activation, up to 50% within the first 24 hours. They are also greatly affected by the presence of heat, moisture, foodstuffs, pH,[66] and also by oral bacteria (Fig. 7.26). Water has certainly been shown to act as a plasticizer in the case of polyurethane,[67] which will have the

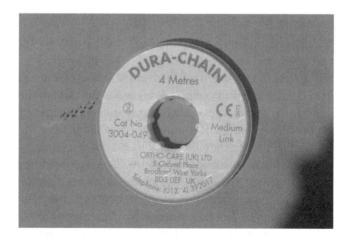

Fig. 7.25 Elastomeric chain on the reel.

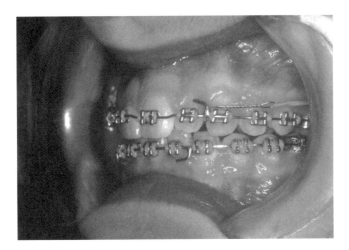

Fig. 7.26 Notice how the elastomeric modules have become swollen in the lower arch due to the poor oral hygiene.

same effect as lowering the glass transition temperature and making the material behave more like a viscous liquid rather than a rubbery solid. All these factors will help to contribute to the dramatic force decay exhibited by elastomeric materials used in orthodontics.

• *Elastomeric thread*—This fine thread can be tied around part or all of a bracket and then tied to the archwire in order to effect movement of a tooth or teeth (Fig. 7.27).

• *Elastomeric tube*—This fine tube is used in the same circumstances as elastomeric thread. In both cases the orthodontist ties one or more knots in

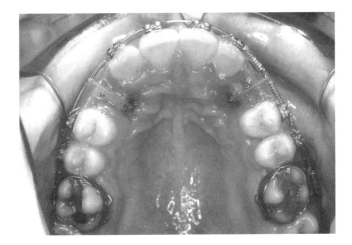

Fig. 7.27 Elastomeric thread used to move palatally positioned canines buccally.

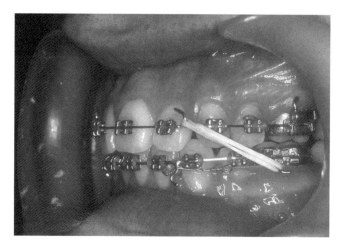

Fig. 7.28 Class II intermaxillary elastics.

the thread/tube during placement. Tubes are thought to offer more resistance to the knot coming undone than thread.

• *Intermaxillary elastics*—These are usually placed and replaced by the patient each day and pass from one arch to the other either as Class II or Class III intermaxillary traction, or sometimes as a cross elastic (Fig. 7.28). They are available in different sizes so that the orthodontist can alter the force applied.

• *Extraoral elastics*—These are used with headgear, either to reinforce anchorage or to apply a distalizing force. Such elastics are still susceptible to stress-relaxation, but being outside the mouth they lose their activation much less rapidly than intraoral elastics. Extraoral elastics should be replaced approximately every 5 days.

7.2.7 Auxiliary components

• *Coil springs*—Coil springs are available as open or closed coils, and are available on a reel or sometimes as individual springs with eyelets on either end. Springs on a reel can be made from stainless steel, cobalt–chromium (Fig. 7.29), or superelastic (austenitic active) nickel–titanium.

• *Auxiliary springs*—Made from stainless steel they are used with the Tip-Edge appliance and occasionally with the Straight-wire® appliance if the bracket has a vertical slot (Broussard slot) behind the archwire slot (Fig. 7.30).

• *Ligatures*—These are made from soft-grade stainless steel and are available in sizes ranging from 0.008 (0.2 mm) up to 0.014 inches (0.35 mm). White ligatures are produced with a Teflon coating in order to improve

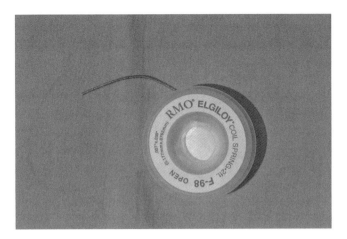

Fig. 7.29 Cobalt–chromium coil spring on the reel.

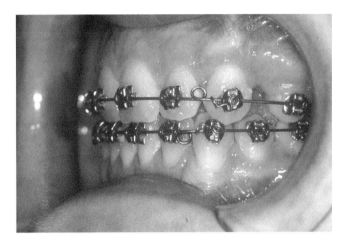

Fig. 7.30 Tip-edge brackets with sidewinder springs slotting in vertical slots within the brackets on the canines.

aesthetics and also to help reduce friction between the archwire and ligature during sliding mechanics.

• *Hooks*—Archwire hooks can be bent into the wire, soldered, screwed, or crimped on to the wire. Soldered hooks are usually made from brass and rectangular steel archwires can be purchased with the two such hooks presoldered in place. The clinician only has to choose the correct interhook distance, using a pair of dividers (Fig. 7.31). Screw hooks consist of a steel tube and a grub screw, which is tightened on to the wire using an Allen key. Screw hooks tend to be rather bulky, but have the advantage that their

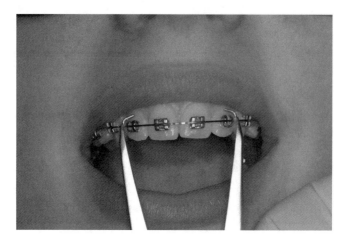

Fig. 7.31 Choosing the correct interhook distance for soldered archwire hooks.

position can easily be changed during treatment. Crimpable hooks are usually open-backed and have a tungsten-carbide coating on the part of the hook that is to be crimped on to the wire. These hooks are very easy to place but require a specifically designed set of crimping pliers to affix them to the wire. Unlike the screw hook they cannot be moved once crimped into position.

7.2.8   Debonding/debanding

Metal bracket removal

Metal brackets are easily removed using bond removing pliers (Fig. 7.32). The beaks of the pliers are placed beneath the tie-wings and above the bracket base and the bracket is gently but rapidly squeezed. It is not necessary to remove the archwires prior to bracket removal. Indeed, it is often easier to leave them in place since it reduces the risk of accidental aspiration/ingestion of the brackets.

Bond failure can occur at a number of sites:
(1) cohesive failure within the bracket;
(2) adhesive failure at the bracket base/bonding agent interface;
(3) cohesive failure within the bonding agent;
(4) adhesive failure at the enamel/bonding agent interface;
(5) cohesive within the enamel;
(6) a mixed mode of failure (usually (2), (3), and (4)).

Failure of metal brackets is usually mixed mode (6), namely sites (2), (3), and (4). However, microscopically, when a diacrylate bonding agent is used to bond the brackets to the teeth, any failure at the enamel interface may involve some cohesive enamel failure. This is due the mechanical interlock created by the acid-etch technique and the bonding resin tags penetrating

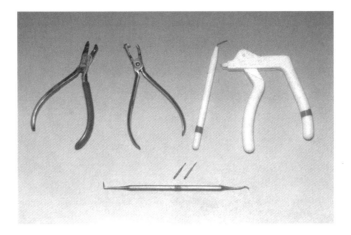

Fig. 7.32 Various instruments used for debanding, debonding, and enamel clean-up.

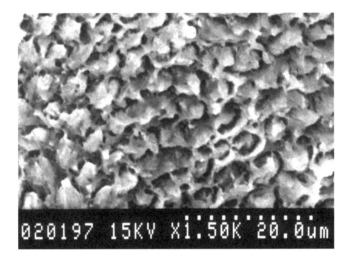

Fig. 7.33 Etched enamel surface prior to bonding. The adhesive resin tags can readily penetrate this surface.

the enamel surface (Fig. 7.33). It has therefore been suggested[68] that failure should be encouraged at sites (2) and (3) in order to preserve the enamel. Thus residual adhesive needs to be removed from this surface following bracket removal.

Ceramic bracket removal

Ceramic brackets are not so easy to remove from the tooth at completion of treatment. When a force is applied to the bracket during the debonding procedure it is hoped that a crack will initiate and propagate along either the bracket base/bonding agent interface (adhesive failure), through the bond-

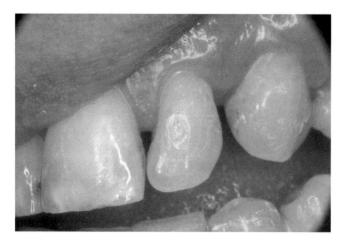

Fig. 7.34 Notice the fractured enamel surface in the centre of the upper lateral incisor tooth following ceramic bracket removal.

ing agent (cohesive failure), or at both sites (mixed mode). In this way the ceramic bracket will come off in one piece and the enamel will remain undamaged. However, the brittle nature of the enamel and ceramic means that both are at risk of fracture during debonding. Surface or bulk imperfections within either material can lead to crack initiation and propagation under an applied load, as occurs during debonding[69] (Fig. 7.34). To reduce this risk of enamel failure, bracket manufacturers have tried to control the site of crack initiation and propagation, restricting it to the bracket base/bonding agent interface or within the bracket itself. Examples include producing a ceramic bracket with a polycarbonate shim base, or an epoxy resin base. At debond the bracket is easily removed, leaving behind the polycarbonate or epoxy resin base on the tooth. It is then simply a matter of removing the base and any bonding agent from the enamel surface using a spiral fluted tungsten-carbide bur in a slow-speed handpiece. An alternative design is to introduce a notch into the ceramic bracket, this will act as a stress raiser and initiate crack propagation within the bracket rather than the enamel.[70] Where no such design features have been incorporated into the bracket, the debonding pliers used with metal brackets can be used to remove the ceramic bracket. Care must be taken to remove any excess composite from around the periphery of the bracket base and the beaks of the pliers must be applied close to the enamel surface at the margin of the bonding material. In this way the bracket and enamel will hopefully remain intact and crack propagation will be within the bonding agent. Other methods of ceramic bracket removal have included electrothermal bracket debonding and chemical action on the bonding resin. With electrothermal debonding, the bracket is gripped by an electrical instrument that softens the adhesive by rapidly heating it to above its glass transition temperature

(T_g). Although preserving the enamel surface, some concern has been expressed that the concomitant rise in the intrapulpal temperature may lead to pulpal inflammation.[71] However, much of the work has been performed on young teeth with large pulps and yet most ceramic brackets are likely to be fitted to older patients with more dentine between the heat source and pulp tissue. Certainly the chances of enamel surface damage are reduced when the electrothermal debonder is used.[72] The use of peppermint oil to plasticize diacrylate bonding resins, and therefore make debonding easier and safer for the enamel, has been suggested. However, it has not been found to be very effective in softening the bonding agent.[73] If it were to be clinically useful, it may take a long time to work if the very small area of exposed bonding agent at the periphery of the bonded joint is considered.

Band removal

Bands are relatively easily removed at the completion of treatment using band-removing pliers. Most of these pliers have a polythene or soft metal stop on one beak, which is applied to the occlusal surface of the tooth, and a sharp beak that is able to engage the edge of the band at the gingival margin. Lower bands should be removed from the buccal surface and upper bands from the palatal surface. This is because the lower buccal and upper palatal surfaces of the teeth are curved, enabling the band to slide off easily. Care must be exercised when using band-removing pliers on teeth with a large restoration. In such instances, a cotton wool roll should be held on the occlusal surface before applying the band-removing pliers. Bands are occasionally used on incisor teeth and anterior band-removing pliers are also available. Even more care is required when removing bands from these teeth. Cotton wool can be applied to the incisal edge to try to protect the tooth. Alternatively, the band can be split using a diamond bur in an air rotor and then more easily removed with the pliers.

Residual adhesive removal and enamel clean-up

Following bracket and band removal, residual adhesive almost invariably remains on the enamel surface. Various methods have been suggested as to how it is best removed, including the use of:
- hand instruments, such as a Mitchell's trimmer or a watch-spring scaler;
- an ultrasonic scaler;
- slow-speed rotary instruments, such as rubber wheels, spiral fluted tungsten-carbide burs, with or without water cooling;
- high-speed rotary instruments, such as diamond or spiral fluted tungsten-carbide burs, with or without water-cooling.

In general, the more lightly filled the diacrylate bonding agent the easier it is to remove the residual adhesive using hand instruments. Heavily filled materials require the use of rotary instruments. The use of rotary instruments leads to more enamel loss than hand instruments, but it is still easy to gouge the enamel surface with the inadvertent use of hand instruments.[74] A spiral fluted, tungsten-carbide bur in a slow-speed handpiece has been shown to be the most useful means of removing residual adhesive.[75] It has the least destructive effect on the enamel surface, although enamel loss will still be in the region of 7–8 μm.[76]

7.3   SUMMARY OF ORTHODONTIC MATERIALS

The materials used in orthodontics include:
1. Removable/functional appliance materials:
   • Acrylic—heat-cured, light-cured, and cold-cured;
   • Wires—stainless steel, cobalt–chromium.
2. Fixed appliance materials:
   • Archwires—stainless steel, nickel–titanium alloy, titanium–molybdenum alloy, titanium–niobium alloy, cobalt–chromium, aesthetic;
   • Bracket/bands—metals, polymers, ceramics;
   • Bonding/banding materials—diacrylates, cyanoacrylates, glass polyalkenoate cement, glass polyphosphonate cement, resin-modified glass polyalkenoate cement, compomers (polyacid-modified resin composites);
   • Elastomerics—separators, ties, chain, thread, tube, intermaxillary and extraoral elastics;
   • Auxiliary components—nickel–titanium springs, hooks, ligatures
   • Debanding/debonding—bracket removal, band removal, and enamel clean-up.

7.4   OBJECTIVES

To understand the following with respect to orthodontic materials:
(1) physical properties
(2) chemical properties
(3) mechanical properties
(4) their application in orthodontics
(5) their interaction with each other and the oral environment.

REFERENCES

1. Read, M. J. F. (1984). The bonding of orthodontic attachments using a visible light cured adhesive. *British Journal of Orthodontics*, **11**, 16–20.
2. Dart, E. C. and Nemcek, J. (1975). *Photopolymerisable composition*. UK Patent 1 408 265.
3. Taira, M., Urabe, H., Hirose, T., Wakasa, K., and Yamaki, M. (1988). Analysis of photo-initiators in visible light-cured dental composite resins. *Journal of Dental Research*, **67**, 24–8.

4. Muira, F., Nakagawa, K. and Masuhara, E. (1971). New direct bonding systems for plastic brackets. *American Journal of Orthodontics*, **51**, 350–61.

5. Kusy, R. P. (1997). A review of contemporary archwires: their properties and characteristics. *Angle Orthodontist*, **3**, 197–207.

6. Brader, A. C. (1972). Dental arch form related with intraoral forces: PR = C. *American Journal of Orthodontics*, **61**, 541–61.

7. Stephens C. D., Houston W. J. B., and Waters N. E. (1971). Multiple-strand wires. *Dental Practitioner*, **22**, 147–9.

8. Buehler, W. J. Wiley, R. C. (1965). Nickel-based alloys, U.S. patent 3,174,851. 23 March 1965.

9. Buehler, W. J. (1963). *Proceedings of the 7th Naval Science Symposium*. Volume 1 unclassified. Washington DC, Office of Naval Research—16. Office of Technical Services. US Department of Commerce, Washington, DC.

10. Buehler, W. J., Gilfrick, J. V. and Wiley, R. C. (1963). Effects of low temperature phase changes on the mechanical properties of alloys-near composition TiNi. *Journal of Applied Physics*, **34**, 1475–84.

11. Buehler, W. J. and Wiley, R. C. (1962). TiNi—ductile intermetallic compound. *Transactions of the American Society of Mechanical Engineers*, **55**, 269–76.

12. Kusy, R. P. (1997). A review of contemporary archwires: their properties and characteristics. *Angle Orthodontist*, **67**, 197–207.

13. Goldberg, A. J., Morton, J., and Burstone, C. J. (1983). The flexure modulus of elasticity of orthodontic wires. *Journal of Dental Research*, **62**, 856–8.

14. Miura, F., Mogi, M., and Ohura, Y. (1988). Japanese NiTi alloy wire: use of the direct electric resistance heat treatment method. *European Journal of Orthodontics*, **10**, 187–91.

15. Okamoto, Y., Hamanaka, H., Miura, F., Tamura, H., and Horikawa, H. (1988). Reversible changes in yield stress and transformation temperature of a NiTi alloy by alternate heat treatments. *Scripta Metallurgica*, **22**, 517–20.

16. Miura, F., Mogi, M., and Okamato, Y. (1990). New application of superelastic NiTi rectangular wire. *Journal of Clinical Orthodontics*, **14**, 544–8.

17. Burstone, C. J., Bai Oin, M. S., and Morton, J. Y. (1985). Chinese NiTi wire. *American Journal of Orthodontics and Dentofacial Orthopedics*, **87**, 445–52.

18. Chang, L. C. and Read, T. A. (1932). *Transactions of AIME*, **191**, 47.

19. Hodgson, D. E., Wu, M. H., and Biermann, R. J. (1999). Shape memory alloys. http://www.sma-inc,com/SMAPaper.html

20. Williams, D. E. (1986). Special Metals Corp, Hartford, NY, private communication. Cited in Kusy, R. P. A. (1997). Review of contemporary archwires: their properties and characteristics. *Angle Orthodontist*, **67**, 197–207.

21. Andreasen, G. F. (1980). A clinical trial of alignment of teeth using a 0.019 inch thermal nitinol wire with a transition temperature range between 31 °C and 45 °C. *American Journal of Orthodontics*, **78**, 528–37.

22. Roberts-Harry, D. P. and Harradine, N. W. (1995). A sectional approach to the alignment of ectopic maxillary canines. *British Journal of Orthodontics*, **22**, 67–70.

23. Dalstra, M., Denes, G., and Melsen, B. (2000). Titanium–niobium, a new finishing wire alloy. *Clinical Orthodontics and Research*, **3**, 6–14.

24. Fillmore, G. M. and Tomlinson, J. L. (1976). Heat treatment of cobalt–chromium alloy wire. *Angle Orthodontist*, **49**, 187–95.

25. Ireland, A. J., Sherriff, M., and McDonald, F. (1991). Effect of bracket and wire composition on frictional forces. *European Journal of Orthodontics*, **13**, 322–8.

26. Zufall, S. W. and Kusy, R. P. (2000). Stress relaxation and recovery behaviour of composite orthodontic archwires in bending. *European Journal of Orthodontics*, **22**, 1–12.

27. Al-Waheidi, E. M. H. (1995). Allergic reaction to nickel orthodontic wires: a case report. *Quintessence International*, **26**, 385–7.

28. Menne, T. (1994). Quantitative aspects of nickel dermatitis. Sensitization and eliciting threshold concentrations. *The Science of the Total Environment*, **148**, 275–81.

29. Menne, T. and Calvin, G. (1993). Concentration threshold of non-occluded nickel exposure in nickel-sensitive individuals and controls with and without surfactant. *Contact Dermatitis*, **29**, 180–4.

30. Feldner, J. C., Sarkar, N. K., Shendan, J. J., and Lancaster, D. M. (1994). *In vitro* torque-deformation characteristics of orthodontic polycarbonate brackets. *American Journal of Orthodontics and Dentofacial Orthopedics*, **106**, 265–72.

31. Swartz, M. (1988). Ceramic brackets. *Journal of Clinical Orthodontics*, **22**, 82–8.

32. Douglass, J. B. (1989). Enamel wear caused by ceramic brackets. *American Journal of Orthodontics and Dentofacial Orthopedics*, **95**, 96–8.

33. Viazis, A. D., DeLong, R., Bevis, R. R., Douglas, W. H., and Speidel, T. M. (1989). Enamel surface abrasion from ceramic orthodontic brackets: a special case report. *American Journal of Orthodontics and Dentofacial Orthopedics*, **96**, 514–18.

34. Gibbs, S. L. (1992). Clinical performance of ceramic brackets: a survey of British orthodontist's experience. *British Journal of Orthodontics*, **19**, 191–7.

35. Angolkar, P. V., Kapila, S., Duncanson, M. G., and Nanda, R. S. (1990). Evaluation of friction between ceramic brackets and wires. *American Journal of Orthodontics and Dentofacial Orthopedics*, **98**, 499–506.

36. Kusy, R. P. and Whitley, J. Q. (1990). Coefficients of friction for arch wires in bracket. *American Journal of Orthodontics and Dentofacial Orthopedics*, **98**, 300–12.

37. Hodges, S. J., Gilthorpe, M. S., and Hunt, N. P. (2001). The effect of micro-etching on the retention of orthodontic molar bands: a clinical trial. *European Journal of Orthodontics*, **23**, 91–7.

38. Barry, G. R. (1995). A clinical investigation of the effects of omission of pumice prophylaxis on band and bond failure. *British Journal of Orthodontics*, **22**, 245–8.

39. Ireland, A. J. and Sherriff, M. (2002). The effect of pumicing on the *in vivo* use of a resin modified glass polyalkenoate cement and a conventional no-mix composite for bonding orthodontic brackets. *Journal of Orthodontics*, **29**, 217–20.

40. Gwinnett, A. J. (1971). Histological changes in human enamel following treatment with acidic conditioning agents. *Archives of Oral Biology*, **16**, 731–8.

41. Retief, D. H. (1973). Effect of conditioning the enamel surface with phosphoric acid. *Journal of Dental Research*, **52**, 333–41.

42. Silverstone, L. M., Saxton, C. A., Dogon, I. L., and Fejerskov, O. (1975). Variation in the pattern of acid etching of human dental enamel examined by scanning electron microscopy. *Caries Research*, **9**, 373–87.

43. Galil, K. A. and Wright, G. Z. (1979). Acid etching patterns on buccal surfaces of permanent teeth. *Pediatric Dentistry*, **1**, 230–4.

44. Brantley, W. A. and Eliades, T. (2001). *Orthodontic materials. Scientific and clinical aspects*. Thieme, Stuttgart.

45. Silverman, E., Cohen, M., Demke, R. S., Silverman, M., and Linwood, N. J. (1995). A new light-cured glass ionomer cement that bonds brackets to teeth without etching in the presence of saliva. *American Journal Orthodontics and Dentofacial Orthopedics*, **108**, 231–6.

46. Council on Dental Materials, Instruments and Equipment (1982). State of the art and science of bonding in orthodontic treatment. *Journal of the American Dental Association*, **105**, 844–50.

47. Hormati, A. A., Fuller, J. L., and Denehy, G. E. (1980). The effects of contamination and mechanical disturbance on the quality of acid etched enamel. *Journal of the American Dental Association*, **100**, 34–8.

48. Bowen, R. L. (1962). *Dental filling materials comprising vinyl silane treated fused silica and a binder consisting of the reaction product of bisphenol and glycidyl methacrylate*. US Patent 066, 112.

49. Watts, D. C. (2001). Orthodontic adhesive resins and composites: principles of adhesion. In *Orthodontic materials, scientific and clinical aspects* (ed. W. A. Brantley and T. Eliades), pp. 189–200. Thieme, Stuttgart.

50. Söderholm, K-J. M. (1985). Filler systems and resin interface. *International symposium on posterior composite resin dental restorative materials*. 3M Co., St Paul, Minnesota.

51. Tavas, M. A. and Watts, D. C. (1979). Bonding of orthodontic brackets by trans-illumination of a light-activated composite: an *in-vitro* study. *British Journal of Orthodontics* **6**, 207–8.

52. Smith, R. T. and Shivapuja, P. K. (1993). The evaluation of dual cement resins in orthodontic bonding. *American Journal of Orthodontics and Dentofacial Orthopedics*, **103**, 448–51.

53. Jeremias, C. G. (1956). *Process for making cyanoacrylates*. U S Patent 2,763,677.

54. Howells, D. J. and Jones, P. (1989). *In vitro* evaluation of a cyanoacrylate bonding agent. *British Journal of Orthodontics*, **16**, 75–8.

55. Crabb, J. J. and Wilson, H. J. (1971). Use of some adhesives in orthodontics. *Dental Practitioner*, **22**, 111—12.

56. Al-Munajed, M. K., Gordon, P. H., and McCabe, J. F. (2000). The use of a cyano-acrylate adhesive for bonding orthodontic brackets: an *ex-vivo* study. *Journal of Orthodontics*, **27**, 255–60.

57. Leonard, F. R., Kulkarni, R. K., Brandes, G., Nelson, J., and Cameron, J. J. (1966). Synthesis and degradation of poly(alkyl α-cyanoacrylates). *Journal of Applied Polymer Science*, **10**, 259–72.

58. Drain, K. F., Guthrie, J., Leung, C. L., Martin, F. R., and Otterburn, M. S. (1984). The effect of moisture on the bond strength of steel–steel cyanoacrylate adhesive bonds. *Journal of Adhesion*, **17**, 71–82.

59. Kvam, E., Broch, J. and Nissen-Meyer, I. (1988). Comparison between a zinc phosphate and a glass ionomer cement for cementation of orthodontic bands. *European Journal of Orthodontics*, **5**, 307–13.

60. Clark, J. R., Ireland, A. J. and Sherriff, M. (2003). An *in vivo* and *ex vivo* study to evaluate the use of a glass polyphosphonate cement in orthodontic banding. *European Journal of Orthodontics*. (In press)

61. Choo, S. C., Ireland, A. J. and Sherriff, M. (2001). An *in vivo* investigation into the use of resin modified glass poly(alkenoate) cements as orthodontic bonding agents. *European Journal of Orthodontics*, **23**, 403–9.

62. Cacciafesta, V., Bosch, C. and Melsen, B. (1999). Clinical comparison between a resin-reinforced self-cured glass ionomer cement and a composite resin for direct bonding of orthodontic brackets. Part 2: Bonding on dry enamel and on enamel soaked with saliva. *Clinical Orthodontic Research*, **2**, 186–93.

63. Gladys, S., Van Meerbeek, B., Braem, M., Lambrechts, P., and Vanherle, G. (1997). Comparative physico-mechanical characterization of new hybrid restorative materials with conventional glass-ionomer and resin composite restorative materials. *Journal of Dental Research*, **76**, 883–94.

64. Millett, D. T., McCluskey, L. A., McAuley, F., Creanor, S. L., Newell, J., and Love, J. (2000). A comparative clinical trial of a compomer and a resin adhesive for orthodontic bonding. *Angle Orthodontist*, **70**, 233–40.

65. Banks, P. A., Chadwick, S. M., Ascher-McDade, C., and Wright, J. L. (2000). Fluoride-releasing elastomerics—a prospective controlled clinical trial. *European Journal of Orthodontics*, **22**, 401–7.

66. Nattrass, C. N., Ireland, A. J., and Sherriff, M. (1998). The effect of environmental factors on elastomeric chain and nickel titanium coil springs. *European Journal of Orthodontics*, **20**, 169–76.

67. Huget, E. F., Patrick, K. S., and Nunez, L. J. (1990). Observations on the elastic behaviour of a synthetic orthodontic elastomer. *Journal of Dental Research*, **69**, 496–501.

68. Retief, D. H. (1974). Failure at the dental adhesive–etched enamel interface. *Journal of Oral Rehabilitation*, **1**, 265–84.

69. Winchester, L. (1992). Methods of debonding ceramic brackets. *British Journal of Orthodontics*, **19**, 233–7.

70. Bishara, S. E. (1997). Evaluation of debonding characteristics of a new collapsible ceramic bracket. *American Journal of Orthodontics and Dentofacial Orthopedics*, **112**, 552–9.

71. Dovgan, J. S., Walton, R. E., and Bishara, S. E. (1995). Electrothermal debracketing: patient acceptance and effects on the dental pulp. *American Journal of Orthodontics and Dentofacial Orthopedics*, **108**, 249–55.

72. Crooks, M., Hood, J., and Harkness, M. (1997). Thermal debonding of ceramic brackets: an *in vitro* study. *American Journal of Orthodontics and Dentofacial Orthopedics*, **111**, 163–72.

73. Larmour, C. J. and Chadwick, R. G. (1995). Effects of a commercial orthodontic debonding agent upon the surface microhardness of two orthodontic bonding resins. *Journal of Dentistry*, **23**, 37–40.

74. Pus, M. D. and Way, D. C. (1980). Enamel loss due to orthodontic bonding. *American Journal of Orthodontics*, **77**, 269–83.

75. Hong Y. H. and Lew K. K. K. (1995). Quantitative and qualitative assessment of enamel surface following five composite removal methods after bracket debonding. *European Journal of Orthodontics*, **17**, 121–8.

76. van Waes, H., Matter, T., and Krejci, I. (1997). Three-dimensional measurement of enamel loss caused by bonding and debonding of orthodontic brackets. *American Journal of Orthodontics and Dentofacial Orthopedics*, **112**, 666–9.

8 Multidisciplinary treatments

CONTENTS

Orthodontic treatment can be performed in combination with a number of other dental disciplines, most notably restorative dentistry, oral and maxillofacial surgery, and paediatric dentistry. Whenever complex multidisciplinary treatment is required, it is advisable to see the patient with a specialist colleague(s) from the other discipline(s) prior to the commencement of treatment. In this way the appropriate aims and objectives will be determined from the beginning of treatment, reducing the risk that inappropriate treatment might be carried out to the detriment of the patient and to the embarrassment of the clinicians involved. It will also clarify the expectations of the patient from the very beginning.

8.1   RESTORATIVE DENTISTRY AND ORTHODONTICS

There a number of instances when multidisciplinary treatment involving the restorative dentist and orthodontist might be appropriate. Examples include:
- relocating or closing space when teeth are absent;
- aligning teeth to provide a path of insertion for a denture, bridge, or crown;
- aligning the roots prior to the provision of an implant;
- realigning periodontally involved teeth prior to permanent splinting.

8.1.1   Relocating or closing space when teeth are absent

Whenever there are missing teeth, whether developmentally or otherwise (e.g. due to caries, periodontal disease, or trauma), a decision has to be made whether to accept, restore, or orthodontically close the resulting space. Factors that will influence the decision whether to reopen the space or to close it include those discussed below.

The patient's motivation towards orthodontic treatment
Total space closure, particularly in the absence of crowding, can mean protracted orthodontic treatment.

The number of missing teeth
If there are multiple missing teeth then complete space closure will not be feasible (Fig. 8.1). Some orthodontic realignment may, however, be necessary prior to the provision of a prosthesis.

The site of the missing tooth/teeth
If it is a posterior tooth that is absent and there are no functional or aesthetic considerations, then the space might be accepted. Alternatively the space may be closed using fixed appliances. If it is an anterior tooth that is missing, it is important to carefully consider the final aesthetic result of

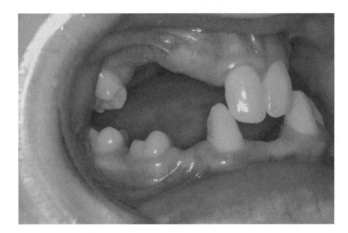

Fig. 8.1 A case with severe hypodontia in which only limited orthodontic realignment can be contemplated.

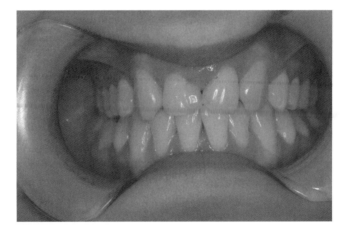

Fig. 8.2 This patient had missing upper central incisors and the lateral incisors were moved mesially and the crowns were built up with composite. Notice how these teeth look wide mesiodistally and short occlusogingivally.

anterior space closure versus prosthetic replacement, perhaps in consultation with a restorative dentistry colleague.

Consider the case of a missing upper central incisor. Can the upper lateral incisor be made to resemble an upper central incisor? The answer will depend somewhat on the relative sizes of the lateral incisor and the tooth it is to replace. It can certainly be difficult to make the lateral incisor big enough to mimic a central incisor. Even when the crown dimensions are changed there are usually large mesiodistal gingival overhangs, which can have detrimental effects on long-term gingival health. In addition, the low level of the labial gingivae on the lateral can be such that it can make the clinical crown of the restored tooth appear very short and yet very wide mesiodistally (Fig. 8.2). Therefore in the case of missing upper central incisors, space will invariably need to be recreated for a prosthetic replacement in order to achieve a satisfactory aesthetic result. Occasionally this may mean extracting further back in the upper arch to facilitate reopening of the space in the upper central incisor region.

In other instances, for example where there is a developmentally absent upper lateral incisor, if the upper canine is relatively small, is of a good colour, and does not have a particularly pointed cusp, it may be perfectly acceptable to approximate the canine and upper central incisor. It may also be possible to reshape the canine by grinding the cusp tip, with perhaps small additions of composite restorative material to make it resemble the incisal edge of the lateral incisor. However, with missing upper lateral incisors another important consideration is symmetry. If only one upper lateral incisor is missing, will complete space closure produce an asymmetrical appearance even after reshaping the approximated upper canine on one side? It is important that the canine on the side of space closure can be made to look like the upper lateral incisor on the opposite side of the same arch. This may not always be possible since the latter tooth in such cases can be quite small. However, it may be possible to close the space on the side of the missing lateral incisor, reshape the canine on this side, and at the same time reopen a small amount of space around the diminutive lateral incisor and restore the size of this tooth using a veneer or crown. If space already exists around the diminutive lateral incisor prior to orthodontic treatment, it is often worthwhile asking the restorative dentist to build this tooth up to the correct size with a composite restorative material first. A fixed appliance can easily be bonded to such a tooth and it takes the guesswork out of where to position the diminutive lateral incisor in relation to its adjacent teeth.

8.1.2 Aligning teeth to provide a path of insertion

If it has been decided to accept and just restore the space where teeth are absent, it is sometimes necessary to align the teeth adjacent to the space to provide a suitable path of insertion. An example would be prior to the provision of a denture or bridge to replace a missing lower molar and where the distal tooth has tipped mesially into the space. This can sometimes be achieved using a sectional fixed appliance, particularly if the rest of the occlusion is to be accepted.

8.1.3 Aligning the roots prior to the provision of an implant

Following on from the work of Bränemark and co-workers,[1] osseointegrated titanium implants have been available for use in restorative dentistry for many years, and their use for single, as well as multiple tooth

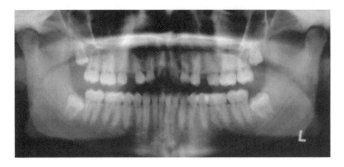

Fig. 8.3(a) This orthopantomogram shows that the root apices of the premolars are too close together for implants to be placed.

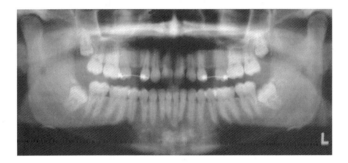

Fig. 8.3(b) Using sectional fixed appliances sufficient space has been created between the apices for implant placement.

replacements appears to be growing in popularity. Patients who may particularly benefit from the provision of one or more implants and who may initially present to the orthodontist are those suffering from hypodontia. Before embarking on any orthodontic treatment for such patients it is worthwhile arranging for them to be seen by a colleague from restorative dentistry. This is to confirm both the suitability of the case for implant placement and the tooth movement required as part of the space management. Orthodontic treatment may be required to relocate space prior to the provision of any prosthesis. However, with implants particular care must be taken to provide space between the roots of the teeth for implant placement (Figs 8.3(a) and (b)). The minimum space necessary for a single tooth implant[2] is 3 mm.

8.1.4 Realigning periodontally involved teeth

Teeth with chronic periodontal disease may drift as a result of a loss of supporting alveolar bone (Fig. 8.4) and the orthodontist may be asked to realign them. However, it is important to ascertain from the restorative dentist/ periodontist that any pre-existing periodontal disease has been brought under control before commencing orthodontic treatment. Otherwise there is a considerable risk of turning what is chronic periodontitis into acute

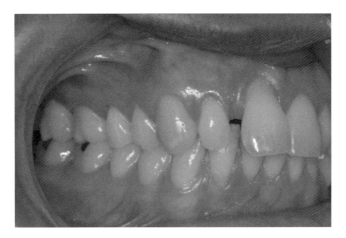

Fig. 8.4 Loss of alveolar bone support has led to this patient's upper right central incisor drifting labially.

periodontitis during tooth movement, hastening both the loss of alveolar bone and the tooth.

Close liaison between the orthodontist and periodontist during orthodontics is essential, with it being appropriate that the periodontist examines the patient during the period of orthodontic care. Good records, particularly clinical records of pocket probing depths, bleeding on probing, and alveolar bone height assessment using long-cone periapical radiographs, both prior to and during treatment, are required. This is necessary in order to monitor any disease progression during orthodontic treatment, especially any loss of alveolar bone.

The reduced alveolar bone support, which caused the tooth/teeth to drift in the first place, means that orthodontic realignment is often reasonably quick. Once a previously periodontally involved tooth has been realigned using fixed or removable appliances, the reduced alveolar bone support will almost inevitably mean that prolonged/permanent retention is required. This may take the form of a bonded multistrand wire (see Chapter 6, Fig. 6.47) or protracted part-time wear of a removable retainer. It could be argued that the requirement for intermittent loading of teeth during function (see Chapter 1), which will be seen with the use of a removable retainer, is eliminated by the use of too rigid a fixed retainer, which may therefore compromise the bony support in the longer term. Certainly there has to be a balance between what is aesthetically acceptable in terms of the final tooth position and the type of retainer to be fitted and what is acceptable regarding the long-term health of the dentition, especially so in the case of an already compromised periodontium.

It may be necessary to discuss retention with the restorative dentist if the patient has a heavily restored dentition, particularly if crown and bridgework is being considered in the region of the retainer.

8.2 ORAL AND MAXILLOFACIAL SURGERY IN RELATION TO ORTHODONTICS

The surgical treatment of orthodontic patients can be divided into two broad categories: minor oral surgery and orthognathic surgery. Patients in the latter group particularly should be seen at a joint consultation clinic with a surgical colleague prior to the commencement of treatment.

8.2.1 Minor oral surgery

A number of minor oral surgical procedures may be carried out in conjunction with orthodontic treatment, and these will now be dealt with in turn.

Extraction of teeth

This is the commonest surgical intervention in orthodontic treatment and teeth are extracted for a number of reasons, as discussed below.

The primary dentition

Extractions may be necessary due to the poor prognosis of one or more teeth. Balancing and compensating extractions may therefore need to be considered in order to preserve centrelines and buccal segment relationships, respectively. This will only be necessary where crowding is likely to be present. Primary incisor loss is not balanced or compensated. The loss of a first primary molar or canine can be balanced with the loss of the first primary molar or primary canine on the opposite side of the same arch. It is unusual to perform compensating extractions for these teeth. The loss of a second primary molar is not followed by a balancing extraction due to: (1) the minimal effect on the centreline; and (2) the rapid space loss due to mesial movement of the first permanent molar and the effect this has on the eruption of the second premolar. For the same reasons the loss of a second primary molar is rarely compensated with the loss of the opposing second primary molar.

The mixed dentition

A primary tooth may require extraction if its permanent successor is showing signs of becoming ectopically positioned. An example is the retained upper primary canine with an ectopically positioned upper permanent canine (Fig. 8.5), or a lingually deflected lower incisor with retained primary incisors (Fig. 8.6). Submerging primary teeth will usually require extraction if they begin to sink beneath the level of the contact points of the adjacent teeth. This can cause the latter teeth to tilt over the submerging tooth[3] (Fig. 8.7). In extreme cases the submerging tooth can disappear from view altogether, making extraction very difficult and usually necessitating removal under general anaesthesia. However, it should be remembered that

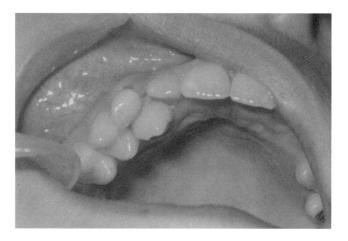

Fig. 8.5 The retained deciduous canine has led to the eruption of the permanent successor in a more palatal position.

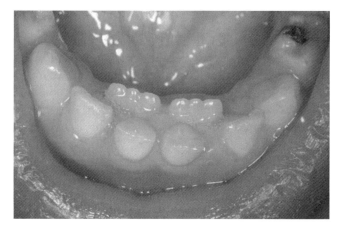

Fig. 8.6 Lower central incisors being deflected lingually by the retained deciduous central incisors. Extraction of the latter would enable the permanent incisors to move into the arch.

submergence of primary teeth is relatively common, with most spontaneously re-erupting before being normally shed. They can sometimes be built up with a composite restorative material to restore the occlusal plane, provided the succeeding tooth is present, in order to preserve the position of the adjacent and occluding teeth until the submerging tooth is naturally shed. First permanent molars may be extracted at this stage if of poor prognosis. The rules governing the extraction of these teeth are covered in *Diagnosis of the orthodontic patient* (see the Further reading list).

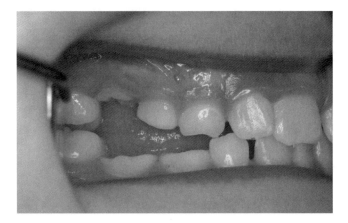

Fig. 8.7 Submerging deciduous molars. Notice how these teeth are below the level of the contact points of the adjacent teeth, which are beginning to tip over them.

Permanent dentition

It is at this stage of dental development that most orthodontic treatment is carried out. Extractions are usually required to relieve crowding prior to the commencement of treatment with fixed or removable appliances. Traditionally, the extractions of choice have been the first premolars, because they are close to the site of any labial segment crowding. However, in recent years there seems to have been a move away from this traditional extraction pattern of four first premolars to either second premolar extractions or non-extraction treatments.[4] Whatever teeth are extracted for the relief of crowding, it is important they be removed as atraumatically as possible in order to preserve the supporting alveolar bone. In this way, the subsequent movement of teeth across the extraction site will be that much easier, facilitating total space closure at the end of treatment. If a small piece of root apex should fracture off during an extraction it is often best to leave it *in situ*. This is particularly so if its removal would require that a mucoperiosteal flap is raised along with the removal of alveolar bone, in order to gain access to the root fragment. A small piece of retained root will rarely interfere with adjacent tooth movement and it may indeed eventually erupt. It can then be simply removed.

Exposure of teeth

Permanent teeth occasionally need to be exposed. This is either to allow spontaneous eruption or to enable the tooth or teeth to be moved into the arch orthodontically. Whichever the case, it is important the surgical procedure is performed with a view to providing the tooth with normal attached gingivae once fully erupted. If the tooth to be exposed is palatally

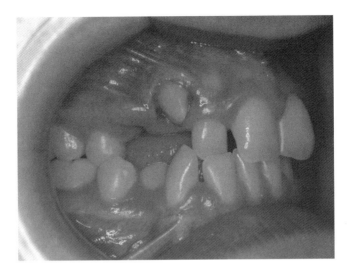

Fig. 8.8 An upper canine exposed using an apically repositioned flap in an attempt to preserve the attached gingivae.

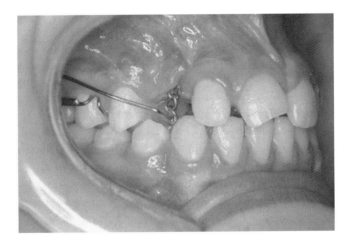

Fig. 8.9 A gold chain has been bonded to the unerupted canine and the mucosal flap replaced. A removable appliance is being used to apply traction to the tooth via the chain.

positioned, surgery will involve exposure through keratinized palatal mucosa. The tooth will therefore erupt through this mucosa and will eventually have a normal attached gingiva. However, in the case of unerupted buccally positioned teeth, if a mucoperiosteal flap is raised through unkeratinized mucosa and the tooth subsequently erupts through this, it will finish up with a gingival margin of unattached mucosa. Buccally positioned teeth are therefore best exposed using an apically repositioned flap (Fig. 8.8). In this way the final gingival margin will consist of keratinized, attached mucosa. Sometimes an ectopically positioned tooth is exposed, a bracket and

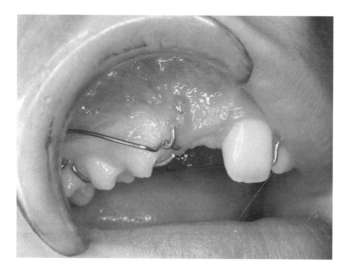

Fig. 8.10 Notice how the gold chain is perforating the attached mucosa overlying this unerupted canine. This may lead to the tooth erupting through unattached mucosa and a less desirable gingival margin when fully aligned.

chain are bonded to the tooth, and the flap is replaced. An orthodontic appliance is then used to apply traction to the tooth to bring it into the line of the arch (Fig. 8.9). Care must be exercised in the placement of the bonded attachment. If the attachment is inappropriately placed, then either the chain or the attachment itself may perforate the unattached mucosa, leading once again to a gingival margin of unattached mucosa. This only applies to buccally positioned teeth, particularly upper incisors or canines (Fig. 8.10). In such cases the attachment is best placed on the palatal aspect of the tooth so that traction is always applied through keratinized mucosa. Alternatively, an exposure should be performed using an apically repositioned flap and the tooth should remain exposed.

During exposure of a tooth it is usual to remove sufficient bone to expose the crown. It is important not to expose the root of the tooth as this may damage the cementum, leading either to reduced periodontal support or possibly ankylosis. Care should also be taken to avoid damaging the adjacent teeth.

Frenectomy

In orthodontics the removal of the upper labial frenum has long been advocated as a means of retaining the closure of a median diastema following appliance therapy. The surgical procedure involves removal of the labial frenum along with the transeptal fibres between the upper central incisors and, where necessary, a recontouring of the associated labial and palatal gingivae.[5] The frenum can either be removed before orthodontic treatment, when access is easier, or following treatment when it might be anticipated that any scar tissue formed would help maintain diastema closure. More

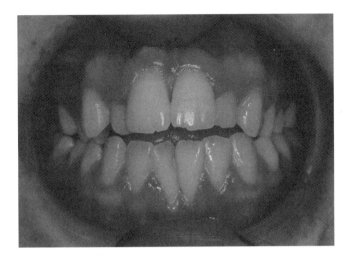

Fig. 8.11 This patient already has labial gingival recession on the lower central incisors. Derotation and pericision around the labial gingival will almost certainly lead to further recession.

recently it has been found that an upper labial frenectomy has little effect on the stability of closure of a median diastema,[6] consequently it is reserved for those cases where the upper labial frenum is either pendulous and unsightly, or where it is attached directly to the gingival margin. In both cases it can adversely affect gingival health, making it difficult to clean or causing the gingival margin to be pulled away from the tooth.

Pericision

Pericision, or circumferential supracrestal fiberotomy, has been recommended in order to minimize rotational relapse once a tooth has been derotated.[7] Under local anaesthesia, a number 11 Bard–Parker blade is inserted into the gingival crevice and the fibres surrounding the tooth are severed to a depth of up to 3 mm below the alveolar crest of bone. This has been shown to reduce rotational relapse by approximately 18–29%.[8,9]

However, it is advisable not to perform pericision on the labial gingivae of the lower incisor teeth. Here the alveolar bone can be particularly thin, with the added possibility of there being a fenestration present within the alveolus. It is therefore recommended that pericision is only performed interdentally and lingually in this region, as it may otherwise lead to the formation of a labial dehiscence (Fig. 8.11). The best time to undertake pericision is as soon as the tooth has been derotated. In this way it will be retained in this position by the orthodontic appliance for the remainder of the treatment, thereby hopefully further minimizing the chances of rotational relapse.

Autotransplantation of teeth

Autotransplantation of teeth from one area of the mouth to another has been practised for many years.[10] Examples include: the transplantation of

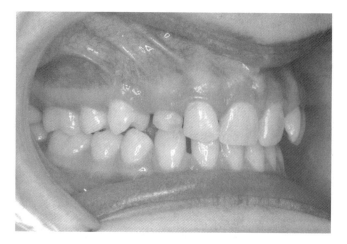

Fig. 8.12(a) This patient has had a small amount of space created around the retained upper deciduous canine in order to accommodate a transplanted upper canine.

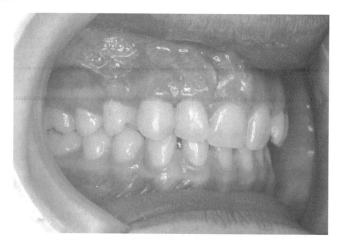

Fig. 8.12(b) The same patient as in Fig. 8.12(a) after transplantation of the ectopically positioned canine.

unerupted third molars to replace missing first permanent molars; premolars to replace upper central incisors;[11] and the transplantation of ectopically positioned canines into their correct position within the arch (Figs 8.12(a) and (b)).

There are really two types of transplantation, requiring two distinct protocols with differing objectives. The first is the transplantation of a tooth with an open apex; the aim is for root apexification to continue (i.e. continued root formation and apex closure) and ultimately for a vital pulp to remain. The second technique involves teeth with closed apices; where the aim is to provide a root-treated and therefore non-vital tooth, which does not show signs of active external root resorption. Both types of transplantation should be deemed successful if there is good periodontal ligament attachment, a tight junction in the region of the gingival crevice, and no active root resorption at the completion of all treatment.

Although there may be two types of transplantation and therefore two protocols, a number of factors are thought to be associated with improved long-term success of a transplanted tooth, namely:

- The root of the transplanted tooth should only be one-half to three-quarters formed, with an open apex.[12–14]
- The surgeon should take care to minimize contact with the root of the tooth during transplantation, preferably only touching the crown.[15]
- The time between removal of the tooth and its reimplantation should be kept to a minimum.[16]
- The recipient site should be of sufficient size to accommodate the transplant and should also be disease-free. Sometimes, if space needs to be created for the transplant and yet the unerupted tooth is preventing such space creation, the latter is temporarily parked elsewhere. It can then be uncovered as a second procedure and transplanted to the desired position once there is sufficient space (Fig. 8.13)
- The transplant should not be root-filled at the time of surgery.
- Postoperative stabilization can be achieved using an orthodontic fixed appliance. Stabilization is only necessary for 1–3 weeks. Longer periods of stabilization may be associated with ankylosis.
- Root treatment may be necessary, beginning 2 weeks after transplantation, if the tooth shows radiographic signs of resorption.

Some of the problems encountered with transplantation include external root resorption, internal resorption, and ankylosis. In one study, ankylosis was observed in 100% of cases,[17] and was probably related to damage to the

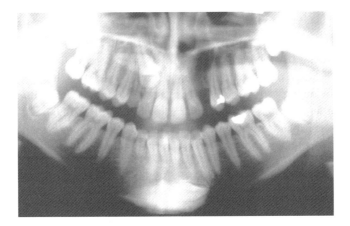

Fig. 8.13 Notice how there are two upper canines on the same side of the arch. The more horizontally positioned of the two has been parked prior to being transplanted to its original side following space creation.

root surface (the layer of cementum) at the time of transplantation and hence the surgeon and surgical techniques used.[18] Since an ankylosed tooth will begin to submerge in a growing individual, transplantation has often been performed in young adults. This, however, means that root formation is likely to be complete and the chances of success are reduced. Not all transplanted teeth necessarily submerge, since rates of ankylosis have been reported to be as low as 2.2%.[11] Indeed, teeth transplanted in growing individuals have been observed to erupt faster than the adjacent teeth, at least initially.[19] Such teeth can also be moved using orthodontic appliances, although it is thought best to delay this until 3–9 months after transplantation.[20]

With the advent of successful endosseous implants it will be interesting to see if autotransplantation continues to be practised to the same extent as in the past. A stated advantage of autotransplantation in the growing individual is that the presence of an erupting tooth within the alveolus will help stimulate bone formation. Therefore, even if the transplant fails after a few years this alveolar bone can ultimately be used to support an implant. However, long-term failures may be relatively few, with recently reported success rates of up to 79% in a series of patients followed for between 17 and 41 years' post-transplantation.[21]

Implants

The orthodontist may become involved in the use of implants in one of two ways:

- As part of a multidisciplinary treatment plan to replace missing teeth (see Section 8.1.3). Orthodontic treatment may be necessary to open space, to relocate space, or to reduce spacing prior to implant placement.
- The implant can be used as a means of reinforcing anchorage during a course of orthodontic treatment.

Anchorage reinforcement can be achieved with one of two types of titanium implant: the endosseous implant; and the subperiosteal implant or onplant. The endosseous implant can be placed in the alveolus, either as a definitive implant (which will eventually receive a conventional superstructure and crown) or as a temporary implant (which will eventually be removed following orthodontic treatment).[22] Short endosseous implants 4–6 mm in length can also be temporarily placed in the midline of the hard palate.[23] A transpalatal arch can then be fabricated which is cemented to the upper first permanent molars but also contacts the implant. Such implants have been found to be successful in preventing mesial movement of the molars during orthodontic treatment.[24] The implant can then be removed at the completion of anchorage reinforcement.

The subperiosteal implant has also been developed as a method of reinforcing anchorage during orthodontic treatment.[25] Like the short endosseous implant it is made from titanium and is placed in the midline of the palate. However, unlike the endosseous implant it is placed subperiosteally but remains on the bone surface. Hence the alternative name of onplant. Where the onplant is in contact with the bone, osseointegration occurs. It can then be used to reinforce anchorage, once again via a transpalatal arch, which here contacts the onplant where it protrudes through the mucosa. The arch is also cemented to the first molar teeth. At the completion of orthodontic treatment the oral surgeon can remove the onplant.

8.2.2   Orthognathic surgery

Orthognathic surgery is usually performed on relatively young adults around 16–20 years of age. These patients can be divided into two main groups, those with:

- *Moderate to severe skeletal or occlusal problems*—In this group the patient's degree of facial deformity is such that orthodontic treatment alone is unable to provide a good occlusion and without detrimental risk to the health of the dentition. The skeletal discrepancy is usually obvious and consequently treatment planning is relatively straightforward and involves orthognathic surgery. This group of problems not only includes anteroposterior skeletal discrepancies, but also vertical occlusal and skeletal discrepancies (Fig. 8.14).

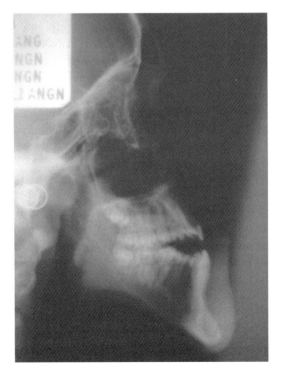

Fig. 8.14 This patient has a combination of anteroposterior and vertical skeletal problems necessitating treatment involving a combined orthodontic/orthognathic surgery approach.

- *Borderline skeletal or occlusal problems*—In this group orthodontic treatment alone could provide a satisfactory occlusion, but the patient might still be unhappy with their facial appearance following such treatment. Such cases often display only a mild skeletal discrepancy and as a consequence it may be more difficult to decide whether to treat using orthodontics alone, or to consider a combined orthodontic/orthognathic surgery approach to treatment.

Surgery can assist in the correction of anteroposterior, vertical, and transverse skeletal and occlusal problems and is usually performed when facial growth is virtually complete.

A number of steps are involved in the diagnosis and treatment of the orthognathic patient, including those discussed below.

Determination of the patient's concerns

The first step in the development of a treatment plan begins with careful questioning of the patient as to their true complaint. It is important to establish whether they are concerned with their skeletal pattern, the position of their teeth, or a combination of the two. There is little point in attempting orthodontic correction of a Class II division I incisor relationship if the patient's principal complaint is their retrusive chin on a moderate to severe Class II skeletal pattern. Conversely, the same patient might only be concerned with the malalignment of their incisor teeth and may wish to opt for simple orthodontic alignment, rather than considering orthognathic surgery to correct the skeletal pattern and increased overjet.

Whatever the course of action, the patient should be made fully aware of the various treatment options, with and without surgery. The advantages, disadvantages, and short- and long-term complications of each of the possible treatment options needs to be discussed. This is not only common sense, but also a legal requirement of informed consent.

Examination of the patient

A detailed extra- and intraoral clinical examination should be performed, as with any potential orthodontic patient.[26] This will help in determining the site and degree of any skeletal discrepancy, along with the amount of dentoalveolar compensation that is already present and which may subsequently need to be reversed prior to surgery.

Special investigations

Good diagnostic records (namely, study models, radiographs, and photographs) should also be obtained. A cephalometric analysis performed on the lateral cephalogram will greatly assist in identifying the skeletal discrepancy, along with the presurgical orthodontic tooth movements required (Figs 8.15(a)–(c)). It is usually at this point that arrangements are made for the patient to attend a joint consultation appointment with the orthodontist and oral and maxillofacial surgeon.

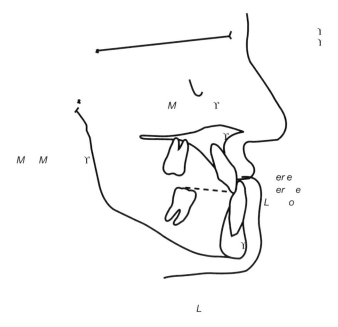

Fig. 8.15(a) A cephalometric analysis can help to identify skeletal and dentoalveolar problems.

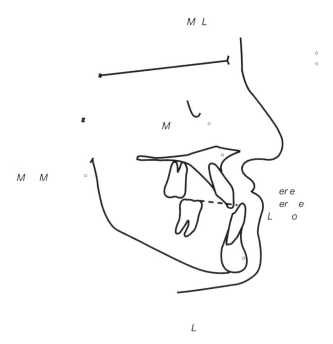

Fig. 8.15(b) The presurgical tooth movements.

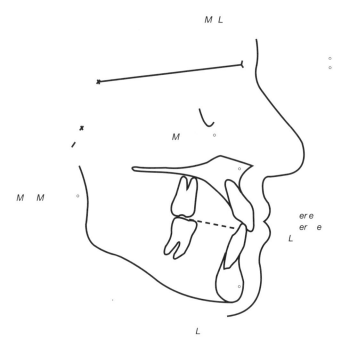

Fig. 8.15(c) Finally the surgery required to treat the patient illustrated in Fig. 8.15(a).

Identification of the possible treatment plans

It has been suggested that the type of jaw surgery planned should be primarily driven by the desired improvement in facial aesthetics, and that this is largely possible following just the extraoral examination.[27] However, it is not always this straightforward, especially in mild cases. A number of different computer software packages are available to aid the diagnostic process, using mainly the lateral cephalogram and a cephalometric analysis. By incorporating the extraoral photographs into the program, it is not only possible to demonstrate the dental and skeletal movements required, but also to give the patient an idea of their likely post-treatment appearance. Care should be exercised when showing a patient such predictions of their post-treatment facial appearance, since the soft tissue movements that occur as a result of surgery do not exactly mimic the bony movements. For instance, it has been demonstrated that the soft tissues over the chin and of the lower lip move to a variable degree with mandibular surgery. At the level of the bony chin the soft tissues are found to move the same amount as the bone, whilst at the level of the lip the movement can range from 0.38 to 0.75 the amount of the surgical bony movement.[28-30] Similarly, movement of the soft tissues at the base of the nose and upper lip following maxillary surgery are also variable, but perhaps less so than in the mandible.[31] Therefore, any prediction of the final extraoral appearance after surgery using computer software may not be entirely accurate,[32] and, in particular, the predicted movements of the lower lip do not necessarily match the surgical outcome[33,34] over the longer term.[35] Although computer predictions do have their limitations, so do other methods, such as hand tracings and the cutting up and manual manipulation of photographs, when predicting facial change postsurgery. Certainly it has been reported that up to 89% of patients are happy that the images predicted using video-imaging were realistic and that the predicted results were generally achieved.[36,37]

Final treatment planning

From the initial examination and diagnostic records it may seem obvious that, for example, the mandible or the maxilla should be advanced or setback following presurgical orthodontics. However, occasionally it is not possible at this initial stage to be specific as to whether the patient requires an operation on one or both jaws or of the amount of surgical movement required. In such cases the final decision is made following the phase of presurgical orthodontics.

Patient expectations of treatment

At each stage of the planning process, from the initial examination of the patient through to the final planning prior to surgery, it is important that the clinicians involved understand the patient's expectations of treatment. This can sometimes be one of the most complex aspects of orthognathic treatment planning. The patient, not necessarily familiar with the examination and subsequent description of facial appearance, may be unable to fully express their concerns or understand the terminology used to describe the problem and its various treatment options. In some cases the perceived problems of the patient do not necessarily coincide with those identified by the clinician. It is essential that not only do the clinicians fully understand the patient's problems and expectations of treatment, but also that the patient understands what treatment options are available, the demands that will be placed upon them if they embark on treatment, the expected outcome, and any risks involved. This is particularly important with orthognathic surgery, which is non-essential, often referred to as 'cold' or elective surgery, in that there is no risk to life if treatment is not undertaken. Attendance at clinics over a number of months is often required to ensure that the expectations of the patient and clinicians coincide. This is time well spent, particularly in an ever-increasingly litigious society, and plays an essential part in obtaining 'fully informed' consent prior to active treatment.

Presurgical orthodontics

In patients with skeletal discrepancies there is usually some degree of dento-alveolar compensation as a result of the action of the soft tissues. In effect, it is nature's way of providing the patient with an occlusion. Therefore in a case with a marked Class III skeletal pattern, the lower incisors might be retroclined and the upper incisors proclined (Fig. 8.16). Conversely, where

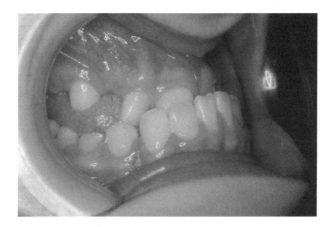

Fig. 8.16 Notice how the lower incisors are very retroclined, compensating to some degree for the marked skeletal III base.

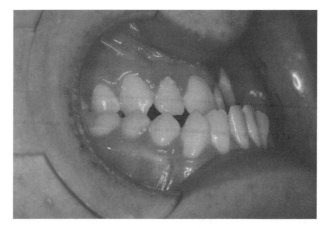

Fig. 8.17(a) Notice how the lower incisors are very retroclined prior to treatment.

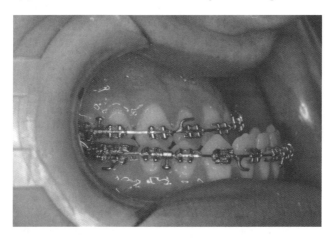

Fig. 8.17(b) Following dentoalveolar compensation in the patient in Fig. 8.17(a), which is just prior to surgery, the Class III incisor relationship has in fact been made worse.

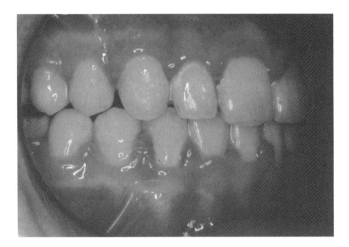

Fig. 8.18 Following dentoalveolar decompensation and surgery the correct occlusal and skeletal results can be achieved.

there is a Class II skeletal pattern the lower incisors might be proclined, although the upper incisors might be markedly retroclined if within lower lip control, or proclined if not controlled by the lower lip. Whatever their position, the aim of presurgical orthodontics is to bring the teeth to a more normal position over their respective skeletal bases. This requires the use of upper and lower fixed appliances. However, the aim is not to improve the occlusal relationship between the upper and lower arch teeth. Indeed, this relationship is often made worse during the presurgical phase of treatment, particularly in Class III and Class II division 2 cases (Figs 8.17(a) and (b)). Only by fully decompensating the teeth can the full surgical correction of the underlying skeletal discrepancy be achieved, along with the production of an ideal occlusion (Fig. 8.18). The consequences of not fully decompensating the arches on the subsequent surgical correction of a Class III skeletal pattern are illustrated in Fig. 8.19.

Although presurgical normalization of tooth positions over their respective skeletal bases is practised in the anteroposterior direction, it is not always performed vertically. In cases where there is an increased overbite and where the anterior lower face height is reduced, one of the aims of the orthodontic/surgical treatment might be to increase this vertical dimension. During the presurgical orthodontic phase it is therefore important to preserve the depth of the overbite by maintaining the Curve of Spee in the lower fixed appliance archwire. In this way the anterior lower facial height is increased as a result of the surgery, although postoperatively the patient will have what is known as a 'three-point landing'. They will only occlude on the incisors and terminal molars. The lateral open bites produced as a result can then be then closed down by extruding the intervening teeth

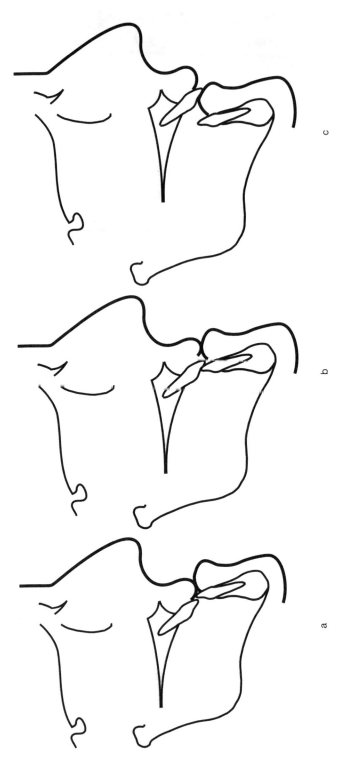

a

b

c

Fig. 8.19 (a) The incisor and skeletal relationship prior to treatment. (b) If no orthodontic decompensation is carried out and surgery is performed to create a normal overjet, the patient will still have a Class III skeletal pattern at the end of treatment. (c) If, however, surgery is used to create a Class I skeletal pattern on the same patient, the overjet will increase and in this case produce a large Class II division 1 incisor relationship.

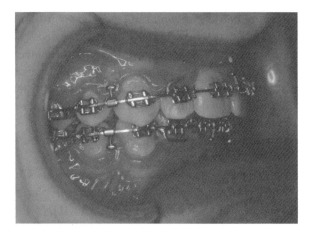

Fig. 8.20(a) Immediately preoperatively both the overjet and overbite are increased in this Class II division 1 incisor relationship.

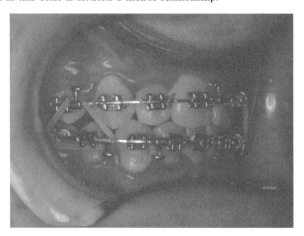

Fig. 8.20(b) Following surgery, the lateral open bites, created as a result of the three-point landing, were closed using intermaxillary triangular elastics.

during the postoperative phase (Figs 8.20(a) and (b)), whilst retaining the increase in anterior lower facial height.

Conversely, in patients with an anterior open bite it is also important to preserve this feature of the occlusion during presurgical orthodontics. If the aim of the surgery is to reduce the anterior lower face height, then it will be important not extrude the incisors during the presurgical orthodontic phase, otherwise face height reduction may not be possible.

When planning the presurgical orthodontic phase of treatment, particularly extractions, the effect of any decompensating tooth movements on space requirements need to be contemplated. Consider, for example, a Class III case where proclination of the lower incisors and retroclination of the upper incisors are planned prior to surgery. Space will be created in the lower arch as proclination occurs and the teeth move on to a larger arc of a circle. Therefore, what may have initially been a crowded lower arch, will not necessarily be crowded following presurgical decompensation (see Figs 8.17(a) and (b)). In the upper arch, retroclination of the upper incisors will move these teeth into a smaller arc of a circle and teeth that may have initially appeared well aligned may end up crowded following retroclination. Inappropriate extractions can lead to problems in trying to close space, and in exceptional circumstances the extracted teeth may require prosthetic replacement.

At the end of the presurgical phase of orthodontics it is usual for the patient to have heavy rectangular stainless-steel wires in place, for example 0.018 × 0.025 inches (0.45 × 0.63 mm), or 0.019 × 0.025 inches (0.48 × 0.63 mm) in a 0.022 × 0.028-inch (0.55 × 0.7 mm) bracket system. The upper and lower arches should be coordinated by this stage so that post-operatively the arches will fit together perfectly. To aid the surgeon during the operation and the orthodontist during the postsurgical phase or ortho-dontics, ball hooks are placed at intervals on these final steel archwires (Fig. 8.21). These open-backed metal hooks are crimped directly on to the archwire using specially designed crimping pliers (Fig. 8.22).

The surgical phase of treatment

Immediately prior to surgery, records should be taken so that the final definitive surgical plan can be confirmed. As a minimum, these records should consist of study models, photographs, and a lateral cephalogram. The surgical plan, anteroposteriorly, can be confirmed using the lateral cephalogram and cephalometric analysis, and the study models can be used to check the anticipated postoperative occlusion. In Class II cases the occlu-sion can also be checked by asking the patient to posture the mandible

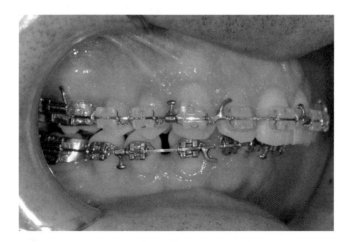

Fig. 8.21 Ball hooks in place prior to surgery.

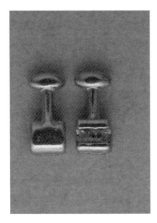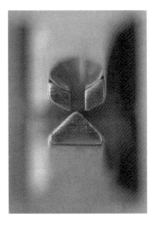

Fig. 8.22 On the left are two ball hooks. The one on the right shows the open back which slips on to the archwire. The ends of the crimping pliers are shown on the far right. These are used to crimp the hooks on to the archwire.

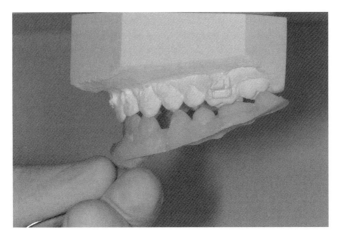

Fig. 8.23 An acrylic model of the lower arch can be held against the upper arch in the patient with a Class III incisor relationship. This is illustrated here by holding the acrylic model against the upper plaster model.

forwards. In Class III cases this is not possible; therefore either study models are required, or an impression can be taken of one arch and an acrylic model made of the occlusal surfaces, with the handle anteriorly, so that it can be checked against the occlusion of the opposing arch in the mouth (Fig. 8.23). In the case of single-arch osteotomies, the study models are also useful in indicating the amount of surgical movement required to achieve the desired occlusion (Fig. 8.24). When surgery is planned in both jaws (bimaxillary osteotomy), or where a vertical movement of the maxilla is going to be performed, it is often advisable to mount the models on a fully adjustable articulator using a facebow record (Fig. 8.25). In this way the precise surgical movements can be performed on the models, the effects

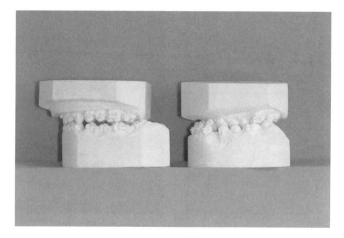

Fig. 8.24 Study models immediately preoperatively. The surgical movement required can be seen by looking at the back of the study models. On the left the occlusion is in the correct postoperative position. Compare this with the position of the models on the right with the preoperative occlusion.

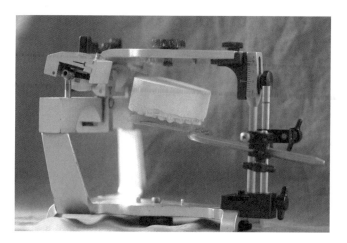

Fig. 8.25 A fully adjustable articulator with the upper model held in place with the positioning jig, the records having been taken using a facebow.

observed, and modifications made where appropriate. Also in such complex cases, the surgeon may ask for intermediate and/or final acrylic inter-occlusal wafers to be constructed from the models. In the case of bimaxillary surgery an intermediate wafer will be used to confirm the new position of the maxilla using the unoperated mandible and mandibular occlusion as a reference during surgery. Once the maxilla is in its new position, the mandibular osteotomy can be performed and the mandible moved into the correct occlusion in relation to the newly repositioned maxilla. A final wafer may be necessary if the occlusal fit is not precise. This might be the case if a three-point landing has been planned (see above Presurgical orthodontics). In such instances the final wafer may be left in position postoperatively until the early postsurgical orthodontic phase.

The surgeon may use the ball hooks (placed earlier by the orthodontist) to hold the jaws in the correct occlusion during the surgery. Powerchain is often used for this purpose, as it is easy to place and then subsequently remove at the end of surgery.

There are very many types of surgical procedures available for use in orthognathic surgery,[38] but those in commonest use are:

- *The bilateral sagittal split osteotomy*—This can be used to advance or setback the mandible.
- *The Le Fort I osteotomy*—This is used to advance the maxilla. A small amount of setback is possible. By removing bone above the osteotomy site it is possible to impact the maxilla. Alternatively, by placing a bone graft at the osteotomy site it is possible to set down the maxilla.
- *The high Le Fort I osteotomy*—This is used to not only advance the maxilla, but more of the anterior wall of the maxilla in cases where presurgically the area of the face either side of the nostrils appears somewhat set back.
- *Genioplasty*—This can be an advancement, setback, or vertical reduction genioplasty.
- *Segmental surgery*—Although this surgery is less common today, it is occasionally useful if only a segment of teeth need to be surgically repositioned.

Whatever the surgery, the bone fragments are usually stabilized using titanium bone plates (Fig. 8.26). It is unusual for the jaws to be wired together using intermaxillary fixation (IMF). The use of bone plates not only improves postoperative stability of the surgical correction,[39,40] but also means the patient can go back to the ward following surgery. Prior to the use of bone plates, in the era of IMF, the patient had to spend the first 24 hours in a high-dependency unit because of the risk to the airway with the jaws wired together.

Envelopes of surgery

There are limits to the degree of jaw movement that can be achieved by orthognathic surgery. The degree of surgical movement is largely determined by the need to provide a pleasing facial appearance following treatment. However, as a general rule, once the amount of anteroposterior movement required for correction exceeds 10 mm, consideration should be given to operating on both jaws (bimaxillary osteotomy), rather than trying to achieve the correction with surgery on one jaw alone (unimaxillary osteotomy). The amount of anterior movement that can be surgically achieved in the maxilla or mandible is approximately 10–12 mm. Exceeding this can be technically difficult, particularly in the maxilla, due to soft tissue

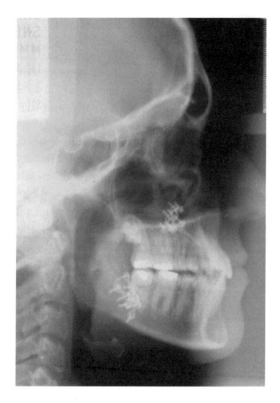

Fig. 8.26 A postoperative lateral cephalogram showing both maxillary and mandibular titanium bone plates in place.

stretch. Care must be taken not to compromise the blood supply by over-stretching the tissues, which could lead to loss of the osteotomized bone. Large surgical movements are also more likely to relapse due to the stretch in the soft tissues.

It is not possible to move the maxilla very far, if at all, posteriorly. Impaction of the maxilla is possible by 5–6 mm, but will be limited by the need to remove the inferior part of the nasal septum and inferior turbinates.

Complications of orthognathic surgery

There are a number of possible complications of orthognathic surgery, excluding the possible anaesthetic risks, and these can be divided into preoperative, intraoperative, and postoperative complications. Examples of such complications include:

(1) *Preoperative* (orthodontic complications):
   - decalcification of the enamel (Fig. 8.27);
   - gingival recession and alveolar bone loss during decompensation (Fig. 8.28);
   - root resorption.

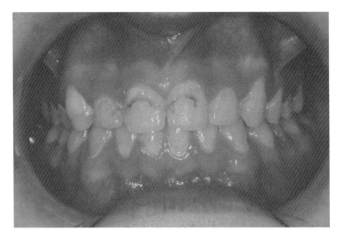

Fig. 8.27 Enamel decalcification following orthodontic and orthognathic surgery due to poor oral hygiene.

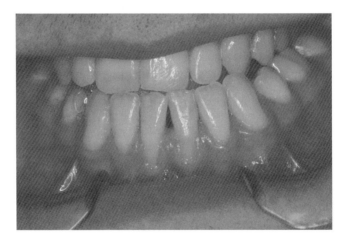

Fig. 8.28 Gingival recession on the labial aspect of the lower central incisors meant decompensation prior to surgery in this Class III case had to stop and the surgical aims revisited.

(2) *Intraoperative*:
- damage to the neurovascular bundle during a mandibular osteotomy leading to paraesthesia—this occurs in up to 32% of patients and can be disturbing for approximately 3% of patients;[41]
- loss of blood supply to part of the maxilla;
- haemorrhage;
- failure of the bone to split cleanly;
- failure to relocate the osteotomized fragments into their correct preplanned position—in particular, care must be taken to maintain the condyles in their fossae during mandibular osteotomies;

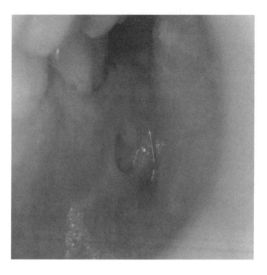

Fig. 8.29 Perforation of the titanium bone plate through the mucosa.

- damage to the teeth adjacent to the osteotomy site, either from the bone cut or the placement of the titanium plates and associated screws.

(3) *Postoperative*:
- failure of the osteotomy to undergo bony union;
- the bone plate perforates through mucosa with chronic infection present (Fig. 8.29);
- relapse towards the preoperative bone position—this can sometimes occur due to condylar resorption, particularly in high-angle cases.[42]

Despite the numerous possible complications, the frequency of severe complications is low and so orthognathic surgery can be considered to be relatively safe.

Postsurgical orthodontics

Following surgery the orthodontist may need to place light intermaxillary elastics in order to detail the occlusion. These are usually placed at around 1–7 days' postoperatively. For patients who have undergone an advancement of the mandible, intermaxillary elastics with a Class II component will usually be worn. Patients who have had a mandibular setback or a maxillary advancement will usually wear Class III intermaxillary elastics. In those cases where a three-point landing has been achieved, or where there was originally an anterior open bite, intermaxillary elastics will be used with a more vertical pull (see Fig. 8.20(b)). In addition, in the arch where most of the vertical tooth movement is required, a more flexible archwire may be used, such as a rectangular nickel–titanium or rectangular braided steel wire. In the opposing arch, where vertical tooth movement is not required, a stiffer rectangular steel wire can remain in place. Whereas a patient may be given intermaxillary elastics to wear within a week of their operation, it is likely to be 3–4 weeks before a lighter archwire can be placed in one of the arches due to postoperative swelling and discomfort.

Sometimes surgery is performed before final orthodontic space closure has been achieved. This is particularly so if teeth are to be extruded postoperatively in order to close a lateral open bite. Space around the teeth to be extruded enables the teeth to move occlusally without interference from their immediate neighbours. It should be noted that space is required when levelling a Curve of Spee (usually performed when reducing an overbite in non-surgical orthodontic cases). Following levelling, final space closure can be performed. The postsurgical orthodontic phase of treatment usually lasts from 2 to 3 months, depending on the degree of presurgical orthodontics already carried out and the success of the surgery in achieving the desired occlusal result. At completion of treatment the fixed appliances are removed and retainers fitted in a similar way as for patients who have only undergone orthodontic treatment. The retention regimen is also no different in orthognathic surgery patients.

Distraction osteogenesis

In recent years there have been numerous reports of mandibular advancement using the technique of distraction osteogenesis.[43] The idea of bony distraction for the correction of dentofacial deformity is not new, it being reported as early as 1948 for the correction of a 2-week-old mandibular fracture.[44] However, it was not until Ilizarov[45–47] utilized the technique for limb lengthening that it found favour in the correction of craniofacial deformities. In general, the technique consists of:

- a corticotomy or partial osteotomy with the periosteum and endosteum preserved to a large degree;
- a latent period of 5–7 days before any distraction;
- distraction of the fragments at a rate of 1 mm/day until the deformity is corrected—this may be in increments of 0.5 mm twice a day.
- fixation in the distracted position for a further 8–10 weeks.

There are problems and questions regarding distraction osteogenesis as a replacement for conventional orthognathic procedures at the present time, and these include:[43]

- The distractor—it should ideally be an intraoral device to minimize extra-oral scarring and distress to the patient. However, such devices are often bulky and it is difficult to apply a distraction force other than in a straight line. This can be a problem in the case of a curved bone such as the mandible where it might be desirable to increase ramal height at the same time as increasing body length.
- What are the long-term effects on facial growth in the younger patient? As yet this is unknown.

- Will there be a slowing of growth in the child patient at the affected site following distraction and so a return of the deformity?
- Will the teeth erupt normally and the alveolus develop normally following distraction?
- Is distraction in the mandible stable in the adult over the longer term?
- What are the limits of distraction?
- If the distraction device is tooth-borne rather than bone-borne will it have any adverse effects on the teeth, their supporting structures, or position?

Many of these questions are as yet unanswered and well-constructed, long-term clinical trials are therefore required. For the foreseeable future, conventional orthognathic surgery will continue to be the principal method used for the correction of dentofacial deformity in combination with orthodontic treatment.[48] However, distraction osteogenesis may have a place for use in cases that are felt to be beyond the scope of conventional orthognathic surgery, due to the need for large bony movements beyond 10–12 mm in each jaw.

8.3 PAEDIATRIC DENTISTRY AND ORTHODONTICS

In most dental disciplines there is invariably some overlap of responsibilities. Depending on local circumstances and the age of the patient, the orthodontist and paedodontist may provide many of the multidisciplinary treatments so far discussed. For example, relocating space prior to prosthetic replacement of a tooth, or extractions during the primary and mixed dentitions. Where the orthodontist and paedodontist, in particular, may undertake multidisciplinary treatment is in the management of dental trauma in the child patient. Examples of which include those mentioned below.

1. *Trauma to the upper incisors but no overt damage visible*—If this occurs in the mixed dentition at around 8–10 years of age and is related to an increased overjet, then a short course of upper removable appliance therapy may be instigated in order to reduce the overjet within the space available, on a non-extraction basis. Orthodontic treatment is best postponed until 3 months after the incident to reduce the risk of inducing irreversible pulpitis. The problems with such orthodontic treatment at around 8–10 years of age are:
(a) the upper lateral incisor may not be fully erupted;
(b) there is a risk of inducing root resorption in the lateral incisor root if it is moved against the crown of the unerupted upper permanent canine;
(c) overjet reduction is likely to relapse due to incompetent lips, either as a result of only partial overjet reduction or because of soft tissue immaturity;
(d) the patient's cooperation towards orthodontic treatment may be used up before they undergo definitive treatment at a later age.

Such trauma in the permanent dentition should also lead to a 3-month postponement of orthodontic treatment. If the patient already has an appliance then it should remain in place but be made passive for this same period.

2.   *Fracture of one or more of the upper incisor crowns*—If there has been a coronal fracture involving dentine and possibly the pulp, then this should be restored as appropriate by the paedodontist. This will not only help to preserve the vitality of the tooth and restore its aesthetics, but it will help to restore the contact points so that subsequent orthodontic realignment will be easier (Fig. 8.30). Failure to restore the contact points will make final restoration of the tooth much more difficult if all the space around it has been closed at the end of orthodontic treatment. This may result in the restored tooth being narrower than it should be, and will be most noticeable in the case of upper central incisors. Once again orthodontic treatment, or continued tooth movement when an appliance is already in place, should not begin until 3 months after restoration of the tooth following trauma.

3.   *Subluxation or avulsion of upper incisors*—Where an upper incisor has been subluxed and has been repositioned within a couple of hours it can be splinted using the adjacent teeth for a period of 1–3 weeks. If a fixed orthodontic appliance is already in place then this can be used to splint the tooth in the correct position. The same applies to avulsed teeth that have been repositioned. Both subluxed and avulsed teeth are prone to external root resorption. Particularly following avulsion it may be necessary for the paedodontist to extirpate the pulp and place a calcium hydroxide root filling, before eventually placing a definitive root filling at a later date. The timing of this will depend somewhat on the length of time the tooth was out of the

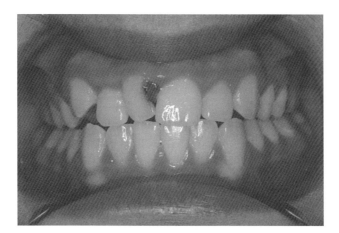

Fig. 8.30 As a result of the fracture of the mesial half of the upper right central incisor there has been rapid space loss.

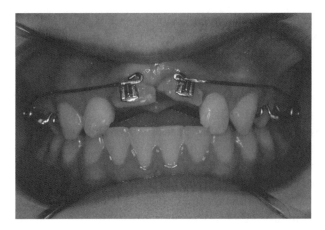

Fig. 8.31 This patient intruded both upper central incisors which then had to be extruded using an upper removable appliance over a period of 2–4 weeks.

mouth before being replaced, its condition, and the stage of root formation. Once root-filled the tooth can then be moved orthodontically. Subluxed teeth that have not been repositioned or avulsed teeth that have been incorrectly replaced can be repositioned orthodontically. If pulpal death occurs, a calcium hydroxide root filling may be placed whilst the orthodontic treatment is used to relatively quickly reposition the tooth. A definitive root filling can be placed at a later date.

4.   *Intruded teeth*—An intruded upper incisor should be extruded orthodontically over a short period of 2–4 weeks. This may mean bonding a bracket to the tooth and using an upper removable of fixed appliance to apply traction to the tooth (Fig. 8.31). Once the majority of the crown is visible it may be necessary for the paedodontist to root-fill the tooth, initially with calcium hydroxide.

5.   *Incisors with a root fracture*—The treatment options available for upper incisors that have suffered a root fracture depend very much on the site of fracture.

(a) If it is close to the apex, the tooth may remain vital and orthodontic tooth movement may not affect this vitality, provided light forces are used. The small apical fragment may not move and so will be left behind.

(b) If the site of fracture is close to the amelocemental junction it will be necessary to remove the coronal portion of the tooth. The root can be filled and a temporary post such as a Dentatus screw can also be fitted. Using this screw, traction can be applied using a fixed or removable appliance to extrude the root so that the margins are supragingival. The tooth can then be restored with a definitive postcrown.

(c) Where the root fracture is in the middle third of the root the prognosis is probably less favourable. There will be insufficient root to support a postcrown if the coronal fragment is removed and the remainder of the root is extruded. Similarly, orthodontic movement of the coronal fragment alone will lead to a tooth with a very reduced root support remaining in the mouth. The only options are either to remove the tooth completely and place a prosthetic replacement, or perhaps transplant a redundant premolar into the site if extractions are to be performed as part of the overall orthodontic treatment. Alternatively, the tooth can be root-treated and a post placed that sits within both the coronal and apical parts of the root, thereby stabilizing the two fragments. The tooth can then be moved orthodontically as a whole, as is necessary.

The above is by no means an exhaustive list of the multidisciplinary treatments that may be undertaken by the orthodontist and paedodontist. Management of the traumatized upper incisor is, however, perhaps the most obvious combined treatment.

8.4   CLEFT LIP AND/OR PALATE PATIENTS

The multidisciplinary treatments so far discussed have centred on two disciplines: orthodontics and one other, such as restorative dentistry or paediatric dentistry. Management of the child with a cleft lip and palate is truly multidisciplinary and involves a much larger multidisciplinary team, namely:

- paediatrician
- feeding nurse
- cleft surgeon
- orthodontist
- speech therapist
- ear, nose, and throat specialist
- paediatric dentist
- general dentist
- clinical geneticist
- clinical psychologist
- restorative dentist.

The reason for such a large team is that the child with a cleft is managed right from the early period as a neonate through to the late teenage years. The presence of a cleft can effect facial growth, facial appearance, dental arch relationships, dental health, speech as well as hearing, and may affect the patient both socially and psychologically. The aim of treatment is therefore to improve dentofacial appearance and function, producing a socially and psychologically well-balanced individual.[49]

Before discussing treatment for the child with a cleft it is worth considering the aetiology, embryology, classification, and incidence of orofacial clefting.

8.4.1   Aetiology

The precise aetiology of cleft lip and palate is as yet unclear, but it is thought to be possibly multifactorial, with there being both genetic and environmental influences. The genetic component is thought to be important, as demonstrated by racial differences in the incidence of clefting[50] (see Section 8.4.4). Up to 63% of clefts may also have another associated defect and half of these may have recognized pattern of anomalies.[51] Clefts are also sometimes seen in more than one individual in a family. It is known, for example, that for parents who are themselves unaffected, but who already have a cleft child, there is an increased risk of having another child with a cleft (approximate 4% chance).[52] Also, if one parent is affected then the risk of having a second cleft-affected child is 10%.[53] However, many clefts are isolated incidents with no previous family history. Therefore the genetic influence is complex, and it is likely that in many cases it operates by altering the response to environmental influences. This genetic influence therefore makes some people more susceptible to specific environmental factors rather than necessarily having a direct genetic effect.[54] Such environmental factors might include the maternal use of anticonvulsant drugs such as phenytoin,[55] benzodiazepines,[56] corticosteroids, and possibly tobacco smoke.[57] In addition, it is possible that a folic acid deficiency in the maternal diet may have an affect on orofacial clefting.[58]

8.4.2   Embryology

The maxilla and mandible arise from the first branchial arches, which begin to fuse in the midline at the 5–6th week *in utero*. In the upper jaw the maxillary process begins to fuse with the frontonasal process, its two median and lateral nasal processes, and the opposing maxillary process (Fig. 8.32). This is thought to lead to the formation of the nasal septum and primary palate, the columella and alae surrounding the nostrils, and the lips, respectively. However, the exact contribution of the frontonasal process and the maxillary processes to the formation of the upper lip is still not clear. It may be that the maxillary processes fuse in the midline to form the upper lip, or possibly that the frontonasal process forms the narrow philtrum of the upper lip to which the maxillary processes fuse from the remainder of the upper lip.[59] A cleft of the lip and alveolus will occur if there is a failure of the maxillary process and the median nasal process to fuse on one or both sides.

The hard palate forms as two lateral palatal processes, which are also derived from the first branchial arch maxillary processes. During the 6th week *in utero* the lateral palatal processes begin to grow down vertically, one on each side of the tongue (Fig. 8.33). At approximately the 8th week *in utero* they move rapidly from their vertical position to lie horizontally above the tongue. Once in this position they then begin to fuse together in the midline, beginning at the incisive foramen and passing posteriorly to the uvula

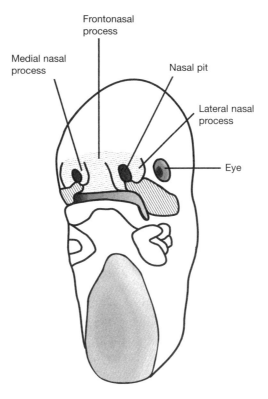

Fig. 8.32 The facial processes during the 5th to 6th week *in utero*.

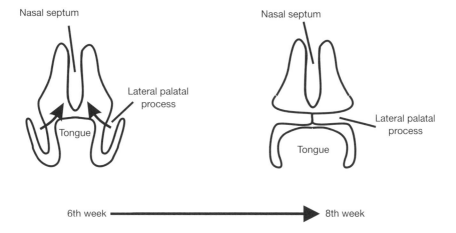

Fig. 8.33 The palatal shelves between the 6th to 8th week *in utero* change form being two vertical shelves either side of the tongue to become horizontal shelves which then fuse in the midline.

of the soft palate, so that by the end of the 10th week fusion is complete. A cleft of the palate may therefore arise either because one or both of the palatal shelves does not move from the vertical to the horizontal,[60] or because of a lack of intimate contact between the two shelves in the midline once both are in the horizontal position.[61]

8.4.3 Classification

There have been many attempts to classify cleft lip and palate.[62,63] However, it has proven difficult to produce a system that is both usable by clinicians in everyday practice and yet is comprehensive enough for use in epidemiological studies on clefting. One of the simplest systems in common usage is that of Kernahan and Stark[64] based on the classification of Veau. Embryologically it is the incisive foramen that is the important structure in describing the nature of the cleft lip and or palate. Therefore clefts are divided into three main types:

1. *Malformation of the primary palate only*—Clefts can range from a simple notch of the lip (Fig. 8.34), right through to a complete cleft of the lip (Fig. 8.35) involving the alveolus as far back as the incisive foramen. They can be unilateral or bilateral and in rare instances, when the premaxilla is missing, it can be median cleft.
2. *Malformation of the secondary palate only*—This can range from a notch in the uvula right through to a complete cleft of the soft and hard palates up as far as the incisive foramen (Fig. 8.36).

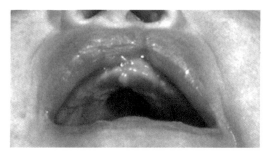

Fig. 8.34 A notch of the lip.

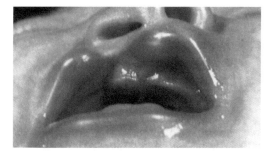

Fig. 8.35 A unilateral cleft of the lip and notch of the alveolus.

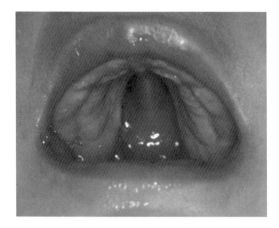

Fig. 8.36 A complete cleft of the secondary palate from the uvula anteriorly to the incisive foramen.

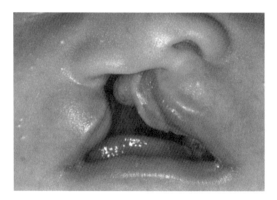

Fig. 8.37 A complete unilateral cleft of the lip, alveolus, and palate.

3. *Malformation of both the primary and secondary palates*—Here the cleft is complete from the lip back to the soft palate and can be unilateral or bilateral (Figs 8.37 and 8.38).

8.4.4 Incidence

The incidence of clefting in the UK is approximately 1 in 700 live births, but from year to year it can show a wide variation from 1 in 1013 to 1 in 540 live births.[65] This variation may be due to inaccuracies in the reporting of cleft births in the UK rather than real fluctuations from year to year. Incidence does vary with race, being more common in Indian and Oriental populations (2.3 per 1000 live births) and least common in Afro-Caribbean populations (0.6 per 1000 live births).[66]

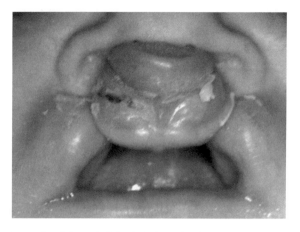

Fig. 8.38 A complete bilateral cleft of the lip, alveolus, and palate.

The distribution of these clefts is reported as follows:[65]
- cleft of the lip with or without cleft of the alveolus—25% (twice as common in males as in females);
- unilateral cleft of the lip and palate—19% (more common on the left side);[67,68]
- bilateral cleft lip and palate—11%;
- cleft of the palate only (including submucous clefts)—45% (twice as common in females).

8.4.5 Treatment

The treatment outline for the cleft patient from prebirth onwards is given below and is summarized in Table 8.1.

Prebirth

Although it may be possible to diagnose cleft lip and palate by 13–14 weeks *in utero*,[69] most ultrasound scans are performed at 18–22 weeks' gestation. However, visualization of a cleft can be difficult due to fetal positioning, particularly as the hands and umbilical chord often lie just in front of the face.[70] Only 40% of isolated clefts may be detected on a routine scan of the face at this time and an isolated cleft palate in particular, can be difficult to detect. Where there is a family history of clefting, repeated scans are therefore performed. Once diagnosed, the parents can be counselled as to the likely outcome and the treatment their child will ultimately receive.

Table 8.1 The multidisciplinary team management of cleft lip and palate

Age	Management	Role of the orthodontist
Prebirth	Fetal ultrasound diagnosis. Parental counselling	—
Birth	**Paediatrician**: assessment	—
Neonate	**Feeding nurse**: establish feeding **Cleft surgeon**: counselling on future treatment	Counselling on future treatment Record taking Presurgical orthopaedics (occasionally)
3–6 months	**Cleft surgeon**: lip and primary palate repair	—
6–18 months	**Cleft surgeon**: soft tissue repair of hard and soft palate	—
>18 months	**Speech therapist**: for assessment **ENT surgeon**: hearing assessment and placement of ventilation tubes (grommets) **Dentist**: dietary and fluoride advice. Fissure sealants as permanent teeth erupt	Record taking at 5 years
7–8 years	—	Procline upper incisors over the bite

Table 8.1 The multidisciplinary team management of cleft lip and palate *continued*

Age	Management	Role of the orthodontist
8–11 years	**Oral and maxillofacial surgeon/cleft surgeon**: alveolar bone graft following orthodontic expansion **Clinical psychologist**: coping strategies	Expand and align the upper arch prior to alveolar bone graft Record taking at 10 years
>12 years	**Restorative dentist**: advice and treatment planning prior to commencement of definitive orthodontic treatment	Definitive upper and lower fixed appliance therapy (in the absence of the need for orthognathic surgery) Record taking at 15 years
16–18 years	**Oral and maxillofacial surgeon**: orthognathic surgery **Restorative dentist**: provision of composite restorations/veneers/crowns/bridges/dentures	Upper and lower fixed appliance therapy to decompensate the arches if orthognathic surgery is required
>18 years	**Cleft surgeon**: rhinoplasty **Clinical geneticist**: genetic counselling	Record taking at 20 years

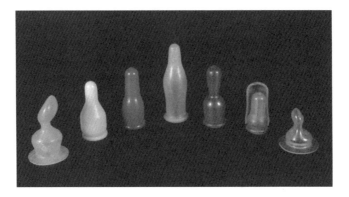

Fig. 8.39 A few examples of the large variety of teats available.

Birth

At birth the baby will be assessed by the paediatrician. Approximately 50% of babies born with a cleft lip or palate will have other congenital defects that may or may not require attention.[71]

Neonatal period

At this time the patient and parents will be visited by the feeding nurse who will give advice. Where possible, the mother will be encouraged to breast-feed, although this often proves difficult. If this is the case, the feeding nurse will advise on the most appropriate bottle and teat combination, various designs of which are available (Fig. 8.39). Presurgical orthodontic plates have been recommended as an aid to feeding, but research has not shown that they confer any such benefit.[72]

The parents and baby will also usually be seen by another member of the cleft team, such as the cleft surgeon and/or orthodontist, who will advise as to the immediate and longer term treatment that will be required (see Table 8.1). A cleft of the lip may be repaired between 24 hours and 6 months after birth, depending upon the preferences of the surgeon. The primary palate (from the lip back to the incisive foramen) is usually repaired at the same time. The argument for an early repair, within days of birth, is for the psychological benefit of the parents. However, research on parents of cleft babies whose lips were either repaired within a few days or around 3 months after birth, failed to demonstrate any difference in the emotional status of the mother.[73] Others have argued for delayed repair so that the surgery does not interfere with the rapid facial growth that occurs soon after birth. Presurgical orthopaedic plates (Fig. 8.40), fitted by the orthodontist, have also been recommended in order to help approximate the two segments of the maxilla over a period of 3–4 months. This is said to make primary

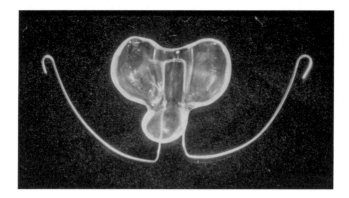

Fig. 8.40 A presurgical orthopaedic plate. This one has a wire facebow so that a headcap can be fitted. This is not required in many cases.

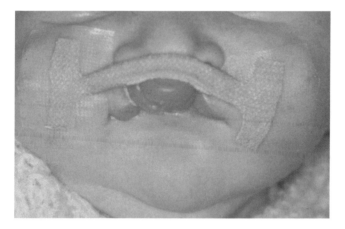

Fig. 8.41 Elasticated strapping is sometimes used to help approximate the segments of the cleft prior to surgical repair.

palate and lip repair easier in both unilateral and bilateral cleft lip and palate cases. However, it is questionable whether repair is made much easier, and certainly there are no measurable long-term benefits from their use on dental arch relationships and facial growth.[74] In the case of bilateral cleft lip and palate babies in particular, strapping is sometimes used, with or without a presurgical orthopaedic plate, to help realign the premaxilla prior to surgical repair (Fig. 8.41).

3–6 months of age
The lip and primary palate are usually repaired during this time. Any repair of the primary palate, including the alveolus, is only a soft tissue repair.

6–18 months

Soft tissue repair of the hard and soft palate may take place at this time, for which there are numerous surgical techniques available. The aim at this stage is to repair the palate to facilitate the development of normal speech.

18 months onwards

Speech therapy may start 18 months and 3 years of age in such patients. The child's hearing will also be assessed by this time and where necessary ventilation tubes (grommets) may be fitted by the ENT surgeons. It is important the child is also seen by a paediatric dentist or by their own local dentist to ensure good dental health. This will involve dietary advice, fluoride supplements,[75] and fissure sealing as appropriate.[76] A pharyngoplasty may be performed to aid speech before the child begins school.

8–11 years

Orthodontic treatment may be started at this time. As the upper central incisors erupt it is not unusual for them to do so in crossbite with the lower incisors (Fig. 8.42). Provided the skeletal pattern is favourable and the upper incisors are retroclined, an upper removable appliance, with posterior biteplanes to free the anterior occlusion, can be used to procline the upper incisors over the bite. Treatment should take no longer than 3–6 months. It is important to keep treatment as short as possible in order not to use up the patient's long-term cooperation for the later orthodontic treatment.

In the case of unilateral and bilateral complete cleft lip and palate cases, orthodontic treatment is performed at this age to facilitate the provision of a bone graft in the alveolar cleft. An upper fixed appliance is fitted along with either a quadhelix or trihelix. The latter is useful if the interpremolar

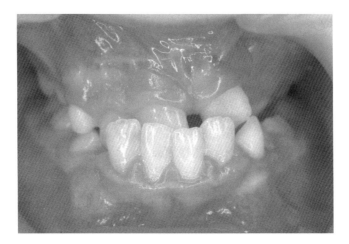

Fig. 8.42 The upper incisors often erupt in crossbite in cleft patients.

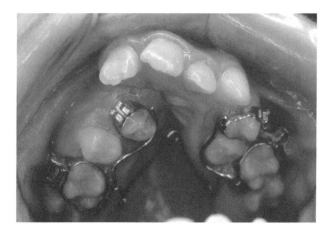

Fig. 8.43 A trihelix used to expand and align the upper arch prior to the provision of an alveolar bone graft in the site of the cleft.

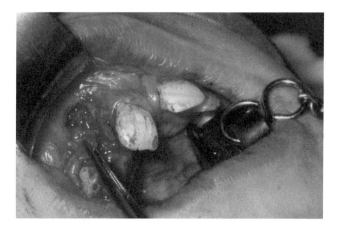

Fig. 8.44 An alveolar bone graft being placed for the patient in Fig. 8.43.

width is particularly narrow (Fig. 8.43). The aim is to expand and round out the upper arch, aligning the teeth to a more normal archform and creating space for the alveolar bone graft at the cleft site. The graft itself is cancellous bone usually taken from the iliac crest of the hip or the fibia (Fig. 8.44). At the time of operation it is important that the nasal floor has been repaired anteriorly to provide a stop for the bone graft and to seal it from the nasal cavity. The presurgical orthodontic treatment and bone graft must be completed prior to the eruption of the upper permanent canine. This tooth should then erupt through the bone graft and into the mouth (Fig. 8.45). The advantages of placing the alveolar bone graft particularly prior to canine eruption are:

1. The maxillary alveolus becomes a single unit without a cleft.

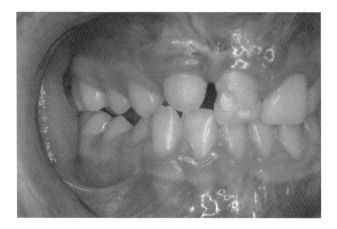

Fig. 8.45 The same patient as in Figs 8.43 and 8.44 where the upper canine has erupted through the alveolar bone graft.

2. The upper canine is more likely to erupt into a normal position with good bone support.
3. The fact that the canine erupts through the graft means this functional bone is likely to remain in place.
4. The bone graft can help to improve facial appearance by supporting the base of the nose.

When the cleft child attends secondary school they may be subject to teasing if the cleft is visible or has an effect on speech. Referral to a clinical psychologist specializing in facial deformity, at around 11 years of age, can help provide the child with strategies to cope with their deformity prior to starting their new school.

12 years onwards

Once the permanent canines and premolars have erupted, the definitive phase of orthodontics, involving upper and lower fixed appliances, may begin. However, the presence of the cleft may have two possible effects on this fixed appliance phase. First, it is not unusual for patients with a cleft to have dental anomalies in the cleft site. This may be in the form of missing, extra, or malformed teeth and their presence or absence may require space to be created or closed during orthodontic treatment, followed by some restorative dentistry. Up to 50% of cleft cases may, for example, have a developmentally absent upper lateral incisor.[77] Advice may therefore need to be obtained from a restorative dentistry colleague at the treatment planning stage and perhaps during active orthodontic treatment. Second, the cleft patient may have a skeletal discrepancy requiring orthognathic surgery and so fixed appliance therapy may be delayed until the patient is 16 years of age.

16–18 years

It is known that the presence of cleft lip and palate has an effect on jaw growth. Certainly such patients have been shown to have a shorter cranial base than normal, with a more retrusive maxilla and nasal complex. Interestingly, they also demonstrate a reduced mandibular length, but with a posterior growth rotation and an increased anterior lower face height.[78] In a study on completely unoperated adult cleft lip and palate patients in Sri Lanka[79] a retropositioned mandible was still seen, but anteroposterior maxillary growth was almost normal. The primary cleft surgery is therefore thought to have a profound effect on subsequent maxillary growth. Why is it though that up to 35–40% of unilateral cleft lip and palate patients in the UK may eventually require an osteotomy for a Class III skeletal relationship in their late teens, when in some other European countries this rate is only 6%?[80] This may be related to differences in care at the time of primary cleft repair. In those countries where the need for a final osteotomy is less, only a few surgeons perform the primary repair and consequently they treat a large number of cases per year (high-volume operators). In the UK, there are more surgeons who individually treat fewer cases per year (low-volume operators). There are also differences in the surgical protocol between the different centres, which may also explain the observed variation in the results. As a result of these and other differences, the Clinical Standards Advisory Group (CSAG) Cleft Lip and Palate Study has recommended centralization of cleft services in order to raise the standard of care in the UK. One of the recommendations is that cleft care should be performed by high-volume operators, both surgeons and orthodontists, working in designated cleft centres. Hopefully, not only will this raise the overall standard of care, but will also ensure that each centre will have sufficient cases to enable a successful audit of their outcomes.[81] Those patients with a cleft who still require orthognathic surgery, due to a Class III skeletal pattern, undergo presurgical orthodontics at this time to decompensate the arches (see Section 8.2.2). This is usually followed by a Le Fort 1 maxillary advancement procedure to correct the underlying skeletal deformity. There are a number of problems with such surgery to advance the maxilla in such patients. Due to previous surgery and the subsequent scarring it can be difficult to advance the maxilla very far anteriorly. Following surgery it can be difficult to stabilize the maxilla in its new position during the immediate postsurgical phase. If surgical advancement is successful there can also be problems with speech if the soft palate is no longer able to adequately meet the posterior wall of the pharynx during function. To reduce this problem it is possible to advance the maxilla and yet leave the soft palate in place.

18 years onwards

Following orthodontic treatment and possible orthognathic surgery, when facial growth is much reduced, the patient may undergo a rhinoplasty to improve the appearance of the nose. Genetic counselling should also be offered due to the increased risk of the patient having cleft children themselves (see Section 8.4.4).

8.4.6 The role of the orthodontist in the management of the cleft patient

The orthodontist is involved in the management of the cleft child from the neonatal period through to the late teenage years. In addition to counselling parents and providing presurgical strapping in perhaps a few instances in the neonatal period, most treatment is performed at three specific times. For the unilateral or bilateral complete cleft lip and palate patient these are:
- Early mixed dentition (6–7 years) when the upper permanent incisors are proclined to correct a reverse overjet.
- Mixed dentition (8–11 years) when the upper arch is expanded prior to an alveolar bone graft.
- Permanent dentition, either as a definitive course of treatment in its own right using upper and lower fixed appliances (12–14 years) to correct the malocclusion, or in combination with orthognathic surgery at around 16–18 years of age.

The exact treatment will depend upon the severity and site of the cleft and the malocclusion. For instance, in the case of an isolated cleft of the lip, or just a cleft of the palate, there will be no need for an alveolar bone graft and the associated orthodontic treatment. An additional role of the orthodontist is to collect records from the neonatal period through to adulthood. This will include photographs, radiographs, and study models so that the results of treatment can be audited and, where necessary, acted upon.

8.5   SUMMARY OF MULTIDISCIPLINARY TREATMENT

Multidisciplinary treatment includes:
1. Restorative dentistry and orthodontics:
    - relocating or closing space when teeth are absent
    - aligning teeth to provide a path of insertion
    - aligning the roots prior to provision of an implant
    - realigning periodontally involved teeth
2. Surgical treatment in relation to orthodontics:
    - minor oral surgery:
        - extraction of teeth
        - exposure of teeth
        - frenectomy
        - pericision
        - autotransplantation of teeth
        - implants
    - orthognathic patients:

3. Paediatric dentistry and orthodontics:
   • traumatized upper incisors
4. Patients with cleft lip and or palate

8.6 OBJECTIVES

Understand the following with respect to multidisciplinary treatment:
1. The ideal time(s) to plan such treatment.
2. When it is likely to be required.
3. The role of the orthodontist in multidisciplinary treatment.

FURTHER READING

Epker, B. N., Stella, J. P., and Fish, L. C. (1995). *Dentofacial deformities. Integrated orthodontic and surgical correction* (2nd edn). Mosby, St Louis.
McDonald, F. and Ireland, A. J. (1998). *Diagnosis of the orthodontic patient*. Oxford University Press, Oxford.

REFERENCES

1. Branemark, P-I., Hansson, B. D., and Adell, R. (1977). Osseointegrated implants in the treatment of the edentulous Jaw. Experience from a 10-year period. *Scandinavian Journal of Plastic and Reconstructive Surgery*, **16**(Suppl.), 18–38.
2. Polizzi, G., Fabbro, S., Furri, M., Herrmann J., and Squarzoni, S. (1999). Clinical application of narrow Branemark system implants for single-tooth restorations. *International Journal of Oral and Maxillofacial Implants*, **14**, 496–503.
3. Becker, A. and Karnei-R'em, R. M. (1992). The effects of infraocclusion: Part 1. Tilting of the adjacent teeth and local space loss. *American Journal of Orthodontics and Dentofacial Orthopedics*, **102**, 256–64.
4. Proffit, W. R. (1994). Forty-year review of extraction frequencies at a university orthodontic clinic. *Angle Orthodontist*, **64**, 407–15.
5. Edwards, J. G. (1977). The diastema, the frenum, the frenectomy: a clinical study. *American Journal of Orthodontics*, **71**, 489–508.
6. Sullivan T. C., Turpin D. L., and A[o]rtun J. (1996). A post retention study of patients presenting with a maxillary median diastema. *Angle Orthodontist*, **66**, 131–8.
7. Edwards, J. G. (1970). A surgical procedure to eliminate rotational relapse. *American Journal of Orthodontics*, **57**, 35–46.
8. Edwards, J. G. (1988). A long-term prospective evaluation of the circumferential supracrestal fiberotomy in alleviating orthodontic relapse. *American Journal of Orthodontics and Dentofacial Orthopedics*, **93**, 380–4.
9. Pinson, R. R. and Strahan, J. D. (1974). The effect on the relapse of orthodontically rotated teeth of surgical division of the gingival fibres—pericision. *British Journal of Orthodontics*, **1**, 87–91.
10. Widman, L. (1915). Om transplantation av retinerade hörntänder. *Svensk Tandläkare Tidskrift*, **8**, 289–96.
11. Czochrowska, E. M., Stenvik, A., Album, B., and Zachrisson, B. (2000). Autotransplantation of premolars to replace maxillary incisors: a comparison with natural incisors. *American Journal of Orthodontics and Dentofacial Orthopedics*, **118**, 592–600.

12. Peskin, S. and Graber, T. (1970). Surgical repositioning of teeth. *Journal of the American Dental Association*, **80**, 1320–6.
13. Guralnick, W. C. (1970). Autogenous and allogenic tooth transplantation. *Journal of Oral Surgery*, **28**, 575–7.
14. Altonen, M., Haavikko, K., and Malmström, M. (1978). Evaluation of autotransplantations of completely developed canines. *International Journal of Oral Surgery*, **7**, 434–41.
15. Skoglund, A., Tronstad, L., and Wallenius, K. (1978). Microangiographic study of vascular changes in replanted and autotransplanted teeth of young dogs. *Oral Surgery*, **45**, 17–28.
16. Northway, W. N. and Konigsbergn, S. (1980). Autogenic tooth transplantation. The 'state of the art'. *American Journal of Orthodontics*, **77**, 146–62.
17. Ahlberg, D., Bystedt, H., Eliasson, S., and Odenrick, L. (1983). Long-term evaluation of autotransplanted maxillary canines with completed root formation. *Acta Odontologica Scandinavica*, **41**, 23–31.
18. Schwartz, O., Bergmann, P., and Klausen, B. (1985). Autotransplantation of human teeth: a life table analysis of prognostic factors. *International Journal of Oral Surgery*, **14**, 245–58.
19. Paulsen H. U. and Andreasen, J. O. (1998). Tooth eruption subsequent to transplantation: a longitudinal study of autotransplanted premolars. *European Journal of Orthodontics*, **20**, 45–55.
20. Paulsen, H. U. (2001). Autotransplantation of teeth in orthodontic treatment. *American Journal of Orthodontics and Dentofacial Orthopedics*, **119**, 336–7.
21. Czochrowska, E. M., Stenvik, A., Bjercke, B., and Zachrisson, B. U. (2002). Outcome of tooth transplantation: survival and success rates 17–41 years posttreatment. *American Journal of Orthodontics and Dentofacial Orthopedics*, **121**, 110–19.
22. Higuchi, K. W. and Slack, J. M. (1991). The use of titanium fixtures for intra-oral anchorage to facilitate orthodontic tooth movement. *International Journal of Oral and Maxillofacial Implants*, **6**, 338–44.
23. Wehrbrein, H., Merz, B. R. and Diedrich, P. (1999). Palatal bone support for orthodontic implant anchorage—a clinical and radiological study. *European Journal of Orthodontics*, **21**, 65–70.
24. Wehrbrein, H., Feifel, H. and Diedrich P. (1999). Palatal implant anchorage reinforcement of posterior teeth: a prospective study. *American Journal of Orthodontics and Dentofacial Orthopedics*, **116**, 678–86.
25. Block, M. S. and Hoffman, D. R. (1995). A new device for absolute anchorage for orthodontics. *American Journal of Orthodontics and Dentofacial Orthopedics*, **107**, 251–8.
26. McDonald, F. and Ireland, A. J. (1998). *Diagnosis of the orthodontic patient*. Oxford University Press.
27. Epker, B. N. and Fish, L. C. (1983). The surgical–orthodontic correction of mandibular deficiency. Part I. *American Journal of Orthodontics*, **84**, 408–21.
28. Lines, P. A. and Steinhauser, W. W. (1974). Soft tissue changes in relationship to movement of hard structures in orthognathic surgery: a preliminary report. *Journal of Oral Surgery*, **32**, 891–6.
29. Quast, D. C., Biggerstaff, R. H., and Haley, J. V. (1983). The short-term and long-term soft tissue profile changes in accompanying mandibular advancement surgery. *American Journal of Orthodontics*, **84**, 29–36.
30. Ewing, M. and Ross R. B. (1992). Soft tissue response to mandibular advancement and genioplasty. *American Journal of Orthodontics and Dentofacial Orthopedics*, **101**, 550–5.

31. Brooks, B. W., Buschang, P. H., Bates, J. D., Adams, T. B., and English, J. D. (2001). Predicting upper lip response to 4-piece maxillary LeFort I osteotomy. *American Journal of Orthodontics and Dentofacial Orthopedics*, **120**, 124–33.

32. Upton, P. M., Sadowsky, P. L., Sarver, D. M., and Heaven, T. J. (1997). Evaluation of video imaging prediction in combined maxillary and mandibular orthognathic surgery. *American Journal of Orthodontics and Dentofacial Orthopedics*, **112**, 656–65.

33. Konstiantos, K. A., O'Reilly, M. T., and Close, J. (1994). The validity of the prediction of soft tissue profile changes after LeFort I osteotomy using the dentofacial planner (computer software). *American Journal of Orthodontics and Dentofacial Orthopedics*, **105**, 241–9.

34. Sinclair, P. M., Kilpeläinen, P., Phillips, C., White, R. P., Rogers, L., and Sarver, D. M. (1995). The accuracy of video imaging in orthognathic surgery. *American Journal of Orthodontics and Dentofacial Orthopedics*, **107**, 177–85.

35. Mobarak, K. A., Espeland, L., Krogstad, O., and Lyberg T. (2001). Soft tissue profile changes following mandibular advancement surgery: predictability and long-term outcome. *American Journal of Orthodontics and Dentofacial Orthopedics*, **119**, 353–67.

36. Sarver, D. M., Johnston, M. J., and Matukas, V. J. (1988). Video imaging for planning and counseling for orthognathic surgery. *Journal of Oral and Maxillofacial Surgery*, **46**, 939–45.

37. Sarver, D. M. (1998). Video-imaging and treatment presentation: medico-legal implications and patient perception. *American Journal of Orthodontics and Dentofacial Orthopedics*, **112**, 360–3.

38. Epker, B. N., Stella, J. P., and Fish, L. C. (1995). *Dentofacial deformities. Integrated orthodontic and surgical correction* (2nd edn). Mosby, St Louis.

39. Rittersma, J., Van Der Veld, R. G. M., Van Gool, A. V., and Kopendraaier, J. (1981). Stable fragment fixation in orthognathic surgery: review of 30 cases. *Journal of Oral Surgery*, **39**, 671–5.

40. Van Sickels, J. E. and Richardson, D. A. (1996). Stability of orthognathic surgery: a review of rigid fixation. *British Journal of Oral Maxillofacial Surgery*, **34**, 279–85.

41. Panula, K., Finne, K., and Oikarinen, K. (2001). Incidence of complications and problems related to orthognathic surgery: a review of 655 patients. *Journal of Oral and Maxillofacial Surgery*, **59**, 1128–36.

42. De Clercq, C. A., Neyt, L. F., Mommaerts, M. Y., Abeloos, J. V., De Mot, B. M. (1994). Condylar resorption in orthognathic surgery: a retrospective study. *International Journal of Adult Orthodontics and Orthognathic Surgery*, **9**, 233–40.

43. Cope, J. B., Samchukov, M. L., and Cherkaskin, A. M. (1999). Mandibular distraction osteogenesis: a historic perspective and future directions. *American Journal of Orthodontics and Dentofacial Orthopedics*, **115**, 448–60.

44. Crawford, M. J. (1948). Selection of appliances for typical facial fractures. *Oral Surgery, Oral Medicine and Oral pathology*, **1**, 442–51.

45. Ilizarov, G. A. (1989). The tension–stress effect on the genesis and growth of tissues: Part I, the influence of stability of fixation and soft tissue preservation. *Clinical Orthopaedics and Related Research*, **238**, 249–81.

46. Ilizarov, G. A. (1989). The tension–stress effect on the genesis and growth of tissues: Part II, the influence of the rate and frequency of distraction. *Clinical Orthopaedics and Related Research*, **239**, 263–85.

47. Ilizarov, G. A. (1990). Clinical application of the tension–stress effect for limb lengthening. *Clinical Orthopaedics and Related Research*, **250**, 8–26.

48. Van Sickels, J. E. (2000). Commentary. Distraction osteogenesis versus orthognathic surgery. *American Journal of Orthodontics and Dentofacial Orthopedics*, **118**, 482–4.

49. Roberts-Harry, D. and Sandy, J. R. (1992). Repair of cleft lip and palate: 1. Surgical techniques. *Dental Update*, **19**, 418–23.

50. Vanderas, A. P. (1987). Incidence of cleft lip, cleft palate and cleft lip and palate among races; a review. *Cleft Palate Journal*, **24**, 216–23.
51. Sphrintzen, R. J., Siegel-Sadewitz, V., Amato, J., and Goldberg, R. B. (1985). Anomalies associated with cleft lip, cleft palate, or both. *American Journal of Medical Genetics*, **20**, 585–95.
52. Curtis, E., Fraser, F., and Warburton, D. (1961). Congenital cleft lip and palate: risk figures for counselling. *American Journal of Diseases of Children*, **102**, 853–7.
53. Harper, P. S. (1998). Oral and craniofacial disorders. In: *Practical genetic counselling*. Butterworth–Heinmann. Oxford.
54. Mossey, P. A. (1999). The heritability of malocclusion: Part 1–genetics, principles and terminology. *British Journal of Orthodontics*, **26**, 103–13.
55. Hill, L., Murphy, M., McDowall, M., and Paul, A. H. (1988). Maternal drug histories and congenital malformations: limb reduction defects and oral clefts. *Journal of Epidemiology and Community Health*, **42**, 1–7.
56. Dolovich, L. R., Addis, A., Vaillancourt, J. M. R., Power, J. D. B., Doren, G., and Einarson, T. R. (1998). Benzodiazepine use in pregnancy and major malformations or oral cleft; meta-analysis of cohort and case-control studies. *British Medical Journal*, **317**, 839–43.
57. Khoury, M. J., Gomez-Farias, M., and Mulinare, J. (1989). Does cigarette smoking during pregnancy cause cleft lip and palate in offspring? *American Journal of Diseases in Children*, **143**, 333–7.
58. Hartridge, T., Illing, H. M., and Sandy, J. R. (1999). The role of folic acid in oral clefting. *British Journal of Orthodontics*, **26**, 115–20.
59. Fitzgerald, M. J. T. (1978). *Human embryology*. Harper & Row, New York, USA.
60. Ferguson, M. W. J. (1981). Development mechanisms in normal and abnormal palate formation with particular reference to the aetiology, pathogenesis and prevention of cleft palate. *British Journal of Orthodontics*, **8**, 115–37.
61. Sun, D., Vanderburg, C. R., Odierna, G. S., and Hay, E. D. (1998). TGFβ3 promotes transformation of chicken palate medial edge epithelium to mesenchym *in vitro*. *Development*, **125**, 95–105.
62. Davis, J. S. and Ritchie, H. P. (1922). Classification of congenital clefts of the lip and palate. *Journal of the American Medical Association*, **79**, 1323.
63. Veau, V. (1931). *Division palatine*. Masson. Paris.
64. Kernahan, D. A. and Stark, R. B. (1958). A new classification for cleft lip and cleft palate. *Plastic and Reconstructive Surgery*, **22**, 435–44.
65. Bellis, T. H. and Wohlgemuth, B. (1999). The incidence of cleft lip and palate deformities in the South-east of Scotland (1971–1990). *British Journal of Orthodontics*, **26**, 121–5.
66. Gorlin, R. J., Cervenka, J., and Pruzinsky, S. (1971). Facial clefting and its syndromes. *Birth Defects*, **7**, 3–49.
67. Jensen, B. L., Kreiborg, S., Dahl, E., and Fogh-Andersen, P. (1988). Cleft lip and palate in Denmark 1976–1981 epidemiology, variability and early somatic development. *Cleft Palate Journal*, **25**, 258–69.
68. Greg, T., Boyd, D., and Richardson, A. (1994). The incidence of cleft lip and palate in Northern Ireland from 1980–1990. *British Journal of Orthodontics*, **21**, 387–92.
69. Cockell, A. and Lees, M. (2000). Prenatal diagnosis and management of orofacial clefts. *Prenatal Diagnosis*, **20**, 149–51.
70. Chitty, L. S. and Griffin, D. R. (2001). *Abnormalities of the fetal lip and palate: sonographic diagnosis in management of cleft lip and palate* In: Management of Cleft Lip and Palate (ed. A. C. H. Watson, D. A. Sell, and P. Grunwell). P. Whurr, London.
71. Shprintzen, R. J., Siegel-Sadewitz, V. L., Amato, J., and Goldberg, R. B. (1985). Retrospective diagnosis of previously missed syndromic disorders amongst 1000

patients with cleft lip, cleft palate or both. *Birth Defects. Original Article Series*, **21**, 85–92.

72. Kuipers-Jagtman, A. M., Prahl-Anderson, B., Prahl, C., Konst, E. M., Severens, J. L., and Peters, H. F. M. (1999). Dutch three-centre randomised prospective clinical trial of presurgical infant orthopaedics. *European Craniofacial Congress*, 1999, Manchester. (Abstract)

73. Slade, P., Emerson, D. J. M., and Freedlander, E. (1999). A longitudinal comparison of the psychological impact on mothers of neonatal and 3 month repair of cleft lip. *British Journal of Plastic Surgery*, **52**, 1–5.

74. Shaw, W. C. and Semb, G. (1990). Current approaches to the orthodontic management of cleft lip and palate. *Journal of the Royal Society of Medicine*, **83**, 30–3.

75. Rivkin, C. J., Keith, O., Crawford, P. J., and Hathorn, I. S. (2000). Dental care for the patient with a cleft lip and palate. Part 1: From birth to the mixed dentition stage. *British Dental Journal*, **188**, 78–83.

76. Rivkin, C. J., Keith, O., Crawford, P. J., and Hathorn, I. S. (2000). Dental care for the patient with a cleft lip and palate. Part 2: The mixed dentition stage through to adolescence and young adulthood. *British Dental Journal*, **188**, 131–4.

77. Ranta, R. (1986). A review of tooth formation in children with cleft lip/palate. *American Journal of Orthodontics and Dentofacial Orthopedics*, **90**, 11–18.

78. Ross, R. B. (1987). Treatment variables affecting facial growth in complete unilateral cleft lip and palate. *Cleft Palate Journal*, **24**, 5–77.

79. Mars, M. and Houston, W. J. (1990). A preliminary study of facial growth and morphology in unoperated male unilateral cleft lip and palate subjects over 13 years of age. *Cleft Palate Journal*, **27**, 7–10.

80. Shaw, W. C., Asher-McDade, C., Brattstrom, V., Dahl, E., Mars, M., McWilliam, J., Molsted, K., Plint, D., Prahl-Anderson, B., Roberts, C., Semb, G., and the RPS (1992). A six-center international study of treatment outcome in patients with clefts of the lip and palate: Part 5. General discussion and conclusions. *Cleft Palate and Craniofacial Journal*, **29**, 413–18.

81. Bearn, D., Mildinhall, S., Murphy, T., Murray, J. J., Sell, D., Shaw, W. C., Williams, A. C., and Sandy, J. R. (2001). Cleft lip and palate care in the United Kingdom—the Clinical Standards Advisory Group (CSAG). Study. Part 4: Outcome comparisons, training, and conclusions. *Cleft Palate and Craniofacial Journal*, **38**, 38–43.

9 Iatrogenic problems

CONTENTS

As a profession we must undertake, wherever possible, to minimize harm to our patients. In a specialty such as orthodontics, which is based largely on improving aesthetics and where there is limited evidence for any increased longevity of the dentition as a result of treatment, we must ensure that the long-term prognosis of teeth is not adversely compromised. At each stage it is essential that consideration be given to the fact that orthodontic treatment can cause damage to a number of tissues. It is fortunate that, in general, such damage is so minimal as to be clinically insignificant with little effect on the long-term prognosis of the dentition. It is a matter of clinical judgement when this damage, or the risk of such damage, outweighs the benefits to be gained by the treatment. All aspects of orthodontic care can produce 'harm' to patients if incorrectly undertaken. These will be considered in this chapter.

9.1   LOCAL DISORDERS

9.1.1   Extraoral

Damage as a direct consequence of trauma
Traumatic injuries can be classified as:
(1) diagnostic injury—radiographs
(2) treatment injury:
    (a) appliances, e.g. headgear
    (b) instruments/materials:
        (i)   cross-infection
        (ii) direct, e.g. trauma/heat.
These will be discussed in turn below.

Diagnostic injury
The most likely source of harm to the patient during the diagnostic process comes from the taking of radiographs. For patients undergoing an orthodontic assessment it is mandatory to have the appropriate radiographs. These might include the dental panoramic (rotational) tomograph (DPT), an upper standard occlusal, and a lateral skull radiograph where there is a skeletal discrepancy, so that a cephalometric analysis can be performed. With an increasing number of adult patients undergoing orthodontic care, consideration should also be given to obtaining other views where there may be a need for accurate and reproducible assessment of the dentoalveolar structures over time. This is particularly so if there is evidence of previous periodontal disease. Equally, this might apply to the child patient with evidence of short roots on one or more teeth. Such views might include the long-cone periapical. As stated earlier, orthodontic treatment almost always causes some minor damage to the tooth or its supporting tissues but is

usually of little consequence in the long term. However, occasionally such damage is more marked and without an accurate pretreatment assessment of these structures, and where necessary during treatment, it will not be possible to monitor the extent and rate of any such damage and therefore modify treatment accordingly.

In recent years there has been some debate over whether the three radiographic views mentioned previously are required for all patients. Clearly, if there is no skeletal discrepancy there is little diagnostic gain from taking a lateral skull radiograph, with the patient being exposed to unnecessary radiation. The dental panoramic tomograph is an important radiograph for use in orthodontic diagnosis to assess the presence, position, developmental staging, and any pathology associated with the dentition. There has been some debate about the usefulness of the upper standard occlusal radiograph in recent years.[1] However, this view is recommended where it is felt that any important structure requiring assessment is outside the focal trough of the DPT. The problem is that, as yet, there are no reliable predictors as to which patients may have pathology in the premaxillary region when the DPT is not of clear diagnostic value. The upper standard occlusal radiograph has a minimal radiation risk, only has to be taken once before a course of treatment, and so it has to be questioned whether a practitioner would be considered negligent if this radiograph was not taken prior to orthodontic treatment.

Currently, there seems to be some confusion regarding the need for radiographic assessment and diagnosis in orthodontics. In addition, the requirement for longitudinal analyses of the effects of treatment has been compromised by well-publicized cases of excessive radiation exposure of patients to 'unnecessary' radiographs. The guidelines detailed by the British Orthodontic Society[2] are specific, in that orthodontic treatment is an indication for appropriate good-quality radiographs.

Incidence

It is reported that there are 1.8 deaths for every million DPT radiographs taken. There is also evidence that the quality of these radiographs in general dental practice is very variable and it is essential that they be assessed rigorously.[3] In one survey of 1800 films as few as 0.8% met the appropriate standard (33% being unacceptable as a minimum standard). The most common faults reported, which contributed to poor-quality radiographs, were anteroposterior positioning errors, low density, and low contrast.

Whilst the risk is low, it is essential that this be taken into account when determining the need for any radiographic investigation. In addition, the risk will exponentially increase if a film, which is deemed necessary, is then of such poor diagnostic quality that it has to be repeated.

Other radiographic imaging techniques are being considered for use in orthodontic diagnosis, e.g. computed tomography (CT). They have been used for the assessment of root resorption, especially in relation to maxillary

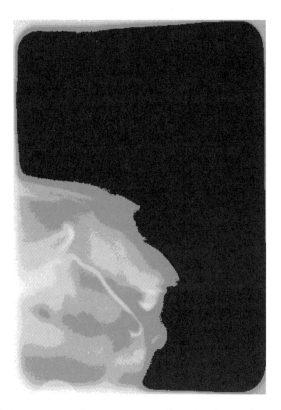

Fig. 9.1 A Scanora view of a cross-section of an alveolus, in this case examining the maxillary labial segment for alveolar bone into which a dilacerated maxillary incisor can be moved.

canines in close proximity to maxillary incisors.[4] However, the radiation dose is high and the additional information beyond that provided by an accurate long-cone periapical radiograph has to be carefully considered. Additional tomographic techniques include the Scanora, which is able to provide clear cross-sections of the alveolus (Fig. 9.1). Another technique is magnetic resonance imaging (MRI), which carries no radiation risk. However, the quality of the image, due to the manner in which the view is produced, may not enhance the clinical diagnosis. Placing children in the imaging equipment could induce claustrophobia and the increased imaging time may fail to produce a clear view. However, for specific soft tissue detail in a compliant patient the additional information can assist clinical diagnosis.[5] This imaging method is currently only available in some hospitals.

Causative agents/pathophysiology
The wavelength of X-ray radiation is such that potential damage can occur either directly to tissues (stochastic tissue damage) or to the genetic tissues,

and in both cases the effects are cumulative. The causes of excessive exposure to radiation in orthodontic diagnosis include:
- faulty X-ray set or processor
- the wrong speed of film
- lack of X-ray beam collimation
- inappropriate radiographs, clear justification
- inadequately trained staff taking and processing the radiographs.

Prevention
The prevention of risks from this aspect of orthodontic care is clearly
detailed in the BOS guidelines[2] and includes:
- accurately positioned and exposed patient
- modern equipment properly maintained
- high-speed films used with the appropriate intensifying screens
- films processed correctly with chemicals that are in the appropriate condition
- the processing equipment should also be maintained to the correct standard.

Every clinician must therefore be sure of the diagnostic information
required before committing the patient to any radiographic investigation.
The radiograph should also be well taken and processed to maximize the
diagnostic yield.

Treatment
Appliances (e g headgear)
Considerable attention has been focused on the potential and actual risk to
extraoral structures from the use of headgear appliances. Of particular concern
is the risk to the eyes. There are a number of tragic and well-publicized cases
where a reported direct injury to one eye, causing perforation, subsequently led
to damage to the contralateral eye via an autoimmune response.[6]

Currently available headgear appliances incorporate a number of safety
devices to minimize the risks associated with their use.[7] These include: locking
facebows; facebows with smooth, large, and blunt ends to the bows
(Fig. 9.2); snap-away spring mechanisms (Figs 9.3(a) and (b)); and safety neck-
straps (Figs 9.4(a) and (b)) to prevent the facebow from inadvertently coming
out of the mouth. The British Orthodontic Society recommends that at least
two safety mechanisms be employed at any one time. If such safety mechanisms are used then the risks from the wearing of headgear are very low.

Instruments/materials
(i) *Cross-infection*—It is essential in any clinical setting that appropriate
     cross-infection control measures are undertaken. The guidelines on
     cross-infection control are covered in many texts, but the legal and
     professional obligations are detailed by the British Dental Association[8]
     and include:
     1. Before patient treatment:
        - ensure all equipment has been sterilized or adequately disinfected

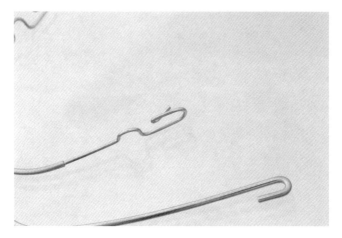

Fig. 9.2 Facebow showing a blunt end to the inner bow to prevent penetrating injuries of the eyes.

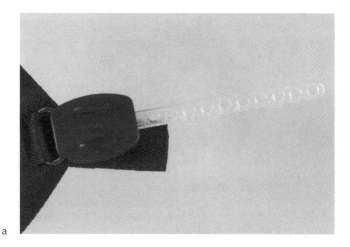

a

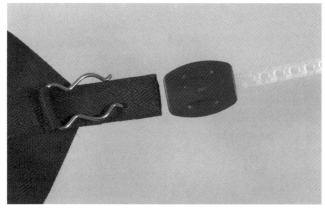

b

Fig. 9.3 A snap-away safety measure, which will disengage when excessive loads are applied (a) attached and (b) disengaged.

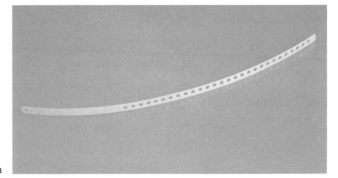

a

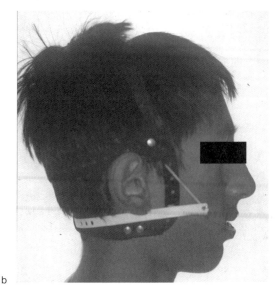

b

Fig. 9.4 A cervical safety neck strap which prevents the headgear from being removed from the mouth (a) as supplied and (b) in place in conjunction with an Interlandii headgear.

- put disposable coverings in place
- place appropriate instruments on the table
- set out all materials and mixing instruments
- update the patient's medical history.

2. During patient treatment:
   - treat all patients as potentially infectious
   - wear gloves, masks, and protective eyewear and clothing where necessary
   - provide eye protection for the patient
   - wash hands before gloving—a new pair of gloves for each patient
   - discard torn or damaged gloves

3. After patient treatment:
- use high-volume aspiration
- handle sharps carefully.

3. After patient treatment:
- dispose of sharps correctly
- clean all instruments and sterilize using an autoclave
- clean and disinfect all contaminated areas
- prepare surgery for next patient.

4. At the end of the session:
- dispose of all clinical waste
- clean and disinfect all work surfaces thoroughly
- disinfect the aspirator, its tubing, and spittoon
- clean the chair and unit.

(ii) *Trauma—heat, chemical*:

- *Heat*—Instruments must be allowed to cool for the correct length of time following their removal from the autoclave. There are isolated reports of damage to the patient's lips caused by instruments that have been used when too hot.[9] It is therefore important the surgery is well equipped with instruments to allow ample time for them to be autoclaved and adequately cooled between patients.

- *Chemical*—Many of the currently available sterilizing solutions are toxic to orofacial tissues. It is essential that instruments are thoroughly rinsed with water and dried before use if they have been immersed in such solutions. Chemical burns can also arise from the use of enamel etchants, such as *o*-phosphoric acid. Care must be taken to ensure the etchant is only placed on the required area of enamel, for there have been reports of lips being burnt from the improper use of these acids.[10] In addition, the simple precaution of using protective glasses for the patient is recommended, particularly when the patient is supine. This not only protects against any corrosive solutions such as sterilizing solution or etchants, but also against any instruments being dropped on the patient. If there is a spillage of any potentially harmful materials, copious amounts of clean water should be used to flush the affected area, an incident report recorded, and, if necessary, further medical advice sought.

Allergies (e.g. nickel sensitivity, acne)

Many of the materials used in orthodontics (see Chapter 7) contain significant amounts of nickel—not only in the nickel–titanium archwires, but also in the more widely used stainless-steel archwires and brackets. The steel used in these products is described as 18:8 steel; the 8 refers to the levels of nickel. Nickel is capable of inducing a type IV immune response, which has been found to occur in almost 1 in 5 individuals.[11] There is a greater reported incidence in females than males (30% versus 3%), and particularly in those with pierced ears (31% compared with 2%). Fortunately, orthodontic treatment only seems to aggravate a condition that already exists,[12,13] with the amount of nickel released from the use of fixed or removable appliances appearing to be lower than is necessary to initiate a hypersensitivity reaction. In orthodontics, reports of a true intraoral nickel allergy are fortunately very rare. Allergic reactions to extraoral appliances are more common and not infrequently seen around the metal studs used in some headgear (Fig. 9.5(a)).[14,15] In addition, patients often show an increase in skin disorders such as acne, which worsen during active treatment (Fig. 9.5(b)) but usually resolve after treatment.

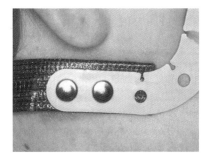 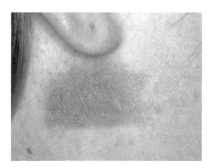

Fig. 9.5(a) A photograph clearly showing the relationship of the nickel-containing studs to the contact area.

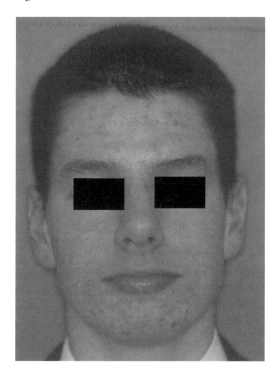

Fig. 9.5(b) An increase in acne is not infrequently found in patients undergoing treatment.

Disorders of the temporomandibular joint

Direct trauma

The application of loads in excess of those encountered in the normal physiology can induce pathology in the temporomandibular joint. The most potent appliance for provoking such damage, due mainly to the nature of loads it produces, is the Herbst appliance.[16] Typically, the head of the mandibular condyle can be flattened, malformed, and there can be areas of erosion identifiable on the articular surface when viewed radiographically (Fig. 9.6). However, it is clear that susceptibility to damage is related to many factors and not just the appliance. Simple orthodontic loads in a patient whose joint is unable to adapt can also provoke pathological changes. In addition, other disorders of the temporomandibular joint can be associated with temporomandibular dysfunction (TMD),[17] including the arthritic change seen in Still's disease,[18] and are unrelated to orthodontic treatment. In those patients at risk of TMD it is mandatory that a history and examination be recorded before treatment commences.

Indirect trauma

Extraction has been a controversial subject for almost as long as the specialty of orthodontics has existed. Some authors believe that the extraction of premolars leads to temporomandibular disorders. This occurs, they say, because the vertical dimension collapses. However, evidence is clear that (1) the vertical dimension cannot be correlated with loss of premolars,[19] and (2) there is no link between orthodontics and TMD; patients are as likely to develop TMD who have not had orthodontic treatment/intervention.[20]

Detrimental change in the patient's profile

There is controversy over the possible effects of orthodontic treatment on facial profile. One group of clinicians attempt to avoid extraction: the extrac-

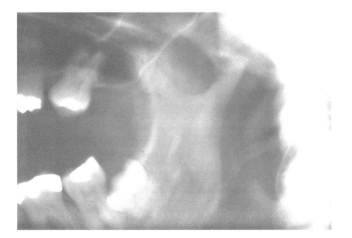

Fig. 9.6 A radiograph showing a condyle clearly resorbed beyond a normal form.

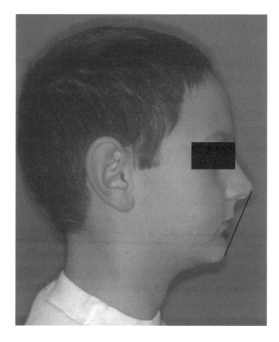

Fig. 9.7 A profile photograph showing a typical retruded facial profile. The upper and lower lips are behind the E line. This is typical of a Class II division 2 incisor relationship.

tion of teeth allegedly leading to a lack of support for the labial soft tissues and producing a typically retruded facial profile (Fig. 9.7). Conversely, the fuller soft tissue profiles are believed to be due to support from the dental structures (Fig. 9.8). This originally derived from work examining American beauty queens,[21] where a factor indicating facial attractiveness was the relationship of the soft tissue profile to the E line (soft tissue tip of nose to the soft tissue pogonion). There are many other considerations regarding the measurement of acceptable facial aesthetics[22,23] and it is this aspect of orthodontics that becomes very subjective in nature. However, progressive flattening of the facial profile has been identified in both extraction and non-extraction patients.[24–27] It has been attributed to maturational changes associated with continued mandibular growth and nasal development and is unrelated to orthodontic extractions. Indeed, there is evidence that such maturational changes in the facial structures continue well into the third decade of life.[28]

9.1.2   Intraoral

Soft tissue damage

Direct trauma and ulceration

There are few patients who have not been able to recall the ulcers and general soft tissue irritation that a fixed appliance can create. Any appliance will

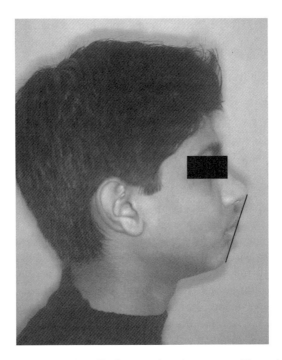

Fig. 9.8 A balanced facial profile showing that the upper and lower lips are slightly in front of the E line.

cause irritation, but this can be reduced by judicial adjustment, removing obviously prominent pieces of wire, and/or polishing areas of acrylic. Otherwise, the discomfort can usually be controlled by the application of wax to the appliance. Patients with a predisposing condition of the mucosa (e.g. xerostomia) or dermatological disorders, such as dystrophic epidermolysis bullosa,[29] may need to be referred for specialist advice prior to treatment, with extra care needed to ensure there are no sharp edges on the appliance and that great care is taken with other factors such as oral hygiene.

Gingival inflammation

The presence of an orthodontic appliance increases both the rate of formation and amount of plaque that develops intraorally.[30,31] As a consequence, the time taken to remove the plaque and the techniques employed vary. Before a course of treatment commences it is essential that the patient's oral hygiene is of an acceptable standard. If not, they must 'prove' themselves capable of maintaining a sufficiently good standard over a sustained period, such as 6 months, prior to starting treatment. It is also important that oral hygiene is monitored carefully throughout orthodontic treatment. This is to prevent enamel decalcification and, in the case of adults with a previous history of periodontal disease, acute periodontitis with rapid alveolar bone loss. The tissues should be observed at each visit and where appropriate pocket depths measured. If a patient is unable to improve their standard of oral hygiene, then serious consideration should be given to stopping the orthodontic treatment.

In a survey of advice given, most specialists (89.5%) gave dietary advice and 84% used disclosing tablets, whilst chlorhexidine mouthwash was recommended by 41.9%. Although the clinician advocates appropriate oral hygiene measures, the efficacy of such methods is determined almost exclusively by the patient's motivation.[32] Even with the most compliant individuals there is still some evidence of alveolar bone loss as a result of orthodontic treatment, and it is imperative that this is kept to a minimum[33] by good oral hygiene.

Apical blood vessels

This area of the periodontal ligament can be readily compressed during orthodontic tooth movement, but it fully recovers in the majority of cases. After the application of orthodontic loads, a period of reduced blood supply has been identified, followed by a 'reactive hyperaemia' to allow full perfusion of the tissues within the pulp chamber.[34] Indeed, the histological changes occurring within the pulp chamber are so consistent that orthodontic forces have been used to study the effects of trauma in detail.[35,36]

There is seldom any long-term damage to the apical blood vessels as a result of orthodontic treatment. Even following orthognathic surgery there is a minimal effect in the long-term blood flow in this region.[37]

Periapical pathology

If there is pre-existing periapical pathology it is important that this is adequately dealt with prior to moving a tooth orthodontically. Failure to do so may lead to an acute flare up of what was a chronic, low-grade infection. During the examination of the patient prior to treatment it is important to look for clues to any possible periapical pathology. These might include obvious caries, a darkened tooth due to pulpal death following trauma, a buccally pointing sinus, buccal expansion of the alveolus, or increased tooth mobility. It may not be possible to see any obvious pathology on a DPT radiograph, and so, where necessary, a long-cone periapical radiograph should be taken of the tooth under suspicion. If root canal therapy is required, then orthodontic tooth movement should be delayed until 3 months after completion of the filling.[38] It is essential that another long-cone periapical radiograph is taken before starting the orthodontic treatment. If there is still evidence of possible periapical pathology with no signs of resolution of the periapical radiolucency on the radiograph, then it is not appropriate to begin orthodontic treatment: otherwise there is the almost certain risk of provoking extensive root resorption.[39] If the radiolucency on the radiograph is still the same or is decreasing in size then orthodontic care can be commenced cautiously, with regular monitoring both clinically and radiographically.

Orthodontic treatment on a previously traumatized tooth requires that a careful history be taken. It is also important to have baseline measurements made on the tooth so that it can be carefully monitored during subsequent orthodontic treatment. Such teeth may be asymptomatic, but orthodontic treatment may compromise the apical blood vessels sufficiently to cause pulpal death. Patients should be made fully aware of any risks prior to starting treatment. The baseline records that should be taken might include:

- vitality testing
- noting the colour of the tooth
- a long-cone periapical radiograph.

If on examination the tooth has an obvious root fracture, then the risks of orthodontic treatment for this tooth need to be explained to the patient. The closer the fracture is towards the amelocemental junction the poorer the prognosis of the tooth, particularly if it is to be moved orthodontically. This probably applies equally to teeth that have a vital pulp or have been root-treated. In most instances, the fragment of root apical to the fracture line will not move with the rest of the crown during orthodontic treatment, unless the tooth has been root-treated and the root filling passes adequately into the apical fragment.[40] The exception to this is when root fractures in vital teeth occasionally show some repair, probably fibrous repair. If the tooth is vital and the coronal fragment is moved orthodontically there is still the risk of pulpal death in this coronal fragment.

If a traumatic episode has only just occurred and both the root and the crown are intact, there are a number of possible outcomes depending on the stage of root formation of the tooth. Therefore the trauma, its likely effects, and treatment can be categorized into:

(1) teeth with open or immature apices
(2) teeth with fully formed or closed apices.

If the tooth has a good local tissue perfusion with an open apex then it is possible the trauma will be of no clinical significance and the root will continue to develop normally. Occasionally the crown is displaced and the root continues to form in the original direction, leading to the creation of a dilacerated tooth. Such teeth can often still be moved orthodontically. If the traumatized tooth has a poor perfusion with a closed apex, orthodontic care may be the final traumatic insult that might induce pulp necrosis with its sequelae of pain and later periapical pathology. However, the tooth can be root-treated and moved orthodontically at a later date.

In addition, there is the potential for surgically induced apical tissue damage when transplanted teeth are used in conjunction with orthodontic treatment. Again, radiographic information, supporting clinical observations of no loss of attachment and acceptable mobility, have to be used in cases where teeth have been transplanted.

External root resorption (inflammatory/replacement)

This type of root resorption has a differing pathophysiology to root resorption induced as a consequence of orthodontic care. In this instance there is often sterile pulpal necrosis, breakdown products of which pass along the dentinal tubules, irritating and destroying the cementoblasts on the external root surface. The role of the cementoblast is to maintain the cementum; necrosis of these cells leads to denudation of the root surface allowing osteoclasts to degrade and destroy the external root surface. This provokes external inflammatory responses, which then lead to inflammatory tissue destroying the tooth, although another sequela is for the tissue to calcify leading instead to ankylosis.[41] Such external root resorption and ankylosis can be seen in the case of teeth with closed apices that have been auto-transplanted.[42] Treatment is aimed at removing the irritant tissues and/or the breakdown products of these tissues before they pass down the dentinal tubules to irritate the cementoblasts. Following extirpation of the necrotic pulp, the tooth is dressed with a mild material such as a non-setting calcium hydroxide. When there is no radiographic evidence of external root resorption then the tooth is definitively root-treated; long-term radiographic monitoring is still essential.

Hard tissue damage

Damage to the apex of the tooth

This region of the tooth is susceptible to loss at all ages. A major problem with bone biology is that cells such as osteoclasts cannot differentiate between bone and tooth substance. As a consequence, there is always some loss of root length following a period of active orthodontic treatment.

Root resorption

There is general agreement that orthodontics can cause root resorption. This is usually of no clinical significance, although when severe it can seriously affect the long-term prognosis of a tooth (Fig. 9.9).

Certain risk factors have been identified that are thought to be related to root resorption.[43-46] One of the most important factors is the duration of any orthodontic treatment. Other factors include the patient's ethnic group (Caucasians are more at risk than other groups) and the type of orthodontic appliance, e.g. the standard Edgewise appliance is worse than the Straight-wire® appliance. Factors that might identify an 'at risk' patient include:[45,46]

- the pattern of resorption in the primary dentition
- anomalies and agenesis in the permanent dentition
- pipette/spindle-shaped roots
- sex—females more prone to root resorption than males
- history of trauma to one or more teeth.

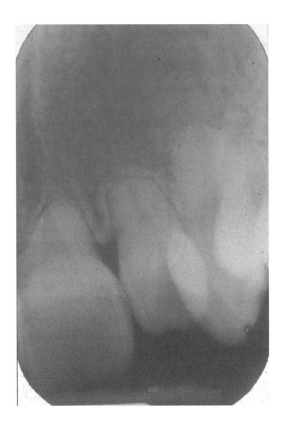

Fig. 9.9 A periapical radiograph showing severe root resorption after protracted orthodontic care (>6 years). The prognosis for the teeth will be compromised by periodontal bone loss.

Complicating the subject of root resorption even further is the new wire technology currently employed with fixed appliances (see Chapter 7). Whilst the loading and unloading characteristics of the newer nickel–titanium alloy wires are claimed to be better than stainless steel, the continuous loads applied over a longer period may compromise the periodontium. It is becoming apparent that the tissues require a phase of repair[47] following orthodontic tooth movement, and that the new wires do not necessarily provide this non-active, resting phase for the tissues. In one study following the treatment of 40 patients, significantly less root resorption was seen in those cases where there was a 3-month pause in the treatment, compared to those cases treated without a pause.[48] Root resorption was assessed using standardized long-cone periapical radiographs.

Considering the risk factors for root resorption mentioned above, who could be considered a high-risk patient and who a low-risk patient?

Patients at risk of root resorption
A Caucasian female with missing lateral incisors, a supernumerary in the premaxillary dentition, and who has been treated with a standard Edgewise

appliance, using nickel–titanium wires, continuously for 4 years. Occurring either immediately before treatment or during treatment, there is a history of a traumatic injury to the dentition.

Persons not at risk of root resorption
An Afro-Caribbean male, treated with the Straight-wire® appliance, using stainless-steel archwires, over a period of 15–18 months. There are no missing or supernumerary teeth, and no history of trauma either before or during treatment.

Habits predisposing to root resorption
There is evidence to suggest that loading of the teeth, other than normal masticatory loading, when superimposed upon orthodontic treatment can induce changes that may predispose to root resorption. Such loading can include nail-biting or trauma. However, despite the evidence, it appears that our ability to predict who is at risk of root resorption is still somewhat limited. To monitor patients appropriately we must have the appropriate start records, followed by the appropriate 'in treatment' records'. There is growing evidence that whilst the DPT for a general overview is good for determining the presence, position, and developmental stage of teeth, it is less useful for determining pathology such as root resorption and root lengths. Suspected pathology is an indication to obtain intraoral radiographs such as bitewings and long-cone periapicals in order to provide more accurate diagnostic information.[50,51]

Damage to supporting alveolar bone

Generalized bone loss
As described previously, orthodontic treatment can enhance plaque accumulation and in so doing cause the patient to develop gingival and subsequent periodontal problems. All patients who undergo orthodontic care will lose some crestal alveolar bone,[52,53] and this has to be accurately monitored in patients who are in 'high risk' groups.[54]

During a course of orthodontic treatment there is a reduction in alveolar crestal bone height of approximately 1.0 mm. This generally does not compromise the longevity of the dentition; but if it is excessive then there is a requirement to stop treatment, allow resolution of the inflammation, eliminate the predisposing factors that might be identifiable, and then, where possible, continue care.

In addition, the possibility of 'early onset' periodontal disease, localized to the first molars and the lower incisors, needs to be considered as these patients risk losing even more bone if they undergo orthodontic treatment.[55] Whilst the bone loss can be dramatic in relatively young patients, the response to treatment can allow successful treatment.

Localized bone defects
In areas where there is already localized alveolar bone loss, it can be exacerbated by orthodontic treatment, even in the presence of good oral hygiene.

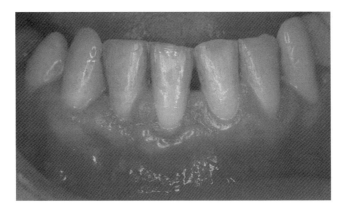

Fig. 9.10 The lower incisor has been proclined through the lower labial plate of bone, and in this case a free gingival graft has been placed to prevent worsening of the gingival health.

The area of most concern is the labial aspect of the lower incisors and this area should be palpated prior to treatment. If the roots are readily palpable and there is a washboard appearance to the alveolus then there is a risk that during the early alignment phase of fixed appliance treatment, with light wires, proclination of the lower incisors may lead to loss of more of the labial alveolar plate of bone (Fig. 9.10).

Linking orthodontic tooth position induced by orthodontic care with gingival health
The concept that the lower incisor position is related to the health of the periodontium appears false, certainly in adolescents. One study[56] examined a group of patients who had undergone orthodontic therapy with a significant amount of lower incisor proclination. However, no link could be identified between the amount of proclination and the health of the periodontium.

Damage to the enamel of teeth
Three terms defining enamel loss can also be associated with enamel damage during orthodontic treatment. They are:
1. *Abrasion*—This is the wear of tooth substance caused by a dissimilar material, e.g. an orthodontic bracket on an opposing tooth.
2. *Attrition*—This involves loss of tooth substance due to wear from the enamel/dentine of an opposing tooth.
3. *Erosion*—This implies loss of tooth substance by a chemical mechanism such as a dietary acid or reflux of acidic gastric contents.

Direct damage
There are a number of ways in which orthodontic appliances and treatment can potentially lead to direct damage of the teeth, including those discussed below.

Direct bonding of teeth

The application of the etchant/primer prior to bonding is designed to condition the enamel to allow the adhesive to attach the orthodontic brackets to the teeth. The etchant, by its very nature, is designed to modify and remove some of the enamel surface.[57] The application of etchant provokes subsurface decalcification into which fluid adhesive can be flowed to produce 'micro-tags' for attachment. If the etched area is not subsequently coated with adhesive it will eventually remineralize due to calcium salts in the saliva.[58] In rare instances, extrinsic stains can be taken up from the diet (particularly from pigmented food, e.g. curry) if ingested within this critical remineralizing period. In order to prevent this, foods should not be consumed within 1 hour of leaving the surgery. Whether the etched enamel remineralizes or is used to bond the bracket to the tooth, inevitably there is still some enamel loss. Attempts have been made to reduce this enamel loss by altering the concentration of orthophosphoric acid from 37% down to as low as 5%, or by reducing the etch time down to as little as 5 seconds. Currently, the most popular concentration is still 37% o-phosphoric acid and used for a minimum of 15–30 seconds. Rather than etch the surface, attempts have been made to grow crystals of gypsum on the enamel in the hope that they would provide a satisfactory mechanical bond with the adhesive. Unfortunately, this has not proved successful.[59,60] More recently, methacrylated phosphoric acid esters (3M Unitek) have been introduced which are capable of etching and priming the enamel surface in 3–4 seconds. The amount of enamel loss using this material is very low at only 0.31 μm.[61] With the commonly used o-phosphoric acid etchants, the degree of enamel loss is still low at 7–50 μm depending on the etch time.[62] Enamel loss can also occur if the enamel is polished with pumice in a rubber cup prior to acid-etching and also at debond when the residual adhesive is removed from the enamel surface with rotary instruments (see Chapter 7).

Abrasion by the opposing orthodontic appliance

Whilst stainless-steel brackets can be seen to abrade teeth (especially to the tips of canine teeth), the material most likely to cause damage is the ceramic used in aesthetic brackets.[63] The areas at greatest risk of this abrasion are the palatal surfaces and incisal edges of the upper incisors in Class I or Class II incisor relationships. For this reason ceramic brackets are not recommended for use on the lower incisors. Less often, wear can also occur on the lingual surfaces and incisal edges of the lower incisors, due to contact with the upper incisor brackets in Class III incisor relationships. This is especially so if ceramic brackets are used on the upper incisors prior to a surgical correction of the incisor relationship. Once surgical correction takes place and the incisor relationship becomes Class I, then the site at greatest risk alters from the lower incisors to the palatal aspect and incisal edges of the upper incisors. Therefore, not only should ceramic brackets not be used

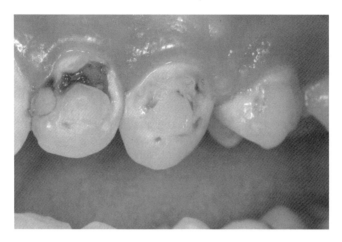

Fig. 9.11 Typical decalcification and white spot lesion seen on the maxillary molar when the oral hygiene is not kept to the ideal level; the patient also had a high 'carbonated drinks' intake and had teeth extracted previously.

on the upper incisors in some Class III cases (particularly surgical cases), but they also should not be used on the lower incisors.

Debonding brackets
Removal of fixed appliances can result in enamel fracture if the cohesive strength of the enamel is less than the cohesive strength of the adhesive, and also is less than the adhesive strength at the bonding agent/bracket base and bonding agent/enamel interfaces. This risk is accentuated when the bracket is hard and brittle, as is the case with ceramic brackets; thermal debonding has been advocated to reduce this risk.[64] It is rarely a problem with metal brackets, which are more easily deformed and peeled from the enamel surface (see Chapter 7, Section 7.2.8).

Indirect damage (i.e. as a consequence of disease processes)
Demineralization of teeth can occur during orthodontic treatment causing loss of enamel, and can range from minor 'white spot' lesions (Fig. 9.11) to actual cavitation. It is most commonly associated with poor oral hygiene, but is also associated with the excessive consumption of chemically erosive foods such as citrus fruits and fizzy drinks.

Incidence
Development of white spot lesions is not unique to orthodontic patients; they develop anywhere where the level of oral hygiene is so poor as to allow plaque to accumulate. Their incidence appears to increase with age.[65] Whilst they are identifiable in patients without a history of orthodontic treatment, there is an increased incidence in the number of lesions and teeth affected following orthodontic appliance therapy. These may still be evident even

5 years after treatment.[66] If the poor standard of oral hygiene is left unchecked, then frank cavitation of the teeth will occur due to caries.[67,68] One of the commonest sites for early white spot lesions to develop during fixed appliance therapy is the labial enamel of the upper lateral incisors. This is most probably due to the position of the hook on the archwire between the upper lateral incisor and canine.[69] A number of techniques have been employed to try to reduce the incidence of white spot formation including:

1. Oral hygiene instruction.[31]
2. Advising the use of fluoride mouthrinses—Fluoride mouthrinses (typically 0.05% sodium fluoride) will help to reduce the incidence of white spot lesions, but in one study of over 200 patients only a 13% compliance rate was identified.[70] However, in those patients where fluoride rinsing was performed, there was a significant reduction in white spot lesions.
3. The use of fluoride-releasing elastomeric modules—See Chapter 7, Section 7.2.6.
4. The use of fluoride-releasing adhesives and cements—These have provided mixed results in reducing decalcification and white spot formation[71,72] (see Chapter 7, Section 7.2.5). The use of the glass poly(alkenoate) cements has certainly reduced the incidence of decalcification beneath molar bands.
5. Checking molar and premolar bands for fit throughout treatment—Once into heavy rectangular archwires it is easy to overlook that a band is indeed loose. Left unnoticed, the protected void beneath the band and adjacent to the enamel surface can lead to plaque accumulation with rapid progression to decalcification and cavitation. In some instances it is advocated to deband a case after 12 months of treatment, take routine bitewing radiographs, and where necessary, organize the appropriate dental care.

If areas of decalcification are present on the teeth prior to commencing orthodontic treatment it is important that good photographic records are obtained in order to prevent future litigation. If decalcification arises during treatment then, in the first instance, photographs should be taken of the clinical problem and the patient informed. The application of topical fluoride at this point can be detrimental, sealing the enamel breaches and preventing slow recalcification of the defective enamel surface. Fluoride, if it is to be applied, should be only be applied 3–6 months after debond.[73]

If the white spots are particularly noticeable then the micro-abrasion technique can be used to improve the appearance. Here a small amount of the enamel surface is removed using 35% phosphoric acid, the etched enamel is then removed with a slurry of pumice in a slowly rotating rubber cup (this removes, on average, 164 μm of surface enamel), and this is followed by calcification of the tooth by the oral fluids.[74]

Areas of decalcification beyond the scope of this technique require either facings or some other form of restorative technique, taking into account the age of the patient.

9.2   SUMMARY

1. Orthodontic treatment can adversely affect the following tissues:
   - enamel
   - dentine/cementum—apical tissues
   - alveolar bone
   - gingivae.
2. There is limited data to correlate orthodontics to:
   - temporomandibular joint disorders
   - adverse profile changes.

9.3   OBJECTIVES

1. Identify the patients at risk.
2. Minimize the risks.
3. Instigate the correct protocol for ensuring treatment problems do not compromise the longevity of the dentition.
4. Counsel patients as to the possibilities of damage and ensure the correct level of informed consent.

REFERENCES

1. Giles, S. A. and Taylor, N. G. (1997). Are anterior occlusal radiographs still indicated for orthodontic assessment? *British Dental Journal*, **183**, 325–8.
2. Isaacson, K. G. and Thom, A. R. (2001). *Orthodontic radiographs—guidelines*. British Orthodontic Society.
3. Rushton, V. E., Horner, K., and Worthington, H. V. (1999). The quality of panoramic radiographs in a sample of general dental practices. *British Dental Journal*, **186**, 630–3.
4. Ericson, S. and Kurol, J. (2000). Incisor root resorptions due to ectopic maxillary canines imaged by computerized tomography: a comparative study in extracted teeth. *Angle Orthodontist*, **70**, 276–83.
5. Cobourne, M., Brown, ??, and McDonald, F. (2002). Analysis of the morbidity of submerged deciduous molars: the use of imaging techniques. *Oral Surgery, Oral Medicine, Oral Pathology, Oral Radiology and Endodontics*, **93**, 98–102.
6. Samuels, R. H. A. and Jones, M. L. (1994). Orthodontic facebow injuries and safety equipment. *European Journal of Orthodontics*, **16**, 385–94.
7. Samuels, R. H. A. (1996). A review of orthodontic face-bow injuries and safety equipment. *American Journal of Orthodontics and Dentofacial Orthopedics*, **110**, 269–72.
8. British Dental Association (2000). *Infection control in dentistry*, Advice sheet A12. BDA.

9. Moore, R. N. and Igel, K. A. (1988). Lip burn from band seater. *American Journal of Orthodontics and Dentofacial Orthopedics*, **93**, 183–5.
10. McGuiness, N. J. (1992). Prevention in orthodontics—a review. *Dental Update*, **19**, 168–70, 172–5.
11. Kerosuo, H., Kullaa, A., Kerosuo, E., Kanerva, L., and Hensten-Pettersen, A. (1996). Nickel allergy in adolescents in relation to orthodontic treatment and piercing of ears. *American Journal of Orthodontics and Dentofacial Orthopedics*, **109**, 148–54.
12. Janson, G. R, Dainesi, E. A., Consolaro, A., Woodside, D. G., and de Freitas M. R. (1998). Nickel hypersensitivity reaction before, during, and after orthodontic therapy. *American Journal of Orthodontics and Dentofacial Orthopedics*, **113**, 655–60.
13. Jia, W., Beatty, M. W., Reinhardt, R. A., Petro, T. M., Cohen, D. M., Maze, C. R., Strom, E. A., and Hoffman, M. (1999). Nickel release from orthodontic arch wires and cellular immune response to various nickel concentrations. *Journal of Biomedical Materials Research*, **48**, 488–95.
14. Lowey, M. N. (1993). Allergic contact dermatitis associated with the use of an Interlandi headgear in a patient with a history of atopy. *British Dental Journal*, **175**, 67–72.
15. McComb, J. L. and King, C. M. (1992). Atopic eczema and orthodontic headgear. *Dental Update*, **19**, 396–7.
16. Paulsen, H. U. (1997). Morphological changes of the TMJ condyles of 100 patients treated with the Herbst appliance in the period of puberty to adulthood: a long-term radiographic study. *European Journal of Orthodontics*, **19**, 657–68.
17. Sari, S. and Sonmez, H. (2002). Investigation of the relationship between oral parafunctions and temporomandibular joint dysfunction in Turkish children with mixed and permanent dentition. *Journal of Oral Rehabilitation*, **29**, 108–12.
18. Pedersen, T. K., Jensen, J. J., Melsen, B., and Herlin, T. (2001). Resorption of the temporomandibular condylar bone according to subtypes of juvenile chronic arthritis. *Journal of Rheumatology*, **28**, 2109–15.
19. McLaughlin, R. P. and Bennett, J. C. (1995). The extraction–nonextraction dilemma as it relates to TMD. *Angle Orthodontist*, **65**, 175–86.
20. Pilley, J. R., Mohlin, B., Shaw, W. C., and Kingdon, A. (1997). A survey of craniomandibular disorders in 500 19 year olds. *European Journal of Orthodontics*, **19**, 57–70.
21. Williams, R. (1969). The diagnostic line. *American Journal of Orthodontics*, **55**, 458–76.
22. Ricketts, R. M. (1968). Esthetics, environment, and the law of lip relation. *American Journal of Orthodontics*, **54**, 272–89.
23. Holdaway, R. A. (1983). A soft tissue cephalometric analysis and its application in orthodontic treatment planning. Part 1. *American Journal of Orthodontics and Dentofacial Orthopedics*, **84**, 1–28.
24. Looi, L. K. and Mills, J. R. (1986). The effect of two contrasting forms of orthodontic treatment on the facial profile. *American Journal of Orthodontics*, **89**, 507–17.
25. Zierhut, E. C., Joondeph, D. R., Artun, J., and Little, R. M. (2000). Long-term profile changes associated with successfully treated extraction and nonextraction Class II division 1 malocclusions. *Angle Orthodontist*, **70**, 208–19.
26. Bishara, S. E. and Jakobsen, J. R. (1997). Profile changes in patients treated with and without extractions: assessments by lay people. *American Journal of Orthodontics and Dentofacial Orthopedics*, **112**, 639–44.
27. DiBiase, A. T. and Sandler, P. J. (2001). Does orthodontics damage faces? *Dental Update*, **28**, 98–102.
28. Driscoll-Gilliland, J., Buschang, P. H., and Behrents, R. G. (2001). An evaluation of growth and stability in untreated and treated subjects. *American Journal of Orthodontics and Dentofacial Orthopedics*, **120**, 588–97.

29. Shah, H., McDonald, F., Lucas, V., Ashley, P., and Roberts, G. J. (2002). A cephalometric analysis of patients with recessive dystrophic epidermolysis bullosa. *Angle Orthodontist*, **72**, 55–60.

30. Zachrisson, B. U. and Zachrisson, S. (1971). Caries incidence and oral hygiene during orthodontic treatment. *Scandinavian Journal of Dental Research*, **79**, 394–401.

31. Zachrisson, S. and Zachrisson, B. U. (1972). Gingival condition associated with orthodontic treatment. *Angle Orthodontist*, **42**, 26–34.

32. Hobson, R. S. and Clark, J. D. (1998). How UK orthodontists advise patients on oral hygiene. *British Journal of Orthodontics*, **25**, 64–6.

33. Zachrisson, B. U. and Alnaes, L. (1973). Periodontal condition in orthodontically treated and untreated individuals. I. Loss of attachment, gingival pocket depth and clinical crown height. *Angle Orthodontist*, **43**, 402–11.

34. McDonald, F. and Pitt Ford, T. R. (1994). Blood flow changes in permanent maxillary canines during retraction. *European Journal of Orthodontics*, **16**, 1–9.

35. Harris, R. and Griffin, C. J. (1972). The ultrastructure of the blood vessels of the human dental pulp following injury. II. *Australian Dental Journal*, **17**, 355–62.

36. Harris, R. and Griffin, C. J. (1973). The ultrastructure of the blood vessels of the human dental pulp following injury. IV. *Australian Dental Journal*, **18**, 88–96.

37. Buckley, J. G., Jones, M. L., Hill, M., and Sugar, A. W. (1999). An evaluation of the changes in maxillary pulpal blood flow associated with orthognathic surgery. *Journal of Orthodontics*, **26**, 39–45.

38. Drysdale, C., Gibbs, S. L., and Ford, T. R. (1996). Orthodontic management of root-filled teeth. *British Journal of Orthodontics*, **23**, 255–60.

39. Parlange, L. M. and Sims, M. R. (1993). A T.E.M. stereological analysis of blood vessels and nerves in marmoset periodontal ligament following endodontics and magnetic incisor extrusion. *European Journal of Orthodontics*, **15**, 33–44.

40. Zachrisson, B. U. and Jacobsen, I. (1974). Response to orthodontic movement of anterior teeth with root fractures. *Transactions of the European Orthodontic Society*, ??, 207–214.

41. Andreasen, J. O. and Andreasen, F. M. (1992). Root resorption following traumatic dental injuries. *Proceedings of the Finnish Dental Society*, **88**(Suppl. 1), 95–114.

42. Czochrowska, E. M., Stenvik, A., Bjercke, B., and Zachrisson, B. U. (2002). Outcome of tooth transplantation: survival and success rates 17–41 years post-treatment. *American Journal of Orthodontics and Dentofacial Orthopedics*, **121**, 110–19.

43. Sameshima, G. T. and Sinclair, P. M. (2001). Predicting and preventing root resorption: Part II. Treatment factors. *American Journal of Orthodontics and Dentofacial Orthopedics*, **119**, 511–15.

44. Mavragani, M., Vergari, A., Selliseth, N. J., Boe, O. E., and Wisth, P. L. (2000). A radiographic comparison of apical root resorption after orthodontic treatment with a standard edgewise and a straight-wire edgewise technique. *European Journal of Orthodontics*, **22**, 665–74.

45. Kjaer, I. (1995). Morphological characteristics of dentitions developing excessive root resorption during orthodontic treatment. *European Journal of Orthodontics*, **17**, 25–34.

46. Sameshima, G. T. and Sinclair, P. M. (2001). Predicting and preventing root resorption: Part I. Diagnostic factors. *American Journal of Orthodontics and Dentofacial Orthopedics*, **119**, 505–10.

47. Brudvik, P. and Rygh, P. (1995). Transition and determinants of orthodontic root resorption–repair sequence. *European Journal of Orthodontics*, **17**, 177–88.

48. Levander, E., Malmgren, O., and Eliasson, S. (1994). Evaluation of root resorption in relation to two orthodontic treatment regimes. A clinical experimental study. *European Journal of Orthodontics*, **16**, 223–8.

49. Odenrick, L. and Brattstrom, V. (1983). The effect of nailbiting on root resorption during orthodontic treatment. *European Journal of Orthodontics*, **5**, 185–8.
50. Rushton, V. E., Horner, K., and Worthington, H. V. (2002). Screening panoramic radiography of new adult patients: diagnostic yield when combined with bitewing radiography and identification of selection criteria. *British Dental Journal*, **192**, 275–9.
51. Leach, H. A., Ireland, A. J., and Whaites, E. J. (2001). Radiographic diagnosis of root resorption in relation to orthodontics. *British Dental Journal*, **190**, 16–22.
52. Alstad, S. and Zachrisson, B. U. (1979). Longitudinal study of periodontal condition associated with orthodontic treatment in adolescents. *American Journal of Orthodontics*, **76**, 277–86.
53. Harris, E. F. and Baker, W. C. (1990). Loss of root length and crestal bone height before and during treatment in adolescent and adult orthodontic patients. *American Journal of Orthodontics and Dentofacial Orthopedics*, **98**, 463–9.
54. Sjolien, T. and Zachrisson, B. U. (1973). A method for radiographic assessment of periodontal bone support following orthodontic treatment. *Scandinavian Journal of Dental Research*, **81**, 210–17.
55. Albandar, J. M., Brown, L. J., and Loe, H. (1996). Dental caries and tooth loss in adolescents with early-onset periodontitis. *Journal of Periodontology*, **67**, 960–7.
56. Ruf, S., Hansen, K., and Pancherz, H. (1998). Does orthodontic proclination of lower incisors in children and adolescents cause gingival recession? *American Journal of Orthodontics and Dentofacial Orthopedics*, **114**, 100–6.
57. Zachrisson, B. U. and Arthun, J. (1979). Enamel surface appearance after various debonding techniques. *American Journal of Orthodontics*, **75**, 121–7.
58. Ogaard, B., Rolla, G., Arends, J., and ten Cate, J. M. (1988). Orthodontic appliances and enamel demineralization. Part 2. Prevention and treatment of lesions. *American Journal of Orthodontics and Dentofacial Orthopedics*, **94**, 123–8.
59. Maijer, R. and Smith, D. C. (1986). Crystal growth on the outer enamel surface—an alternative to acid etching. *American Journal of Orthodontics*, **89**, 183–93.
60. Jones, S. P., Gledhill, J. R., and Davies, E. H. (1999). The crystal growth technique—a laboratory evaluation of bond strengths. *European Journal of Orthodontics*, **21**, 89–93.
61. Hosein, I. (2002). An investigation into enamel loss following orthodontic bonding, debonding and clean up. Unpublished MSc dissertation. University of Bristol.
62. Pus, M. D. and Way, D. C. (1980). Enamel loss due to orthodontic bonding. *American Journal of Orthodontics*, **77**, 269–83.
63. Viazis, A. D., DeLong, R., Bevis, R. R., Rudney, J. D., and Pintado, M. R. (1990). Enamel abrasion from ceramic orthodontic brackets under an artificial oral environment. *American Journal of Orthodontics and Dentofacial Orthopedics*, **98**, 103–9.
64. Rueggeberg, F. A. and Lockwood, P. E. (1992). Thermal debracketing of single crystal sapphire brackets. *Angle Orthodontist*, **62**, 45–50.
65. Ogaard, B. (1989). Prevalence of white spot lesions in 19-year-olds: a study on untreated and orthodontically treated persons 5 years after treatment. *American Journal of Orthodontics and Dentofacial Orthopedics*, **96**, 423–7.
66. Ogaard, B., Artun, J., and Brobakken, B. O. (1986). Prevalence of carious white spots after orthodontic treatment with multibonded appliances. *European Journal of Orthodontics*, **8**, 229–34.
67. Rytomaa, I., Meurman, J. H., Koskinen, J., Laakso, T., Gharazi, L., and Turunen, R. (1988). *In vitro* erosion of bovine enamel caused by acidic drinks and other foodstuffs. *Scandinavian Journal of Dental Research*, **96**, 324–33.
68. Ireland, A. J., McGuinness, N., and Sherriff, M. (1995). An investigation into the ability of soft drinks to adhere to enamel. *Caries Research*, **29**, 470–6.

69. Gorelick, L., Geiger, A. M., and Gwinnett, A. J. (1982). Incidence of white spot formation after bonding and banding. *American Journal of Orthodontics*, **81**, 93–8.

70. Geiger, A. M., Gorelick, L., Gwinnett, A. J., and Benson, B. J. (1992). Reducing white spot lesions in orthodontic populations with fluoride rinsing. *American Journal of Orthodontics and Dentofacial Orthopedics*, **101**, 403–7.

71. Akkaya, S., Uner, O., Alacam, A., and Degim, T. (1996). Enamel fluoride levels after orthodontic band cementation with glass ionomer cement. *European Journal of Orthodontics*, **18**, 81–7.

72. Norris, D. S., McInnes-Ledoux, P., Schwaninger, B., and Weinberg, R. (1986). Retention of orthodontic bands with new fluoride-releasing cements. *American Journal of Orthodontics*, **89**, 206–11.

73. Ogaard, B., Rolla, G., Arends, J., and ten Cate, J. M. (1988). Orthodontic appliances and enamel demineralization. Part 2: Prevention and treatment of lesions. *American Journal of Orthodontics and Dentofacial Orthopedics*, **94**, 123–8.

74. Pourghadiri, M., Longhurst, P., and Watson, T. F. (1998). A new technique for the controlled removal of mottled enamel: measurement of enamel loss. *British Dental Journal*, **184**, 239–41.

Index